Clinical Dental Medicine 2020

Nairn H.F. Wilson

Clinical Dental Medicine 2020

Edited by

Nairn H.F. Wilson

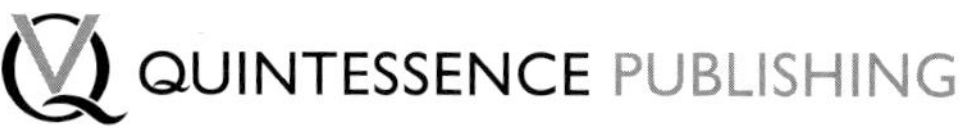

London, Berlin, Chicago, Tokyo, Barcelona, Beijing, Istanbul, Milan, Moscow, New Delhi, Paris, Prague, São Paulo, Seoul and Warsaw

British Library Cataloguing in Publication Data
Clinical Dental Medicine 2020.
1. Dentistry
I. Wilson, Naim H. F.
ISBN 13: 978-1-85097-189-4

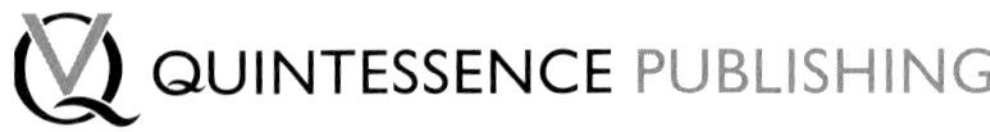

Quintessence Publishing Co. Ltd.
Quintessence House
Grafton Road, New Malden
Surrey KT3 3AB, United Kingdom
www.quintpub.co.uk

Production:
Les Streater, Quintessence Publishing Co. Ltd.
Editorial coordination: Elizabeth Ducker,
Quintessence Publishing Co. Ltd.
Printing: freiburger graphische betriebe, Freiburg, Germany

Printed in Germany

Preface

This book was commissioned as one of the initiatives to mark 60 years of publishing by Quintessence. It provides authoritative commentaries by international opinion leaders on the state of the art and science of dentistry, and looks forward, scoping anticipated developments in the major areas of clinical practice. The essence of many of these developments is captured in the title of the book – ***Clinical Dental Medicine 2020***; dentists and other members of the dental team of the future are anticipated to be as much oral physicians as dental surgeons.

Not all aspects of the present or anticipated future clinical practice of dentistry can be covered in this book. The areas collectively considered constitute the majority of the clinical practice of dentistry, both currently and, it is predicted, for the foreseeable future, specifically through to 2020. While developments in other aspects of dentistry will be as exciting and important as those discussed in this book, ***Clinical Dental Medicine 2020*** sets the scene for the major elements of the clinical practice of dentistry over the second decade of the 21st century.

Predicting the future is not an exact science. Unforeseen events and ground-breaking scientific discoveries, and the way society responds to an ever-changing world will, as in the past, fashion the future as much as, if not more than, predictable developments and trends. But envisioning the future, based on what is known and can be expected, is important: better to have a vision to revise and refine than to be blind to what probably lies ahead. To think only of today and the past is two- rather than three-dimensional thinking.

By looking to the future, it is hoped that this book will inspire the next generation of practitioners, students, teachers, researchers, opinion leaders and authors in dentistry. In this way, it is hoped that ***Clinical Dental Medicine 2020*** will be an inspirational insight into what should transpire in dentistry between now and 2020. If you think the last ten years has been a time of unprecedented change and development, prepare yourself for the impact of an increasing number and range of even greater life-changing innovations in the next ten years. Whatever happens, dentistry in 2020 will be very different from what it is today.

Working with the illustrious teams of contributors to this book has been a pleasure and an honour. I have learnt a great deal from the authoritative insights and predictions of the renowned authors. Indeed, editing this book has given me a new perspective of the priorities and enormous opportunities to be grasped in the further development of dentistry and oral healthcare provision. ***Clinical Dental Medicine 2020*** looks beyond the present horizons at the next 10 years of new, practice-changing frontiers in dentistry.

Nairn Wilson

Contributors

Per Axelsson	Emeritus Professor in Preventive Dentistry, School of Dentistry, University of Göteborg, Sweden
Efthimia K. Basdra	Associate Professor, Department of Histology and Embryology, Craniofacial Development Unit, University of Athens Medical School, Athens, Greece
Steven E. Eckert	Professor of Dentistry, College of Medicine, Mayo Clinic, Program Director, Prosthodontics, Mayo Graduate School of Medicine
Roland Frankenberger	Associate Professor, University Medical Center Erlangen, Dental Clinic 1 - Operative Dentistry and Periodontology, Gluckstrasse 11, D-91054 Erlangen, Germany
Kishor Gulabivala	Professor and Head of Endodontology and Training Programme Director for Restorative Dentistry, UCL Eastman Dental Institute, London, UK
Keith Horner	Professor of Oral and Maxillofacial Imaging, School of Dentistry, University of Manchester, Manchester, UK
J. Thomas Lambrecht	Professor and Chairman, Department of Oral Surgery, Oral Radiology, Oral and Oral Medicine, University of Basel, Basel, Switzerland
William R. Laney	Professor Emeritus, Division of Prosthodontics, Department of Dental Specialties, Mayo Clinic College of Medicine, Rochester, MS 55905, USA
Yuan-Ling Ng	Clinical Lecturer in Endodontology and Programme Director for Masters Degrees in Endodontology, UCL Eastman Dental Institute, London, UK
Mariano Sanz	Dean of the Faculty of Odontology and Chair of Periodontology, University Complutense of Madrid, Madrid, Spain
Nairn H. F. Wilson	Dean and Head of King's College London Dental Institute and Professor of Restorative Dentistry, King's College London, London, UK

Contents

CHAPTER 1

Dentistry today

Nairn Wilson

Introduction

Dentistry today is a complex healthcare science. Looking back over the twentieth century, dentistry remained largely unchanged during the first half but experienced a growing rate of change in the latter half, particularly over the last 20 years. This rate of change has continued to accelerate in the first decade of the twenty-first century and, according to all predictions, is set to continue to gain momentum for at least the foreseeable future. As a consequence, dentistry today is constantly changing, and we may look forward to an exciting future of new developments and challenges. With such prospects come opportunities to realize new heights in the art and science of dentistry.

Dentistry in transition

For existing members of the dental profession, their clinical practice of dentistry is evolving as it adapts to change. For some, they see the beginning of a trend towards dental practitioners becoming as much oral physicians as dental surgeons. For others, clinical practice is becoming much more specialized and sophisticated than previously. If nothing else, the clinical practice of dentistry is increasingly becoming patient-centered and contributing to 're-connecting the mouth to body.' This is part of a drive to better meet the ever-increasing expectations of patients and thereby help to promote and enhance their general well-being and health.[1] Current trends in the clinical practice of dentistry are being driven by a complex set of circumstances. This includes new understanding of the importance of oral health,[2] demand for care increasingly replacing the need for treatment with clinical care involving as much, if not more prevention and maintenance than interventive procedures; tooth-colored restorative systems and associated adhesive procedures replacing traditional restorative materials and operative procedures; implant dentistry growing at the expense of traditional prosthodontics, let alone influencing aspects of treatment planning in endodontics and peridontology; and the exponential growth in esthetic dentistry and related cosmetic techniques. Of particular importance to patients, many of whom will live much longer than their predecessors, is the increasing adoption of the philosophy of 'teeth for life' underpinned by the practice of minimally interventive dentistry: 'the maintenance and monitoring of oral health through continuous care, comprising comprehensive preventive management, a longitudinal approach to the risk assessment and diagnosis of chronic disease and a minimally invasive approach to any necessary operative intervention.'[3] In years to come, complete dentures (Fig. 1-1) and dentitions heavily restored with metallic restorations, often in less than ideal oral environments (Fig. 1-2), should become much less common – a trend that is already well advanced in certain countries, notably in Scandinavia, as detailed in Chapter 2. Such trends are to be warmly welcomed and fully embraced, if for no other reason than, for the benefit of patients. If the outcome of a lifetime of care is an extensively restored, typically compromised dentition, with the prospect of high maintenance, including repeat dentistry as restorations and prostheses fail, the needs of the patient have not been met.[1] Oral healthcare of the future must have better outcomes, as may be seen in cases where prevention has prevailed and been effective through a working partnership between the patient and their oral healthcare support team (Fig. 1-3).

Inequalities in oral health

Although there has been a general reduction in the incidence and severity of dental caries and periodontal disease in many countries in recent years, individuals in lower socioeconomic groups may not have benefited a great deal, if at all, from these improvements. This has resulted in more pronounced health inequalities around the world. This trend poses an enormous challenge to healthcare systems, with the situation being aggravated by policies to have individuals assume more responsibility for their own health: new responsibilities for self-help are difficult or impossible for many individuals on the wrong side of the health-inequality

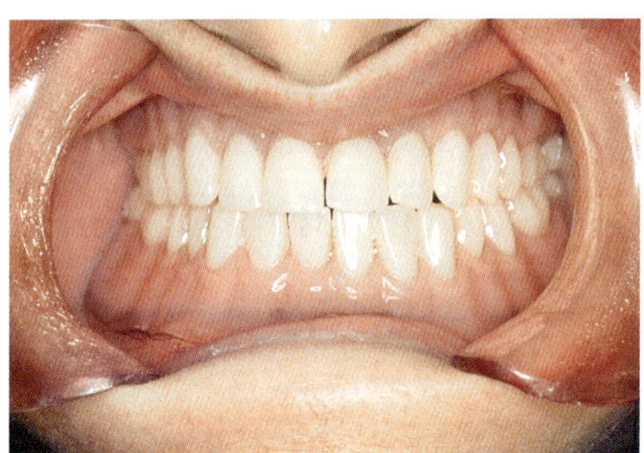

Fig. 1-1 Complete dentures in clinical service. (Courtesy of Dr David Radford, King's College London Dental Institute, London, UK)

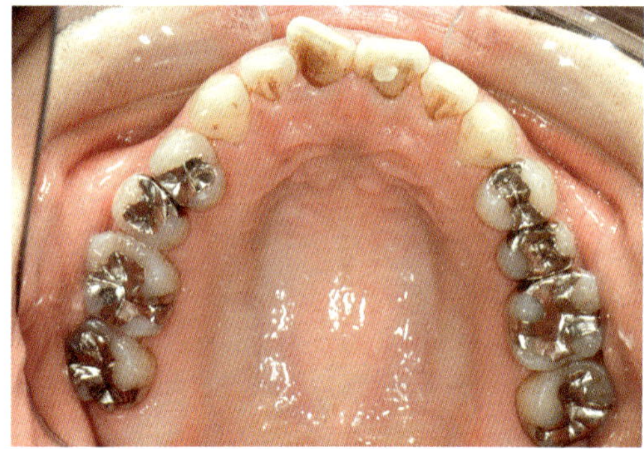

Fig. 1-2 A dentition heavily restored with metallic (dental amalgam) restorations in a less than ideal oral environment.

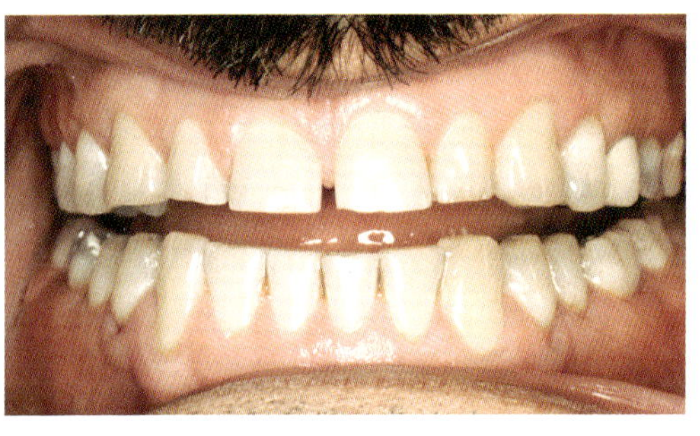

Fig. 1-3 Dentition of a mature adult in whom prevention, including actions to limit progressive wear, has been effective through a partnership between the patient and his oral healthcare support team.

divide. Crossing the divide is not simply a matter of resources; there are barriers to be overcome in terms of acquired behavior, attitude and understanding.[4]

Evidence-based dentistry

Evidence-based care has been a major driver in transforming healthcare provision in recent times. The provision of evidence-based oral healthcare requires an integrated approach, encompassing the patient's needs, preferences, values and expectations, the clinician's expertise and skills, and the best available research evidence. Evidence-based oral healthcare is not 'cookbook style' treatment, assuming the best researched approach is most appropriate in all situations. Patients must be treated as individuals, applying the best research evidence according to the circumstances. In the absence of appropriate evidence, best available knowledge must be applied. This approach should result in consistency, efficiency, effectiveness and quality and safety in the provision of care.[5] Analyses of the impact of evidence on patient care outcomes in oral healthcare are, however, limited.[6] There is, therefore, a need to put more emphasis on evidence-based care in primary and subsequent dental education.[7]

Recent times have seen the introduction and development of evidence-based oral healthcare resources and databases, many online. Examples include the Cochrane Oral Health Group, Centre for Evidence-Based Dentistry, Pan-American Centers for Evidence-Based Dentistry (Evidentista) the International Centre for Evidence-based Oral Health and the Oral Health Specialist Library. These resources, which provide much-needed, invaluable syntheses of best available evidence, should be a frequent source of information for students and be central to continuing professional development for existing members of the dental team. In making such statements,[7] it is accepted that there is limited evidence that evidence-based oral healthcare works in practice; however, there is widespread acceptance that evidence-based oral healthcare, integrated with modern skills of caring, is an important key to improving the health and well-being of patients and, in turn, enhancing their communities. Patients deserve a caring, scientific approach to their treatment. This requires practitioners to practice more from what is known rather than from what they have been led to believe through anecdote and custom and practice passed on from one generation to the next.

Esthetic dentistry

The last decades of the twentieth century will come to be associated with a new era in patient expectation and demand for dental attractiveness.[8] This development has fuelled the remarkable growth and expansion of esthetic dentistry and related cosmetic procedures. Elements of esthetic dentistry are non-invasive and do little, if any, damage to teeth and adjacent soft tissues, while at the other end of the spectrum certain procedures used in so-called dental makeovers are very invasive, with a substantial risk of iatrogenic, tooth-threatening effects, let alone the legacy of subsequent cost consequence.[9] Notable in the exponential growth of esthetic dentistry has been bleaching or, as it is possibly more accurately referred to, 'tooth whitening,' given the opacifying effect bleaching agents tend to have on dental enamel.[10] Beauty is in the eye of the beholder, who in present day society tends to be influenced more by the so-called Hollywood smile than by the natural beauty of intact well-maintained teeth.

The dental team

In an increasing number of countries, the dental workforce is being expanded to include a range of dental care professionals, including dental hygienists and various forms of therapists, not to forget clinical dental technicians (denturists).[11] In addition, dental nurses (chairside assistants) tend to have an increasing range of roles and responsibilities, typically including clinical procedures such as routine intraoral radiography, recording impressions for study models and the placement of rubber dam. This, many would say, long overdue development of the dental team shares certain features with the ways in which the medical workforce developed in the twentieth century, and continues to evolve to this day, allowing the doctor, as the leader of the medical team, to focus on roles, procedures and innovations that cannot be delegated.[12] Medicine views its team approach, which involves things that were once the sole domain of doctors being undertaken by other healthcare professionals, as a strengthening rather than a diminution of medical care. As in medicine, dentists should no longer work alone but in teams in which the various members of the team contribute in different ways to the holistic, high-quality care of patients, with synergy of expertise, skills and knowledge.[11] This creates opportunity for the dentist, as the leader of the dental team, to focus on the overall care of patients, advanced and complex skills and procedures, the introduction of new technologies and the delivery of effective oral healthcare. With the further development of the dental team, dentistry will justify a prominent role in modern healthcare provision. For many, the time has already passed when dentists can claim to have acquired and to be maintaining all the skills and competencies necessary for the clinical practice of dentistry in its many diverse forms. As discussed below, such thinking has profound implications for dental education at all levels.

The impact of new technologies

There have been huge technological advances in dentistry in recent times. The full impact is yet to be realized in respect of osseointegration, the introduction of adhesive technologies, modern imaging systems and computer-assisted design/computer-assisted manufacture (CAD/CAM), let alone the transforming influences of the many other significant technological innovations of recent times. Indeed, many would claim that the profession has, at best, seen only the 'tip of the (new technology) iceberg' to date. Notwithstanding the transforming impact of new technologies on patient care and the provision of dental services, there are other far-reaching consequences, spanning the continuum of dental education, the shape, structure and operation of professional bodies and specialist interest organisations, the direction of travel of the dental trade and manufacturing industry, and the position of oral sciences in the scientific community. Future projections are often overoptimistic; however, as set out in the various chapters of this book, there is every reason to anticipate ground-breaking innovations in respect of drugs, genetics, bioengineering and biomaterials, miniaturization including nanotechnology, and e-oral health and teledentistry, to list but a few areas of real promise for new frontiers.

Although certain new technologies have had a positive impact on the cost of provision of care, new technologies tend to contribute to an increase in expenditure overall. Such expenditure must, however, be viewed in the context of enhanced clinical outcomes, heightened levels of patient satisfaction and, in many cases, the opportunity for reduced retreatment costs. Osseointegrated implant-retained prostheses are a case in question. Implant dentistry, as discussed later in this book, is invariably a much more expensive treatment modality than alternative forms of prosthodontic care, notably removable prosthodontics. Once successfully completed, however, the prognosis for fixed implant-supported prostheses tends to be much more favorable than that for removable prostheses, which, in addition, may cause more iatrogenic damage than implant-supported alternatives.

By way of a cautionary note, some new technologies involving, for example, the use of stem cells and genetic modification procedures are anticipated to pose social and ethical dilemmas, while others may be questioned in terms of cost benefits. Dentistry must learn from experiences, such as the difficulties encountered in the widespread introduction of water fluoridation, and apply different techniques to win over public support to translate new science into clinical practice. This is a challenge that must be tackled today rather than put off until tomorrow.

Dental education

In many countries dental education has not moved with the times. Indeed, dental students of a century ago would recognize much of what goes on in dental schools today, albeit in a changed environment. More of the same will not suffice in the future, let alone attract students of the best quality.[13] The concept of the continuum of dental education, starting from the time of entering dental school and running through to retirement is already well established and accepted. What is less well accepted is the need for revalidation, possibly involving periods of retraining at intervals in the professional lives of all members of the dental team. Dental education is available in many forms, both traditional and making use of modern technologies, and many more members of the dental team are participating in lifelong learning than ever before. Regrettably, for many in the profession, education continues to be viewed as a means to an end rather than a professionally rewarding indulgence. That said, as in all other aspects of present-day dentistry, attitudes and behaviors are changing.

Research

Research in dentistry is growing year on year, both in volume and diversity. The range of this research is immense, yielding more outcomes than can be assimilated by teams of experts, let alone individual members of the profession. Systematic reviews are of assistance in distilling down new and existing knowledge, but such publications cover a mere fraction of the new information and understanding generated by research. There are great stockpiles of useful research findings, conclusions and recommendations, but with limited means to translate this information into benefits, particularly for patients. At the same time, there are many priorities and unanswered questions in dental research that need to be addressed. In taking matters forward, much more research in dentistry needs to be practice based, or otherwise designed to be of immediate practical relevance to practitioners. Furthermore, it is a matter of concern, as indicated earlier in this chapter, that so little of what is done for patients in the present provision of oral healthcare is evidence-based.[6] Current research priorities in dentistry are many and varied. They include, among others, improving the health of populations, reducing inequalities, widening access to care, enhancing the quality and cost benefits of services and outcomes, developing more efficient and effective procedures and processes, and developing materials and devices to reduce technique sensitivity. Funding and delivering such a broad range of research is challenging. It is important to the future development of dentistry, however, that ways and means are found to sustain high levels of research in dentistry of international quality and relevance. It is considered most encouraging that research in dentistry has become increasingly multidisciplinary and more international in its approach, with individuals and centers around the world coming together to tackle common problems and goals.

Provision of care

Dentistry, as discussed in this chapter, is changing, together with treatment needs and demands of populations.[1] Where state funding is available to support the provision of dental services, it tends to be targeted to provide for selected groups, often the young, the older patient and those with special needs, let alone to deal with dental health inequalities. As a consequence, private and insurance-based care, together with the market for, in particular, over-the-counter oral hygiene products, continues to grow around the world as many more people, despite ethnic and cultural differences, realize the importance and benefits of good, well-maintained oral health. In consumer societies, dental teams, unlike their medical counterparts, are now increasingly engaging in promoting their skills and services and responding to demand-driven markets. For many practitioners, unaccustomed to such ways of working to ensure the financial viability of their practices, developments in the business of dentistry are unsettling, if not threatening. But such are the pressures for dentistry and other essential elements of healthcare provision in modern healthcare systems.

In considering present and possible future patterns of provision of care, it is important to understand the attitudes and motivation of the potential providers: the future dental workforce. It would appear that future healthcare workers are attracted to dentistry as they perceive it to be a financially lucrative contained career option, with professional status, job security and the opportunity to work flexibly.[14] The long-term expectations of new members of the dental team have been shown to be closely linked with a vision of a favorable work-life balance.[9]

An overview

Dentistry today could be considered to be in a state of flux. Dentistry has, however, come a long way in recent times, building on an illustrious history to become a very dynamic, multifaceted, forward-looking healthcare profession. This, together with the increasing awareness of the importance of oral health to general health and well-being, and increasing interests in and demands for dental attractiveness, makes dentistry an appealing, important healthcare profession. Being a member of the dental profession today carries many responsibilities, including being a lifelong learner - a student for life - and being able to change with the times, but such responsibilities are far outweighed by the opportunities for personal and professional reward and fulfillment. As a consequence, dentistry remains a popular career choice.

For the patient, dentistry today offers so much more than was previously possible. With modern materials, techniques and procedures, there is a real prospect of 'teeth for life,' and choice in the ways in which this goal may be achieved. In retaining teeth for life, they should function well, look good, give people confidence and, very importantly, contribute to health and well-being through the various phase of adulthood and into old age.[15] This, however, assumes that the patient takes ownership of the day-to-day care and maintenance of their oral health, with their dental practitioner providing occasional help, support and, when necessary, minimally interventive operative care.

Dentistry today is on the cusp of change, which will hopefully surpass the expectations of patients. When change is inevitable, you 'go with the flow' or get left behind. Dentistry is too important to be left trailing the rest of modern healthcare provision, and must, therefore, be proactive in embracing the inevitable change that is coming its way.

References

1. Inge R. Institute for Oral Health: advancing dental care innovation. Dent Abstr 2008;53:228-229.
2. Williams RC, Barnett AH, Claffey N, Davis M, Gadsby R, Kellet M et al. The potential impact of periodontal disease on general health: a consensus view. Curr Med Res Opin 2008;24:1635-1643.
3. Wilson NHF (ed). Minimally Invasive Dentistry. London, Quintessence, 2007.
4. Shanley D, Manogue M (eds). Global Congress on Dental Education III: composite congress papers and reports. Eur J Dent Educ 2008;12(special issue):3-197.
5. Sackett DL, Straus SE, Richardson WS, Rosenbeg W, Haynes RB. Evidence-based medicine: how to practice and teach EBM. New York: Churchill Livingstone, 2000.
6. Richards D, Clarkson J. Evidence-based Dentistry: Managing Information for Better Practice. London: Quintessence, 2008.
7. Winning T, Needleman I, Rohlin M, Carrassi A, Chadwick B, Eaton K et al. Evidence-based care and the curriculum. Euro J Dent Ed 2008;12(Suppl 1):48-63.
8. Bartlett D, Brunton PA. Aesthetic Dentistry. London, Quintessence.
9. Gallagher J, Wilson NHF. The future dental workforce? Br Dent J 2009; in press.
10. Haywood VB. Tooth Whitening: Indications and Outcomes of Nightguard Vital Bleaching. Hanover Park, IL: Quintessence, 2007.
11. Dyer TA, Robinson PG. Exploring the social acceptability of skill-mix in dentistry. Int Dent J 2008;58:173-180.
12. Slater M (ed). Dental Team Companion. London: Quintessence, 2009.
13. Eaton KA, Reynolds PA, Grayden SK, Wilson NHF. A vision of dental education in the third millennium. Br Dent J 2008;205:261-271.
14. Gallagher JE, Clarke W, Eaton KA, Wilson NHF. Dentistry: a professional contained career in healthcare. A qualitative study of vocational dental practitioners' professional expectations. BMC Oral Health 2007;7:16 (www.biomedcentral.com/1472-6831/7/16).
15. Kadelman D, Peterson PE, Ueda H. Oral health, general health, and quality of life in older people. Spec Care Dentist 2008;28:224-236.

CHAPTER 2

Needs-related preventive programmes based on risk prediction

Per Axelsson

Definitions

Prevention may be primary, secondary or tertiary.

- *Primary prevention.* The aim of primary prevention programs is to prevent the initiation and development of periodontal diseases and dental caries. Primary prevention should be targeted towards those with healthy periodontal tissues and teeth promptly after the eruption of primary and permanent teeth. If efficient primary prevention is established in young children, neither secondary nor tertiary prevention should be necessary as adults.

- *Secondary prevention.* Secondary prevention is aimed at preventing the recurrence of disease after successful treatment and is achieved through supportive (maintenance) care programs.

- *Tertiary prevention.* Tertiary prevention is the elimination of disease through treatment, usually using non-surgical or surgical periodontal treatment methods and remineralization or restoration of caries lesions. Worldwide, only a small percentage of adolescents, adults and, particularly, the elderly has had no experience of dental caries and periodontal diseases. Consequently, approximately 80–90% of the world's population should receive tertiary prevention and/or secondary prevention. The variation between provision of tertiary prevention and secondary prevention is substantial among different countries, age groups and individuals.

Caries preventive methods

For efficient prevention and control of dental caries, needs-related combinations of the following methods should be implemented:

- plaque control
- use of fluorides
- use of fissure sealants in erupting permanent molars
- reduction of fermentable carbohydrate intakes, reduction of sugar clearance times
- salivary stimulation.

Prevention and control of periodontal diseases

Efficient prevention and control of periodontal diseases must be based on plaque control. The most successful plaque-control programs are based on a combination of:

- mechanical plaque control by self-care and professionals (professional mechanical tooth cleaning [PMTC])
- chemical plaque control by self-care and professionals.

Etiology

Dental caries and periodontal diseases are infectious and transmissible diseases caused by different species of microorganisms colonizing on the tooth surfaces forming plaque (so-called biofilms). Subgingivally, even non-attaching microorganisms may act and sometimes invade the soft periodontal tissues.

Modifying factors

The onset and progression of dental caries and periodontal diseases may be modified by external (environmental) and internal (endogenous) factors. The so-called plaque hypothesis considers that there are non-specific, specific and ecological factors leading to plaque formation. Therefore, from a cost-effectiveness view, plaque control has to be supported by elimination or reduction of the modifying factors that increase the risk for onset or progression of dental caries and periodontal diseases.

Historical milestones

Dental caries

It has been demonstrated that germ-free animals do not develop caries even with frequent sugar intake; however, all animals in such a group rapidly develop caries lesions when human cariogenic bacteria (mutans streptococci) are introduced into the mouth of one animal. Therefore, caries is a transmissible infectious disease, and sugar is not an etiologic factor but an external modifying risk factor.[1,2]

The Vipeholm study was conducted in Sweden over a five-year period (1946 to 1951). The aim was to clarify the relationship between sugar intake and caries incidence.[3] The subjects were institutionalized, mentally handicapped or retarded adults, with a mean age of 32 years at the baseline examination. Because of their poor oral hygiene (fewer than 20% brushed their teeth regularly), they had abundant amounts of plaque, an important prerequisite for caries development. The subjects were, therefore, not representative of the general population.

The stated objective was to study the relationship between sugar consumption and caries activity by varying the cariogenic substrate (present or absent), the amount of sugar (less than, equal to, or double the normal intake), the form of sugar (non-sticky or sticky) and the frequency of sugar intake (only at meals or at and between meals).

In this study, the total sugar consumption by the subjects was about twice that of the normal Swedish diet, and their plaque accumulation was far heavier than normally found today.

Other caries-modifying variables (absence of oral hygiene and use of fluoride) were also different 60 years ago. The results, therefore, should not be extrapolated directly to modern societies. The main conclusions from the Vipeholm study were as follows.

1. Consumption of sugar, even in large quantities, was associated with only a small increase in caries incidence, provided that ingestion was limited to mealtimes, at most four times a day.
2. In subjects with no or poor oral hygiene and no use of fluoride, consumption of sugar both between meals and at meals was associated with a marked increase in caries incidence.
3. Under uniform experimental conditions, the increase in caries incidence varied widely from person to person.
4. Caries activity subsided once sugar-rich foods were withdrawn from the diet.

5. In subjects with poor oral hygiene, caries lesions occurred despite the avoidance of sugar.

In a classic study of experimental caries in humans,[4] it was shown that clinical signs of enamel caries developed within three weeks in the absence of oral hygiene (ie with free accumulation of plaque) and rinsing nine times a day with a sucrose solution. When the same research team repeated the study, but introduced chemical plaque control (rinsing twice a day with 0.2% chlorhexidine solution), the subjects did not develop caries, even though they rinsed with sucrose solution nine times a day for three weeks.[5] In other words, when the etiologic factor was suppressed or eliminated, the precondition for caries did not exist and no lesions developed, despite the subjects having very frequent exposure to sucrose.

In the Turku sugar studies from 1972 to 1974,[6] the objective was to study the effect on caries incidence of almost total substitution of sucrose with either fructose or xylitol in a normal diet. The caries incidence was reduced by approximately 30% and 70% in the fructose and xylitol groups, respectively, compared with the sugar group.

Using the telemetric method for measurement of the 'true' pH fall beneath undisturbed plaque on the tooth surface after rinsing with, for example, 10% sucrose solution, it has been shown that three-day-old plaque on the approximal surfaces rapidly undergoes a critical pH fall to 4.5, while maximum 12-hour-old plaque on the lingual surfaces shows almost no pH reduction.[7] In tooth-brushing populations, three-day-old plaque may only be found on approximal surfaces of the posterior teeth. That is why these surfaces are most frequently the sites of decay in such populations. Using the Plaque Formation Rate Index (PFRI),[8] which is based on de novo plaque accumulation over 24 h after PMTC, it has been shown that most plaque is reaccumulated on approximal surfaces, followed by the lingual surfaces of the mandibular molars.

The caries-reducing effect of fluoride has been known for approximately 65 years. For 30 to 40 years following the pioneering work by Dean and co-workers,[9] it was generally believed that the most significant caries-preventive effect of fluoride was preeruptive. Recommendations for use were based on the assumption that incorporation of fluoride in the enamel apatite lattice would confer on the enamel a resistance to acid dissolution; that is, a high intake of fluoride during tooth formation and mineralization would result in enamel that was rich in fluoride, with enduring resistance to dental caries.

Preventive measures based on this assumption included fluoridation of public water supplies to the 1 mg/L level or supplying fluoride in salt or milk, or in form of a tablet to children. In a review of the old water-fluoridation studies, it was estimated that there was a 40–70% reduction in caries.[10]

There is general agreement today among those who research fluoride action that the caries-preventive and caries-controlling effects of fluorides are almost exclusively posteruptive, mainly by enhancing remineralization and retarding demineralization.

In the early 1960s, supervised mouthrinses with 0.2% NaF once a week resulted in a 25–40% caries reduction in Swedish schoolchildren.[11,12] It must be observed, however, that no efficient fluoride dentifrices were available, and regular tooth cleaning by self-care was not an established habit. As a consequence, caries prevalence was very high in Scandinavia. Twenty years later, a three-year randomized controlled double-blind study showed no difference between rinsing once per week with NaF solution and rinsing with distilled water, when fluoride dentifrice was used daily in Swedish schoolchildren with well-established oral hygiene habits.[13]

In the 1960s and 1970s, chalk was the most common abrasive in dentifrices. This inactivates NaF; however, neutral sodium monofluorophosphate is efficient in the presence of chalk.[12] Therefore, efficient fluoride dentifrices containing neutral sodium monofluorophosphate plus chalk abrasives have been available since the late 1960s. In the 1970s, dentifrices with silica abrasives compatible with NaF, SnF_2 or aminofluoride were also introduced. Based on meta-analyses, the caries-preventive effect of fluoride dentifrices ranges from 20% to 30%. The effect is correlated with the fluoride concentration. Fluoride denti-

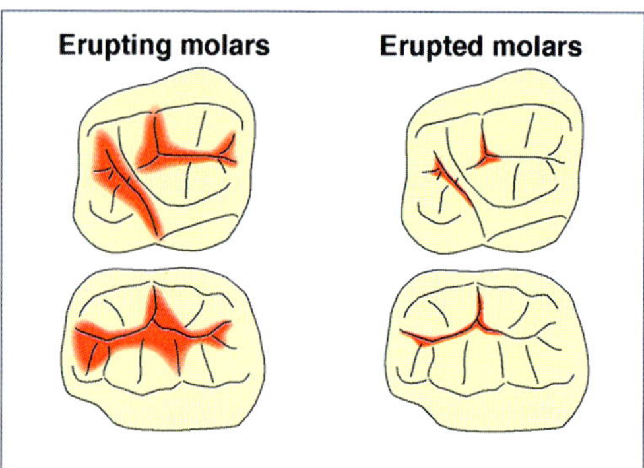

Fig. 2-1 Reaccumulation of plaque (red areas) at 48 h in partially and fully erupted molars. (Modified from Carvalho et al. [1989][18]).

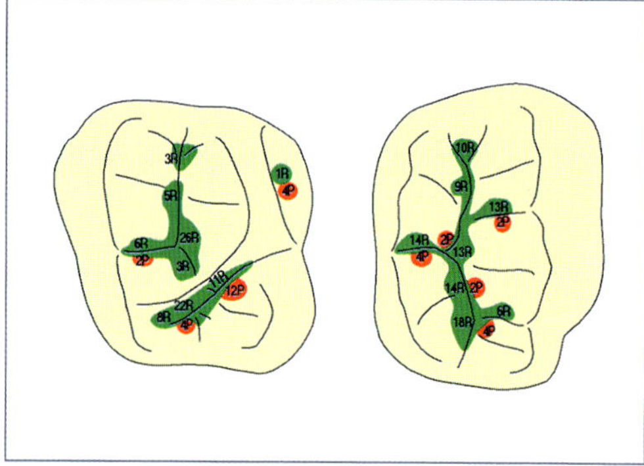

Fig. 2-2 Development of occlusal enamel caries in children in a non-invasive preventive program. Green [R], arrested caries; red [P], enamel caries that has not progressed to cavitation. (Modified from Carvalho et al. [1992][19]).

frices are the most frequently used fluoride materials in the world.

The first studies on painting teeth with neutral 2% NaF were conducted in children in the early 1940s. After thorough PMTC, the teeth were isolated with rubber dam and dried. Then, all tooth surfaces were painted with 2% neutral NaF solution, which was allowed to dry for at least three minutes. This technique, modified and described by Knutson,[14] took an average of 15 to 20 min per treatment, including PMTC, placement of rubber dam and application and drying of the NaF solution. In 1948, the US Public Health Service recommended a series of four-weekly applications of 2% NaF at age 3, 7, 11 and 13 years, to coincide with the eruption of new groups of teeth, because tooth surfaces are especially caries susceptible during and just after eruption, before the so-called secondary maturation phase. The average caries reduction achieved with such a regimen was approximately 30%.

Fluoride varnishes have been available for professional use in Europe since the late 1960s. Fluoride varnishes are regarded as slow-release fluoride agents applied at needs-related intervals on 'key-risk' surfaces in individuals with caries risk.

Historically, several methods have been used for prevention and preventive treatment of occlusal caries. In fact, there had been a long-standing interest in sealing as a method of preventing occlusal caries for more than 100 years. While investigating different methods of improving the marginal seal of acrylic resin restorative materials, Buonocore[15] decided to test the effect of etching the tooth surface with an acid solution before application of the restorative material. This alteration in technique had a dramatic effect on the adhesion of the acrylic resin to the tooth, and acid-etching techniques were soon introduced to the field of fissure sealing.[16,17]

Close to 100% of all fissure caries is initiated during the eruption of the first and second molars, in particular in the distal and central fossae. This occurs because plaque reaccumulates much faster on the occlusal surfaces of erupting molars than on fully erupted teeth with functional wear (Fig. 2-1).[18] In a three-year clinical trial in selected children with high caries risk, Carvalho and co-workers[19] showed that fissure caries could be almost totally prevented and controlled without fissure sealants if daily tooth cleaning by the parents using fluoride dentifrice was supplemented at needs-related intervals by PMTC and painting with 2% NaF solution during eruption of the molars; 80–90% of active caries lesions were remineralized or inactive after three years and there was no progression into dentin (Fig. 2-2). These principles are being successfully implemented on a large scale in different regions of Denmark. This has resulted in an increase of caries-free

12 year olds from 30% to 90% over 10 years.[20] Slow-release fluoride agents such as fluoride varnish or glass-ionomer cements could be successful substitutes for the 2% NaF solution.

To date, the relative caries-preventive effect on accessible tooth surfaces of tooth brushing and fluoride dentifrice has not been evaluated in a high-caries activity, non-tooth-brushing population within a correctly designed randomized controlled, longitudinal study, with a standardized quality of daily tooth brushing with a placebo or fluoride dentifrice, and a comparison group that is a true negative control group. For ethical reasons, it is now probably too late to conduct such a study because the use of fluoride dentifrice is so widespread. That means that most of the supervised tooth-brushing studies conducted in schools are irrelevant, as none had a true negative control group, because the controls could have their teeth brushed at home by self-care or by the parents more frequently and efficiently than the test groups.

Interproximal tooth cleaning is not an established habit among teenagers, which is why the approximal surfaces of the posterior teeth are frequently decayed in tooth-brushing teenagers. In the Dorchester split-mouth study,[21] the approximal surfaces on the test sides were cleaned daily with quality control. Compared with the contralateral control sides, test sides had approximately a 50% reduction in caries.

In a three-year longitudinal study, 12-year-old schoolchildren in Sao Paulo, Brazil, were randomly assigned to two test groups and one control group. All the children had a well-established habit of daily tooth brushing with fluoride dentifrice. In addition, all children were exposed to fluoridated drinking water and supplied with fluoride dentifrices.

Children in test group I were trained and motivated to identify sites with inflamed gingivae, which had the potential to heal, and sites with enamel caries, which had the potential to remineralize. By using the PFRI as a guideline, they deduced how frequently they needed to clean their teeth and which sites required special attention during tooth-cleaning procedures. Based on the linking method,[22] the children were motivated and trained

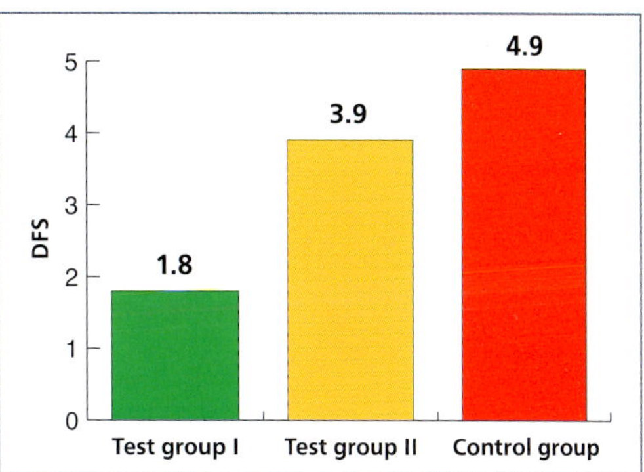

Fig. 2-3 Mean values of new approximal decayed and filled surfaces (DFS) in molars and premolars per child over three years in test group I, test group II and the control group. See the text for explanation of the groups. (From Axelsson et al. [1994][23] with permission.)

to apply fluoride dentifrice to the approximal surfaces of molars and premolars first. After these surfaces had been meticulously cleaned with dental tape, used in a rubbing technique, they then carefully cleaned the lingual and buccal surfaces with a toothbrush and fluoride dentifrice. After three initial visits at short intervals, the children were recalled for a monthly checkup during the first four months, and then every three months, for re-evaluation of the results based on self-diagnosis.

The children in test group II were trained, both on models and in their mouths, to clean every tooth surface meticulously, using dental tape, fluoride dentifrice and toothbrush. They were recalled for reinstruction at the same intervals as test group I.

During the three-year period, the children in test group I developed 54% and 63% fewer new posterior approximal lesions of dentin, per individual, than did children in test group II and the control group, respectively ($P < 0.001$) (Fig. 2-3).[23] The following conclusions were drawn from this study.

1. In a tooth-brushing population using fluoride dentifrice and fluoridated drinking water, a highly significant reduction in the incidence of approximal caries will be achieved with an oral hygiene education program based on self-diagnosis and the linking method.

2. In such a population, frequent repetition of meticulous oral hygiene training is almost redundant.[23]
3. The effect on plaque and gingivitis was also significantly higher in test group I than in test group II and the control group.[24]
4. Because all three groups had the same exposure to fluoride from dentifrice and drinking water, the greater reduction in caries found on the approximal surfaces in test group I compared with test group II and the control group must be the effect of improved interdental plaque control.

The cost-effectiveness (cost savings) of large-scale implementation of the system used in this low-cost, low-technology study based on self-care is almost inestimable.

Studies by Nyvad and Fejerskov[25] in elderly patients with active root caries lesions have also shown that improved oral hygiene converts active lesions to inactive lesions. Even root caries lesions with deep cavities could be successfully converted to inactive lesions by improved plaque control and use of fluoride.

Recent meta-analyses of well-controlled longitudinal studies show that the average caries-preventive effect of fluoride dentifrice is approximately 20–30%, while chemical plaque control by daily use of chlorhexidine results in 40–50% caries reduction. Plaque control is more effective because it targets the etiology of dental caries (ie the cariogenic plaque), while fluoride exerts a modifying effect on the demineralization and remineralization processes.

Periodontal diseases

In 1965, Löe and co-workers[26] conducted a pioneering study of experimental gingivitis in humans. When dental plaque was allowed to accumulate undisturbed, students with healthy gingiva developed clinical signs of gingivitis within two or three weeks; on resumption of oral hygiene, the inflammation subsided within a week.

In a six-week study in students, Lang and co-workers[27] showed that no clinical signs of gingival inflammation appeared if plaque was thoroughly removed at least every second day; with less-frequent plaque removal, only every third or fourth day, gingivitis developed. Bosman and Powell[28] induced experimental gingivitis in a group of students: gingival inflammation persisted if plaque removal occurred only every third or fifth day, whereas healing occurred within 7 to 10 days in the two groups who cleaned their teeth at least every second day.

These studies provided evidence that prevention of gingivitis should be based on plaque control: thorough mechanical cleaning of all tooth surfaces every second day is more effective than daily cosmetic brushing of the buccal and lingual surfaces that are not at risk. Animal studies have shown that untreated plaque-induced gingivitis can eventually progress to periodontitis.[29,30] In humans, although gingivitis is very common, progressive periodontitis develops in only a minority of individuals and sites. At the 1st European Workshop on Periodontology,[31] consensus was reached that periodontitis is always preceeded by gingivitis. Prevention of gingivitis should, therefore, also prevent periodontitis.

The importance of the patient's oral hygiene efforts, as well as regular recall for PMTC and debridement, to the long-term maintenance of periodontal health was first examined in a study of gingival conditions in 1428 individuals, 20 to 60 years of age, in an industrial company in Oslo, Norway.[32] Over a five-year period of regular recall (two to four times a year) for education in oral hygiene, PMTC, debridement and scaling, gingival conditions improved by approximately 60%. Loss of teeth was reduced to approximately 50% of what would otherwise have been expected. No surgical treatment of periodontal pockets was undertaken; satisfactory results were very difficult to achieve in pockets more than 5 mm deep. However, there was marked improvement in the periodontal health, even in patients whose oral hygiene remained substandard during the five years of the trial.

Suomi and co-workers[33] measured loss of periodontal support in young adults with gingivitis or with only minor loss of periodontal attachment.

The experimental group received education in oral hygiene measures, PMTC, debridement and scaling every third month over a three-year period. Plaque accumulation and gingival inflammation were significantly reduced, and the mean value for clinically measurable loss of attachment was only 0.08 mm per surface during the observation period. Loss of attachment in the control group, in which no special measures were taken to improve oral hygiene, was 0.30 mm (0.10 mm per year).

Frequent PMTC has been successfully used for secondary prevention following initial non-surgical or surgical treatment of marginal periodontitis. In a study by Rosling and co-workers,[34] patients with a high prevalence of infrabony pockets were randomly allotted to a test or a control group. After initial open-flap surgery, scaling and root planing, the test group received PMTC every two weeks for two years. At the re-examination, approximately 95% of the infrabony pockets had healed, and the condition of the gingiva was excellent. Among the patients in the control group, there were some non-responders with very significant loss of periodontal attachment and some lost teeth.[35,36]

In an investigation by Nyman et al[35] of 20 surgically treated patients with advanced periodontitis, an experimental group subsequently received thorough PMTC and oral hygiene education every two weeks. No further clinical loss of attachment could be demonstrated after two years. The patients in the control group received the same initial treatment, including surgery, and were recalled for debridement and scaling six months after surgery but no other attempts were made to maintain gingival plaque control. After two years, the control patients exhibited an average clinical loss of attachment of approximately 2 mm. This very rapid periodontal destruction suggests that periodontal surgery may, in fact, do more harm than good in the absence of proper supportive care based on excellent gingival plaque control. In the control group, probing depth two years after surgery was approximately the same as before surgery; in the experimental group, the probing depths were maintained at the immediate postoperative level.

In a split-mouth study, Lindhe and co-workers[37] found excellent healing of marginal periodontitis irrespective of the initial treatment method (non-surgical or different types of flap surgery) when this was followed by frequent PMTC for two years. Even in patients with aggressive periodontitis, no recurrence was observed over a five-year period when initial non-surgical or surgical treatment was followed by frequent PMTC during the first two years.[38]

In the pioneering split-mouth clinical studies by Ramfjord,[39-44] the long-term effect of three different treatment procedures was evaluated:

- subgingival curettage: based on the description, this procedure should be regarded as closed subgingival scaling, debridement and root-planing (ie 'non-surgical' treatment)
- modified Widman flap surgery: pocket reduction procedures without bone removal and repositioning of the flap with interdental covering and suturing
- pocket elimination surgery: reversed bevel flap, bone contouring, apical positioning of the flap and gingivectomy in patients where no bone removal was needed for pocket elimination.

The patients were then maintained on a program including repeated oral hygiene education and debridment (including PMTC) once every three months. The effect on pocket depth and periodontal attachment level was analyzed after five years[40] and eight years.[43,44] The results showed that pocket depth in moderate and deep pockets was reduced over eight years for all three methods. Only curettage and modified Widman flap surgery resulted in significant gain of periodontal attachment in moderately deep pockets. In deep pockets (7–12 mm), the gain of attachment was greatest after the modified Widman flap surgery.

The claim that treated pockets with a long junctional epithelium could predispose to repocketing has been refuted by research. The results from one study[42] suggest that resistance to progression of periodontal disease is similar for a long epithelial attachment and a connective tissue attachment.

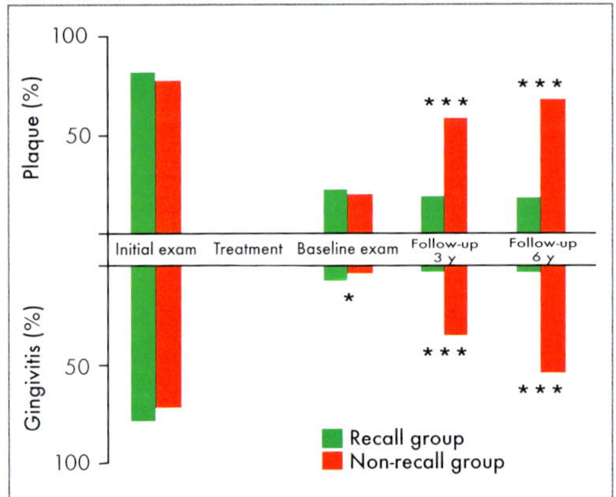

Fig. 2-4 Percentage of tooth surfaces with plaque and inflamed units in the two groups of patients at the initial, baseline and follow-up (three and six years after the baseline) examinations. See the text for explanation of the groups.
*$P < 0.05$; ***$P < 0.001$.
(Modified from Axelsson and Lindhe [1981][49] with permission.)

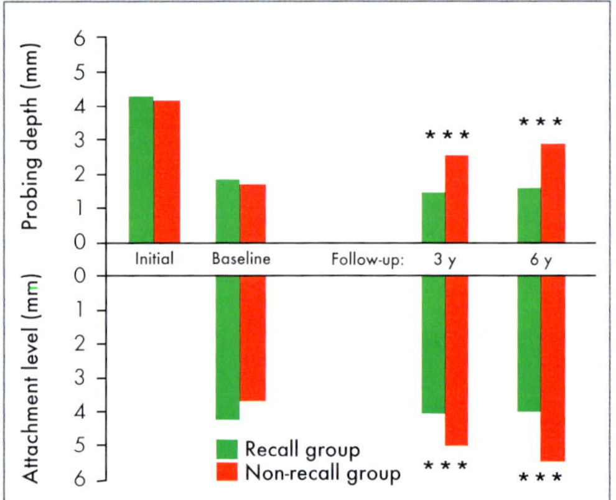

Fig. 2-5 Individual mean pocket (probing) depth and periodontal attachment level data from the initial, baseline and follow-up (three and six years after the baseline) examinations.
See the text for explanation of the groups.
***$P < 0.001$.
(Modified from Axelsson and Lindhe [1981][49] with permission.)

A higher percentage of shallow pockets (< 3 mm) lost more than 2 mm of attachment over five years compared with deeper pockets, mostly as an iatrogenic effect on buccal surfaces. Consequently, there appears to be no justification for forceful penetration of the junctional epithelial attachment at recall. If there is no calculus, tightly adapted pocket walls without appreciable subgingival spread of plaque biofilms and inflammation, the sites should be treated only by PMTC and cautious debridement.

Several studies using a study design that included subgingival instrumentation and assessment of subgingival recolonization have incidentally allowed investigation of the influence of gingival plaque control on subgingival recolonization.[45] It is, however, acknowledged that some bacteria may persist at the pocket sites following such instrumentation. Mousqués and co-workers[46] reported a positive correlation between low supragingival plaque scores and a subgingival flora resembling that associated with health in 14 individuals who had received thorough scaling and root planing but no oral hygiene instruction.

Magnusson and co-workers[47] observed that, in the presence of supragingival plaque, a subgingival flora with large numbers of motile rods and spirochetes reformed in four to eight weeks after subgingival instrumentation, whereas sustained reductions in motile rods and improved periodontal conditions were achieved following subgingival debridement plus supervised oral hygiene and PMTC. Similarly, Sbordone and co-workers[48] reported that subgingival debridement without gingival plaque control was insufficient to maintain a healthy subgingival microflora.

Axelsson and Lindhe[49] also demonstrated the value of a carefully designed secondary prevention program, based on meticulous gingival plaque control by self-care and PMTC, for patients who had been treated for advanced periodontal disease: 77 patients were examined before treatment, two months after the last surgical procedure, and after three and six years. Two thirds of the patients (n = 52) were placed on a supervised maintenance program that included oral hygiene education, meticulous PMTC and needs-related debridement every two months for the first two years and every three months for the last four years of the observation period (recall group). The remaining 25 patients resumed care by the referring dental clinician, who was informed of the importance of checking their oral hygiene, calculus formation and gingival and periodontal conditions (non-recall group).

The data from the second examination showed the positive effect of the initial treatment in both groups. Subsequently, the recall patients were able to maintain excellent gingival health and unaltered attachment levels as an effect of proper oral hygiene and supportive PMTC. In the non-recall group, plaque scores increased markedly from the baseline values, as did the number of inflamed gingival units (Fig. 2-4). Concomitantly, there were obvious signs of recurrent periodontitis. The mean values for probing depth and attachment levels at the three- and six-year examinations were higher than at baseline (Fig. 2-5). Approximately 99% of the tooth surfaces showed improvement, no change or < 1 mm of attachment loss in the recall group, compared with 45% in the non-recall group. In the latter group, 55% of the sites showed 2–5 mm of further attachment loss at the six-year examination, and 20% of the pockets were > 4 mm deep.[49]

Cortellini and co-workers[50] reported the long-term maintenance results in 23 patients undergoing guided tissue regeneration treatment of 40 deep infrabony pockets. After one year of stringent maintenance, a marked gain of attachment was registered in all patients. The patient sample was then divided: one group was enrolled in a strict maintenance program based on gingival plaque control by self-care and PMTC, while the other group received only sporadic care during the subsequent four years. In the well-maintained group, the gained attachment levels remained stable, and the subjects had significantly lower complete-mouth plaque and bleeding scores. In the sporadically treated group, there was loss of attachment compared with pretreatment levels. The study showed that stability of gained clinical attachment was associated with stringent gingival plaque control; this was more predictably enforced by a regular supportive periodontal care program. In another study, Gottlow and co-workers[51] reported that clinical attachment gained by guided tissue regeneration can be maintained for up to five years if there is meticulous gingival plaque control by self-care and PMTC.

In a study of 75 patients with extremely advanced periodontitis who had been successfully treated for the disease through initial cause-related therapy and modified Widman flap procedures, recurrent infection occurred in only very few sites during a 14-year period of effective secondary prevention by so-called supportive periodontal treatment (SPT).[52] However, it has to be understood that recurrent periodontitis was noticed at completely unpredictable time intervals but was concentrated in approximately 25% of the patient population (15 out of 61). This suggests that, in a periodontitis-susceptible risk population, the majority of patients can be 'cured' provided an optimally organized secondary prevention program is performed, while a relatively small proportion of patients (20–25%) will suffer from occasional episodes of recurrent periodontal reinfection. It is obviously a challenge for the diagnostician to identify such patients with very high disease susceptibility and to monitor the dentitions for recurrent periodontitis on a long-term basis.

Rosling and co-workers[53] evaluated the effect of SPT in a group of 225 subjects with 'normal' and a group with high susceptibility (n = 109) to periodontal disease (based on baseline data). Baseline examination was carried out one year after initial non-surgical therapy (tertiary prevention). SPT including oral hygiene education, PMTC and needs-related subgingival debridement occurred three to four times per year. After 12 years, mean periodontal attachment loss was only 0.04 mm/tooth surface per year in the normal group, compared with 0.06 mm in the group with high susceptibility.

Microbiology has been used to determine the frequency of recalls. Listgarten and co-workers[54,55] reported data from a longitudinal study of patients with treated periodontitis who were on two maintenance program schedules. The control schedule was standard and consisted of recall every three months with professional prophylaxis. The experimental group followed the same program but the decision for active prophylaxis was determined by the outcome of subgingival plaque analysis. In the experimental group, SPT intervals could be increased from an average of 4.5 months after one year to 20.1 months after four years.[54,55] The authors concluded that recalls every three months may not be adequate

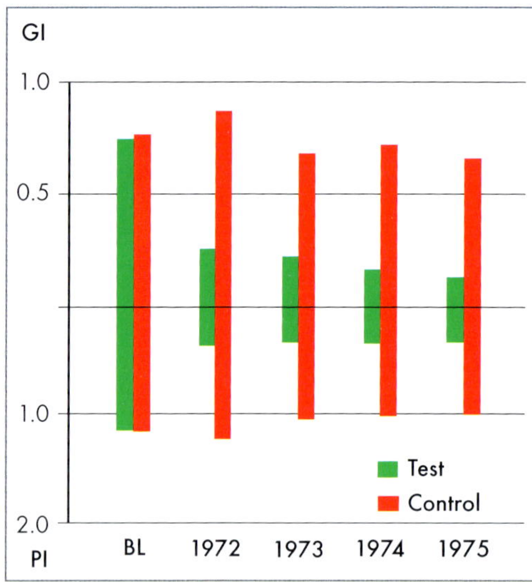

Fig. 2-6 Annual variations in mean Gingival Index (GI) and mean Plaque Index (PI) for children in test and control groups (see text). The average values for groups 1, 2 and 3 have been used. BL, baseline.
(Modified from Axelsson and Lindhe [1977][57] with permission.)

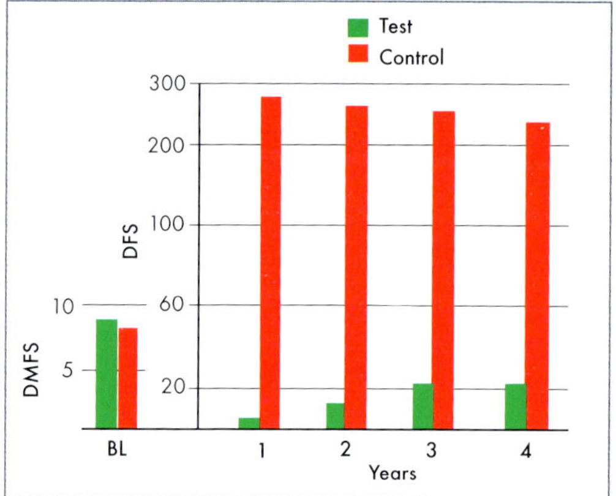

Fig. 2-7 The mean number of new caries lesions or filled surfaces in the three control groups compared with the three test groups during the four-year trial. See the text for explanation of the groups. DFS, decayed and filled surfaces; DMFS, decayed, missing or filled surfaces; BL, baseline. (Modified from Axelsson and Lindhe [1977][56] with permission.)

for all patients, and that some patients may still do well even with longer intervals.[55]

The intervals of SPT in the test groups in most of the above reviewed studies have been three to four times per year or even more frequent irrespective of the individual need. Even for subjects with high susceptibility for periodontal disease, this frequent interval seems to be efficient. However, in subjects with low susceptibility and high standard of gingival plaque control by self-care, three to four SPT per year should be regarded as overtreatment. Therefore, from the cost-effectiveness point of view, materials, methods and intervals for SPT must be based on the individual needs.

Dental caries and periodontal disease

In 1971, a longitudinal clinical trial was initiated to test the hypothesis that gingivitis and dental caries do not develop in schoolchildren maintained on an oral hygiene program that includes PMTC and oral hygiene education once every two weeks. The subjects were 216 children, aged 7–8, 10–11 and 13–14 years at the beginning of the study. All children were from the same elementary school in the city of Karlstad, Sweden, and all had the same socioeconomic background. All were randomly assigned to a test or a control group. During a four-year period, a preventive dentistry assistant carried out PMTC on the test group 16 times a year for the following two years, and then four to six times a year in the following two years. The control group received ordinary dental treatment once a year, supervised tooth brushing using the Bass method and fluoride rinsing 10 times a year for the entire trial period. Thus, there was no true negative control: for ethical reasons the subjects in the control group were maintained on the regular dental care schedule.

The effect of treatment on the amount of plaque was assessed using the Silness and Löe Plaque Index (PI), and the development of gingivitis using the Löe and Silness Gingival Index (GI) (Fig. 2-6).[56] There were no differences between the two groups at baseline. After one year, there was a marked reduction in both plaque and gingivitis in the test group, but scores on both indices remained persistently high in the control group. The test group succeeded in maintaining low scores for the following three years, but the high plaque and gingivitis scores in the control group did not improve. More pronounced was the effect on the development of dental caries (Fig. 2-7). During the entire four-year trial, the test group developed only 62 new decayed and filled surfaces (DFS) in all, while the control group developed 941.[56,57]

The long-term benefits of this early introduction of a program of meticulous mechanical plaque control on dental caries and the standard of self-performed oral hygiene and gingival health should not be underestimated. The long-term caries-preventive effect of frequent PMTC in young children was later reconfirmed in another Swedish study.[58]

This study was followed up with other clinical trials to compare the separate effects of PMTC on caries and gingivitis with other preventive measures such as oral hygiene training, chemical plaque control and topical use of fluorides. In all these studies, frequent PMTC was superior to the other measures.[59-61] In reviews of almost 20 studies based on PMTC, with or without oral hygiene education, the range of caries reduction was 35–95%.[17,62,63]

The overall goals for maintenance programs in randomized samples of adults should be to prevent tooth loss and the recurrence of dental caries and periodontitis after initial active treatment of the diseases (ie secondary prevention and control). However, for cost-effectiveness, such programs must be based strictly on individual needs.

There are very few longitudinal clinical studies in adults on the prevention of recurrence of both periodontal disease and dental caries. In 1971 and 1972, a clinical study was initiated in the city of Karlstad, in the county of Värmland, Sweden, to determine whether the development of caries and the progression of periodontitis could be prevented in adults, and whether a high level of mechanical plaque control could be maintained by regularly repeated self-care education based on self-diagnosis, PMTC and needs-related subgingival debridement. An attempt was also made to study the progression of dental disease in individuals who did not receive special self-care education but who regularly received conventional dental care.

Two groups of subjects from the same region were recruited for the study. Of these, two thirds (n = 375) were assigned to test groups and one third (n = 180) to control groups, stratified by age: 20–35 years (group 1), 36–50 years (group 2) and 51–65 years (group 3). The baseline examination included the following variables:

- Plaque Index (% according to O'Leary)
- gingival and pocket bleeding indices (%)
- Community Periodontal Index of Treatment Needs (CPITN): periodontal depth (mm), calculus and restoration overhangs
- clinical periodontal attachment loss
- alveolar bone loss
- numbers of decayed, missing or filled teeth and surfaces
- history taking, for example general diseases, medications, socioeconomic condition, body mass index, lifestyle, dental care and oral hygiene habits, and dietary and smoking habits.

During the first six-year period, the control patients were examined regularly once a year for conventional dental care. After initial scaling and root planing, the test group participants were recalled every second month during the first two years and once every third month during the following four years of the study for education in self-care and for PMTC and needs-related subgingival debridement by a dental hygienist. The oral hygiene training program was carried out with emphasis on self-diagnosis and interproximal cleaning with wooden, triangular-tipped toothpicks and fluoride dentifrice on the approximal surfaces of the posterior teeth. At each visit, a plaque-disclosing tablet was used to detect any residual gingival plaque. Supplementary interdental probing was used for the posterior teeth. After discussion with the patient about any sites with residual plaque, needs-related PMTC was carried out. The first step after plaque disclosure was the application by syringe of fluoride-containing prophylaxis paste to the interdental areas of the mandibular posterior teeth followed by the maxillary teeth. This was followed by careful approximal PMTC with a prophylaxis contra-angle handpiece and a reciprocating triangular flexible pointed tips. The PMTC usually also included use of a rotating rubber cup and prophylaxis paste, particularly on the lingual surfaces of the mandibular posterior teeth, and was supplemented, as necessary, by non-aggressive subgingival debridement or topical application of fluoride to specific key-risk surfaces.

The subjects were re-examined toward the end of the third and sixth years of the study. After six years, the number of new caries surfaces per subject was 14.0 in the control groups and only 0.2 in the test groups. On average, patients in the control groups lost 1.2 mm of periodontal attachment during the six-year period, while those in the test groups had an average gain of 0.2 mm. It is important to note, however, that most of the subjects and sites in the control groups did not lose any periodontal attachment, or had very limited loss; the mean data indicated that there were a number of extreme 'downhill' patients and sites (high risk patients and sites that developed disease much more than average patients).[64]

After the six-year re-examination, the control groups were disbanded: for ethical reasons, these subjects were also offered needs-related preventive programs, and most accepted. The few subjects in the test groups who developed new caries lesions and/or lost periodontal attachment during the six-year period were classified as high-risk or at-risk individuals for caries and/or periodontitis. During the following years, up to the 15- and 30-year re-examinations, all subjects in the test groups received a needs-related maintenance program from the same dental hygienist. To ensure maximum cost-effectiveness, the recall intervals, as well as the preventive measures used, were based strictly on individual need. Approximately 60% visited the dental hygienist only once a year, 30% twice a year and 10% (the at-risk and high-risk individuals) three to six times a year. The average annual number of visits for age groups 1, 2 and 3 was 1.2, 1.5, and 1.8, respectively. The patients were re-examined by a dental clinician on an average of only once every two to four years, including the compulsory 15- and 30-year re-examinations.

At the 15-year (1987)[65] and 30-year (2002)[66] re-examinations, 317 and 257, respectively, of the original 375 test subjects from the baseline examination in 1972 were available for re-examination. Fewer than 10 subjects were unwilling to continue in the study, confirming high patient acceptance of the maintenance program. The main reason for drop-outs in group 1 (50–65 years of age in 2002) and group 2 (66–80 years of age in 2002) was moving to other areas of Sweden. In group 3 (81–95 years of age in 2002), most were lost to follow up through death. Only 0.2 teeth per individual were lost over 15 years. During the same period, it was estimated that the randomized samples of the Swedish adult population lost, on average, four teeth per individual.[67] From 1978 until 1987, the total cost per individual per year in the test groups was approximately 50% of the cost per Swedish adult recall patient. From 1978 until 1987, the mean treatment time by a dental clinician (including examination) was less than 20% of the average for recall patients in Sweden.[65]

As an effect of self-care education based on self-diagnosis, supplemented with needs-related intervals of PMTC, stained plaque was almost non-existent at the 30-year re-examination compared with the baseline examination.

Effect on tooth loss

The mean number of teeth per individual in age groups 1, 2 and 3 and in all groups at the baseline examination in 1972 and at the 30-year re-examination in 2002 is shown in Fig. 2-8.[66] Because third molars were excluded, the maximum number of teeth was 28. At the 30-year re-examination, groups 1, 2 and 3 were 50–65, 66–80 and 81–95 years old. On average, groups 1, 2 and 3 lost only 0.4, 0.7 and 1.8 teeth, respectively. Over 60% of these few lost teeth were lost because of root fractures in teeth with posts. In comparison, randomized samples of Swedes aged 45–50 years showed a loss of almost 3 teeth per subject over 11 years (ie about

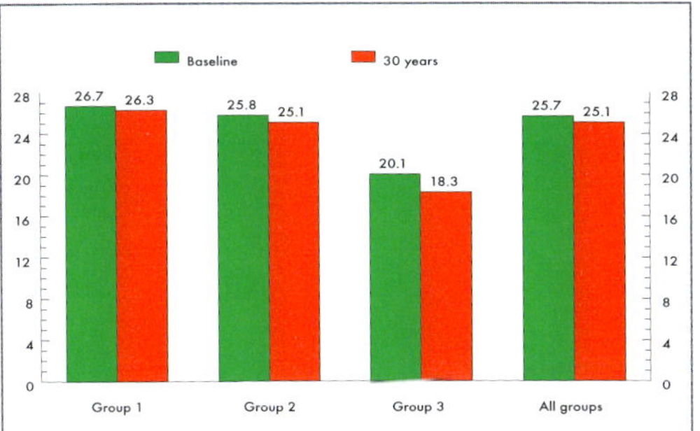

Fig. 2-8 Mean number of teeth (third molars excluded) per individual in age groups 1, 2 and 3 and all groups at the baseline examination and at the 30-year re-examination. See the text for explanation of the groups. (Modified from Axelsson et al. [2004][66] with permission.)

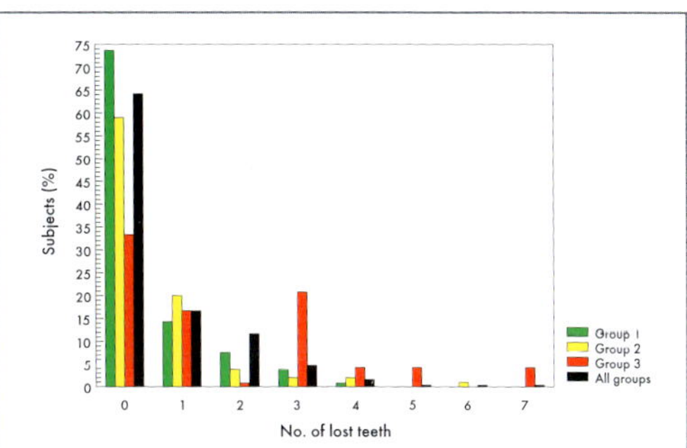

Fig. 2-9 Frequency distribution of lost teeth over 30 years in age groups 1, 2 and 3 and all groups. See the text for explanation of the groups. (Modified from Axelsson et al. [2004][66] with permission.)

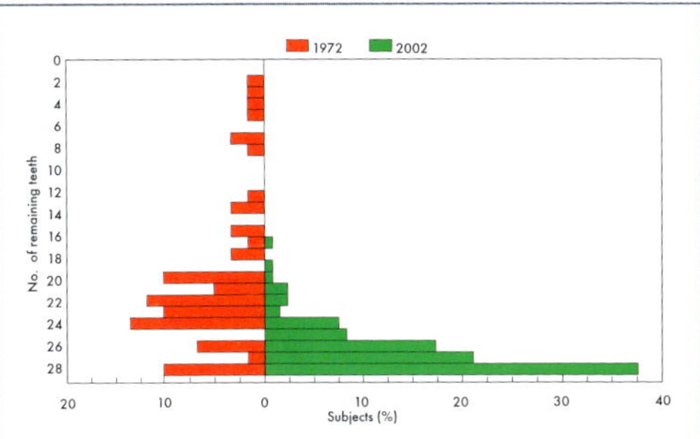

Fig. 2-10 Frequency distribution of remaining teeth in subjects aged 51–65 years in 1972 compared with subjects aged 50–65 years in 2002. (Modified from Axelsson et al. [2004][66] with permission.)

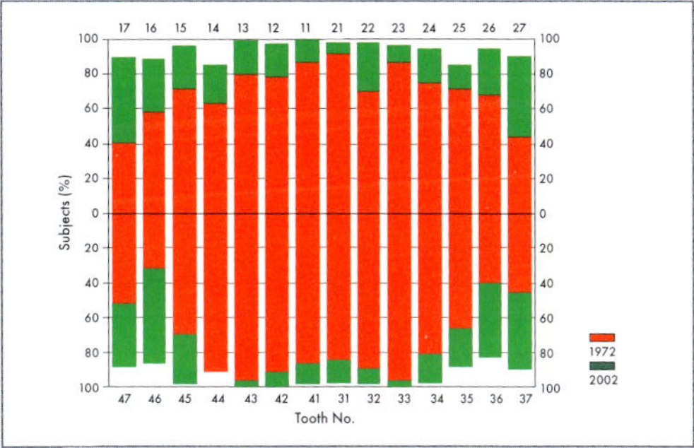

Fig. 2-11 Mean percentage of remaining individual teeth (Fédération Dentaire Internationale tooth-numbering system) in subjects aged 51–65 years in 1972 compared with subjects aged 50–65 years in 2002. (Modified from Axelsson et al. [2004][66] with permission.)

8 teeth over 30 years).[67] Almost 75% of subjects in group 1 and 60% in group 2 did not lose a single tooth, and 15–20% lost only one tooth during the 30-year trial (Fig. 2-9). In contrast, among a randomized sample of adults aged 35–55 years, in the county of Stockholm, Sweden, during a 20-year study, the mean number of lost teeth was 5 (ie 7.5 lost teeth per subject over 30 years). Only 27% did not lose any teeth; 38% lost 1 or 2 teeth; 18% lost 3 or 4 teeth; 7% lost 5 or 6 teeth; 3% lost 7 or 8 teeth; 15% lost between 9 and 16 teeth, and 2% lost > 16 teeth.[68]

For ethical reasons, the control groups were offered needs-related preventive dentistry after six years, as mentioned above. Therefore, the baseline data of group 3 (51–65 years in 1972) were used as a cohort control group for group 1 (50–65 years in 2002) at the 30-year examination. In 2002, group 1 exhibited an average of 26.3 remaining teeth (third molars excluded) compared with only 20.1 in subjects in group 3 in 1972. The frequency distribution of remaining teeth in subjects aged 51–65 years in 1972 and 50–65 years in 2002 is shown in Fig. 2-10. Approximately 30% of those aged 51–65 years in 1972 had 24 to 28 remaining teeth, compared with approximately 95% in those aged 50–65 years in 2002. The pattern of remaining teeth in subjects aged 51–65 years in 1972 and 50–65 years in 2002 is shown in Fig. 2-11.

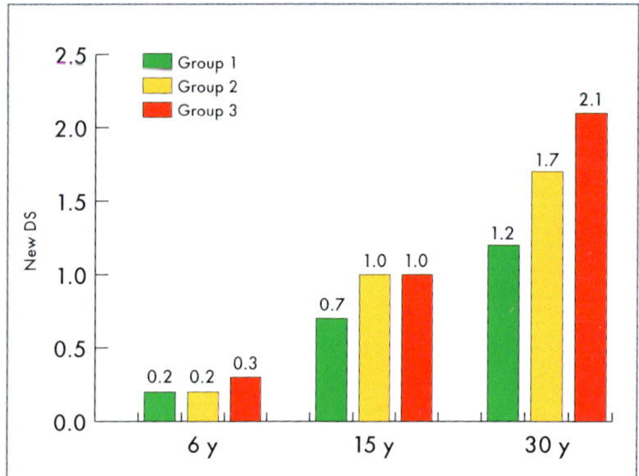

Fig. 2-12 Mean caries incidence after 6, 15 and 30 years, by age group: group 1 (50-65 years in 2002); group 2 (66-80 years in 2002); group 3 (81-95 years in 2002). DS, decayed surfaces. (Modified from Axelsson et al. [2004][66] with permission.)

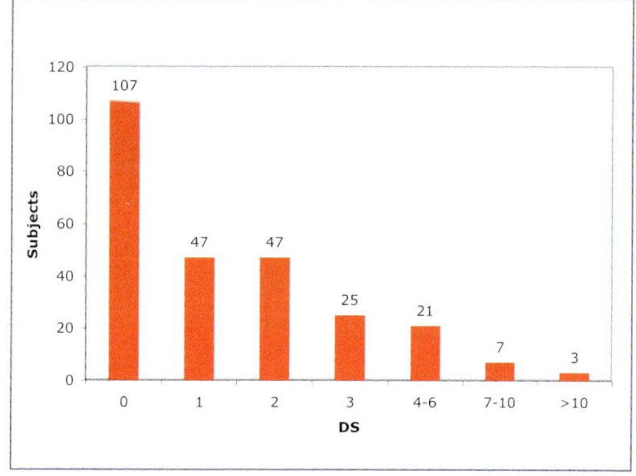

Fig. 2-13 Frequency distribution of new caries lesions/filled surfaces among the 257 subjects from 1972 to 2002. (Modified from Axelsson et al. [2004][66] with pemission.)

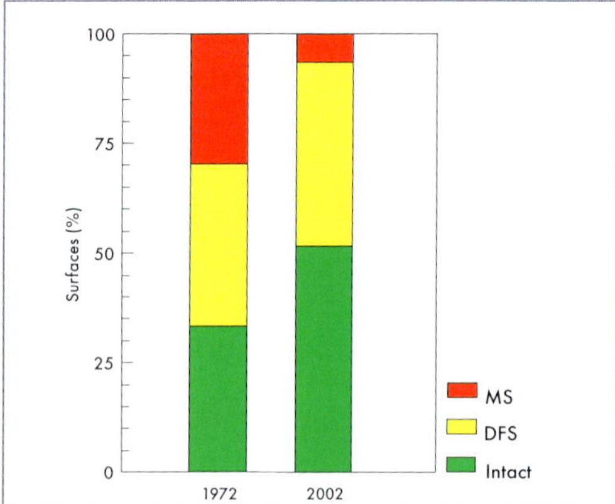

Fig. 2-14 Caries prevalence in subjects aged 51-65 years in 1972 compared with those subjects 50-65 years of age in 2002. DFS, decayed and filled surfaces; MS, missing surfaces. (Modified from Axelsson et al. [2004][66] with permission.)

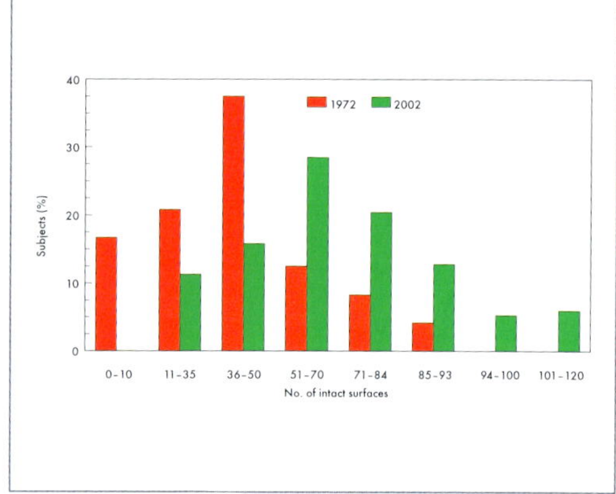

Fig. 2-15 Frequency distribution of subjects with specific numbers of intact tooth surfaces aged 51-65 years in 1972 compared with subjects aged 50-65 years 2002. (Modified from Axelsson et al. [2004][66] with permission.)

Effect on dental caries

The mean values of new carious surfaces per subject after 6, 15 and 30 years is shown in Fig. 2-12. In each age group, recurrent caries predominated. Of 257 subjects, 107 developed no new caries lesions; 47 developed only one new caries lesion and 47 developed two new caries lesions. Only 10 subjects exhibited more than six new decayed surfaces (Fig. 2-13). In this context, it must be realized that Swedish subjects who are not enrolled on preventive programs experience a much higher incidence of caries than carefully maintained patients. Fure[69] showed that in randomized samples of subjects aged 55, 65 and 75 years from the city of Göteborg, Sweden, the average number of new coronal DFS during a 10-year interval were 6.0, 3.8 and 1.8, respectively, while the mean number of root caries lesions in the same period amounted to 5.5, 8.1 and 14.3, respectively.

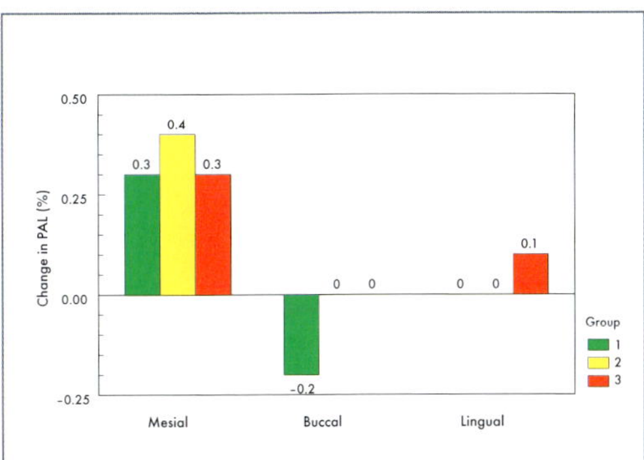

Fig. 2-16 Mean periodontal attachment loss (PAL) changes in the three age groups at mesial, buccal and lingual sites from 1972 to 2002.
(Modified from Axelsson et al. [2004][66], with permission.)

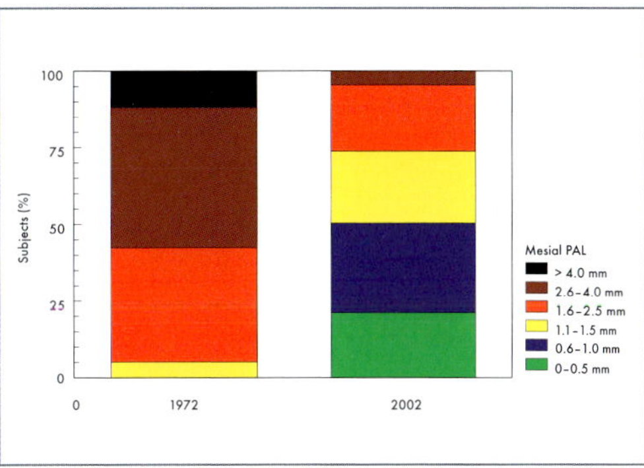

Fig. 2-17 Frequency distribution of subjects aged 51–65 years (1972) and 50-65 years (2002) with specific mean periodontal attachment loss (PAL) mesially in.
(Modified from Axelsson et al. [2004][66] with permission.)

The percentage of intact and missing teeth and DFS in subjects aged 51–65 years in 1972 compared with those 50–65 years of age in 2002 is shown in Fig. 2-14. In particular, the percentage of intact surfaces increased from < 35% to > 50% and the percentage of missing surfaces was reduced from almost 30% to only approximately 5%. The frequency distribution of subjects with specific numbers of intact tooth surfaces aged 51–65 years in 1972 was compared with subjects aged 50–65 years in 2002 and is shown in Fig. 2-15.

Effect on periodontal disease

Except for a mean loss of 0.2 mm on the buccal surfaces in group 1 as an iatrogenic effect, there was no marked change in periodontal attachment level on the buccal and lingual surfaces; however, on the approximal surfaces, gains ranging from 0.3 to 0.4 mm were recorded in the three age groups (Fig. 2-16). Most likely, several approximal intrabony pockets at baseline had been 'repaired' during the study. Although there was an overall gain of attachment in the sample, further attachment loss of > 2 mm had occurred on a few of the sites (2–8%), mainly buccally, as an iatrogenic effect of frequent mechanical cleaning. For comparison, the annual mean loss of periodontal support was 0.1 mm in an 11-year longitudinal study in a randomized sample of Swedish adults[67] and two 20-year longitudinal studies in adults in the counties of Jönköping[70] and Stockholm[68] in Sweden (ie an average of 3 mm of periodontal support loss over 30 years). The buccal surfaces exhibit the most attachment loss, which can be explained by a combination of erosion and iatrogenic trauma caused by mechanical cleaning, as discussed above. Therefore, to eliminate the iatrogenic effects on periodontal attachment loss, only approximal periodontal attachment loss should be presented as resulting from periopathogens.

The frequency distribution of subjects aged 51–65 years and 50–65 years with specific mean mesial periodontal attachment loss in 1972 and 2002 respectively is shown in Fig. 2-17 and that for mesial sites with different levels of periodontal attachment loss in Fig. 2-18. The pattern of periodontal attachment loss mesially in subjects aged 51–65 years in 1972 compared with subjects aged 50-65 years in 2002 is shown in Fig. 2-19. Most improvement was achieved in the maxillary teeth and mandibular posterior teeth.

Missing sites and teeth do not have any periodontal treatment needs. Therefore, periodontal treatment needs should take into account missing sites when the 'true' treatment need is estimated. The frequency distribution of sites according to CPITN score 0 to 4 and missing sites in subjects

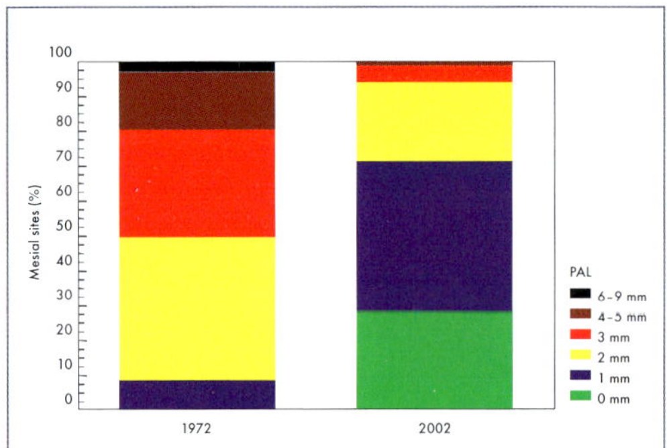

Fig. 2-18 Frequency distribution of levels of mean periodontal attachment loss (PAL) on mesial sites in subjects aged 51-65 years (1972) and 50-65 years (2002).
(Modified from Axelsson et al. [2004][66] with permission.)

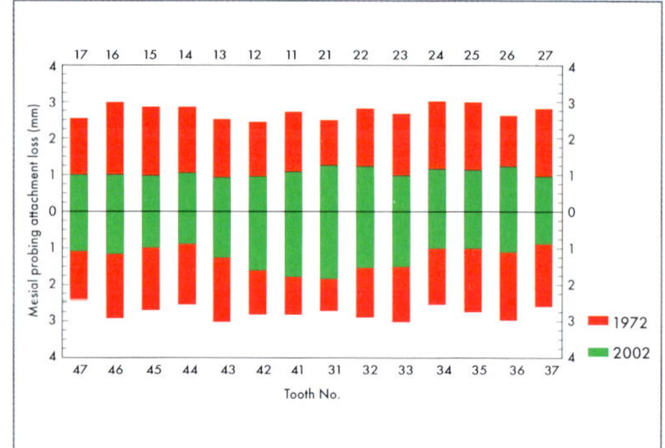

Fig. 2-19 Pattern of mesial mean periodontal attachment loss in subjects aged 51-65 years (1972) (red) and 50-65 years (2002) (green). (FDI tooth-numbering system).
(Modified from Axelsson et al. [2004][66] with permission.)

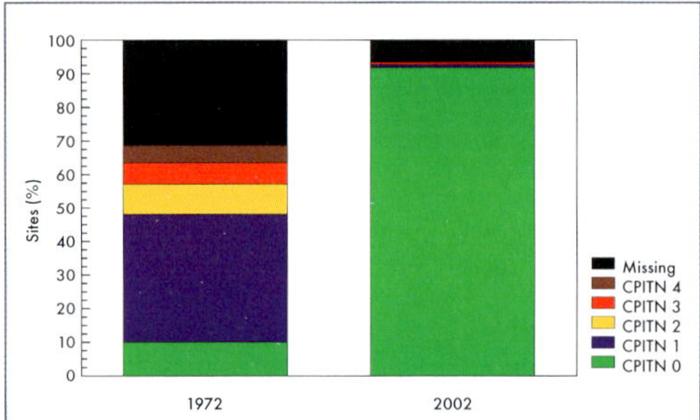

Fig. 2-20 Frequency distribution of missing sites and sites with Community Periodontal Index of Treatment Needs (CPITN) scores 0 to 4 in subjects aged 51-65 years (1972) and 50-65 years (2002). (Modified from Axelsson et al. [2004][66] with permission.)

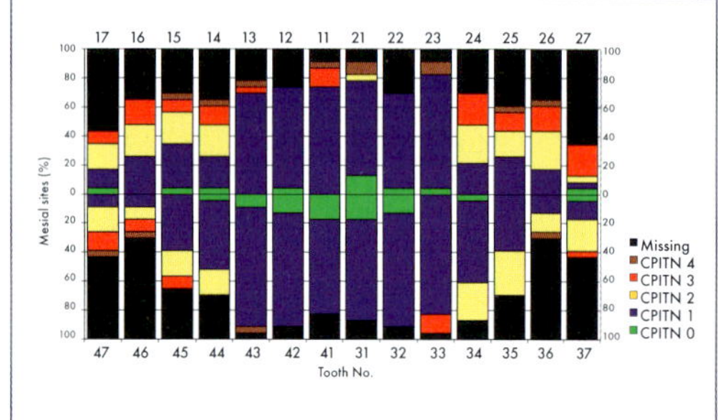

Fig. 2-21 Pattern of missing sites and sites with Community Periodontal Index of Treatment Needs (CPITN) score 0 to 4 mesially in subjects aged 51-65 years in 1972.
(Modified from Axelsson et al. [2004][66] with permission.)

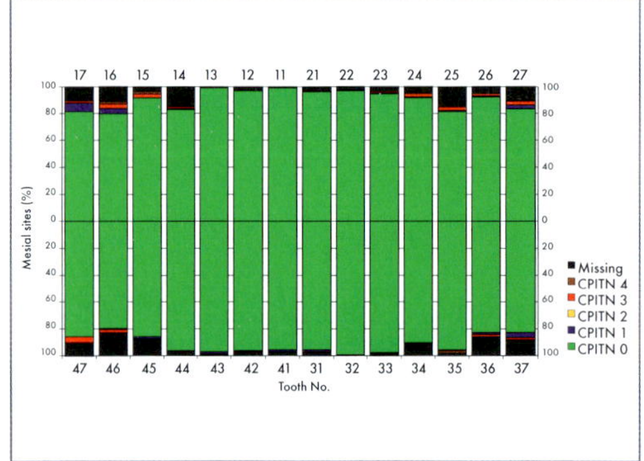

Fig. 2-22 Pattern of missing sites and sites with Community Periodontal Index of Treatment Needs (CPITN) score 0 to 4 mesially in subjects aged 50-65 years in 2002.
(Modified from Axelsson et al. [2004][66] with permission.)

aged 51-65 years in 1972 compared with subjects aged 50-65 years in 2002 is shown in Fig-2-20.

Almost 95% of the sites were healthy and only 5% were missing in 2002, compared with only 10% of sites healthy and more than 30% of sites missing in 1972. In 2002, more than 75% of the subjects had a CPITN score of 3, compared with only 23% in 1972. The pattern of missing sites and sites with CPITN score 0 to 4 mesially in subjects aged 51-65 years in 1972 and 50-65 years in 2002 is shown in Figs 2-21 and 2-22. In 1972, most missing sites were found in the maxillary and anterior mandibular molar regions; most CPITN scores 3 and 4 sites were found approximally in the maxillary posterior teeth, and most CPITN score 2 (calculus) sites were found lingually in the mandibular anterior teeth. By comparison, in 2002, almost 100% of all sites were healthy. In conclusion, this study showed that a well-trained dental hygienist, supervised by a dental clinician and using established professional preventive measures to complement improved self-care, was able to prevent further loss of periodontal attachment and reduce the development of new caries lesions to less than two caries surfaces per subject over 30 years, irrespective of age. It was also shown that excellent self-care habits, including self-diagnosis, can be successfully established in adults; age does not matter. At the 30-year re-examination, 92% brushed their teeth two or more times per day and 8% either in the morning or before going to bed. In addition, 70% used toothpicks daily, 44% used dental tape daily and 35% used interdental brushes daily. In addition, the percentage of smokers was reduced from 46% in 1972 to only 10% in 2002.[66]

Treatment concepts

The effect of needs-related preventive programs for children and young adults

Based on the experiences from our clinical research studies on different preventive methods and risk prediction, a preventive program was designed in 1978. This program is continuously updated and improved.

The large-scale implementation of our needs-related preventive program for all aged 1 to 19 years in the county of Värmland, Sweden has resulted in a dramatic reduction of caries prevalence. The goals for the subjects following the program from birth to the age of 19 years were:

- to have no approximal restorations
- to have no occlusal amalgam restorations
- to have no approximal loss of periodontal attachment
- to be motivated and encouraged as individuals to assume responsibility for their own oral health.

The effect of the program is evaluated once a year on almost 100% of all those 3–19 years of age in a computer-aided epidemiologic program initiated in 1979. Most of the individualized preventive program is carried out by dental hygienists or prophylactic dental assistants at clinics in the elementary schools.

Effect on primary teeth

As a result of the preventive program gradually introduced at the health centers for expectant mothers and the child welfare centers in the 1970s, the percentage of caries-free three year olds increased from 35% in 1973 to 97% in 1993 and is still maintained at this level, which is suboptimal. In 1999, the mean values of primary teeth that were decayed, extracted owing to caries or filled in children aged three, four and five years were only 0.07, 0.3 and 0.4, respectively. The percentages of teeth that were caries free in children aged three, four, five and six years were 97, 90, 83 and 76%, respectively.

Effect on permanent teeth

Caries prevalence in the county of Värmland expressed as mean DFS for all surfaces and approximal surfaces per individual in 1979 and 1999, in all age groups from 7 to 19 years old is shown in Fig. 2-23. The average caries reduction ranged from 85 to 95%. The mean total number DFS per individual aged 12, 16 and 19 years, respectively, declined from 6, 12 and 24.3 DFS in 1979 to 0.3, 1.15 and 2.1 DFS in 1999. In the same age groups, DFS on the approximal surfaces represented 20–25% of the total in 1979, declining from 1.1, 3.0 and 5.0, respectively, in 1979 to 0.1, 0.6 and 1.1 DFS, respectively, in 1999. The frequency distribution of DFS in the different age groups in 1999 showed that the percentages of caries-free individuals from ages 7 to 19 years were 98, 96, 94, 92, 91, 86, 81, 77, 72, 71, 66, 64 and 60%, respectively (Fig. 2-24).

Caries incidence in permanent teeth

Compared with 1979, the mean number of new decayed surfaces per individual per year was also reduced by 85 to 95% in 1999, including all surfaces, as well as the approximal surfaces, in the different age groups. In those aged 7, 12 and 19 years,

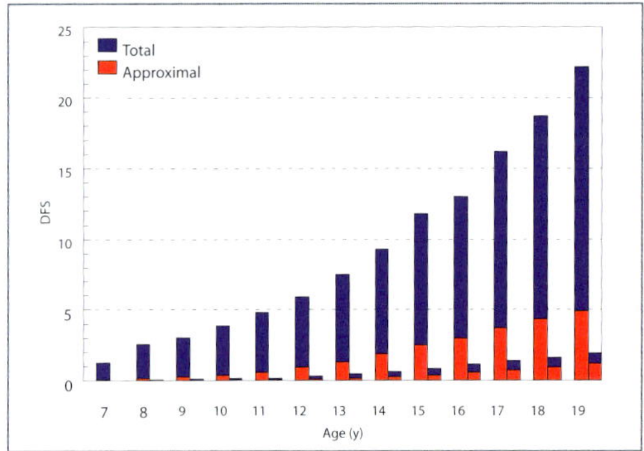

Fig. 2-23 Mean number of decayed and filled surfaces (DFS) for all surfaces and approximal surfaces in 1979 (left bar) and 1999 (right bar) in individuals aged 7 to 19 years in the county of Värmland, Sweden. (from Axelsson et al. [2004][17] with permission.)

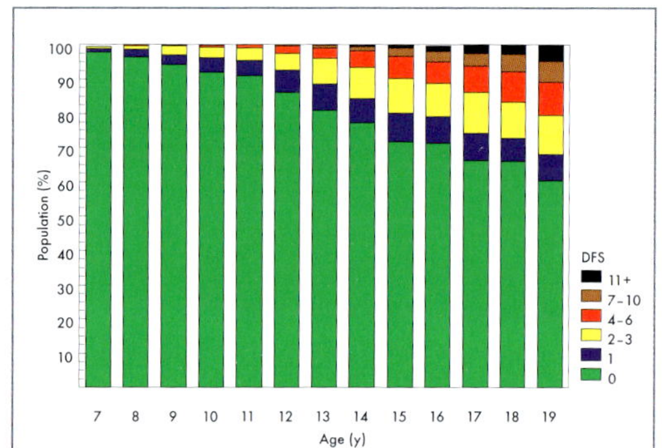

Fig. 2-24 Frequency distribution of decayed and filled surfaces (DFS) in individuals aged 7 to 19 years in the county of Värmland, Sweden, in 1999. (from Axelsson et al. [2004][17] with permission.)

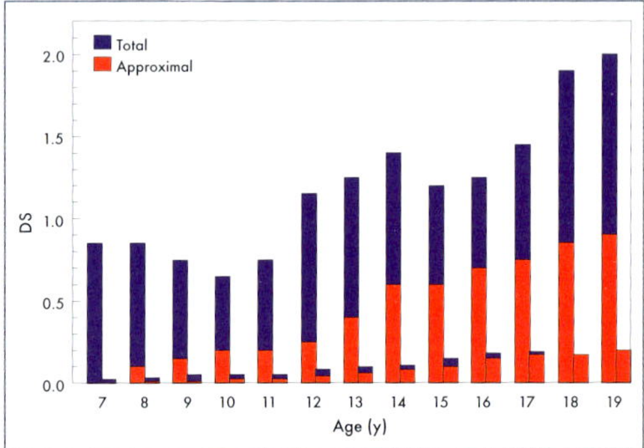

Fig. 2-25 Mean number of total new decayed surfaces (DS) and approximal new DS in 1979 (left bar) and 1999 (right bar) in individuals aged 7 to 19 years in the county of Värmland, Sweden. (from Axelsson et al. [2004][17] with permission.)

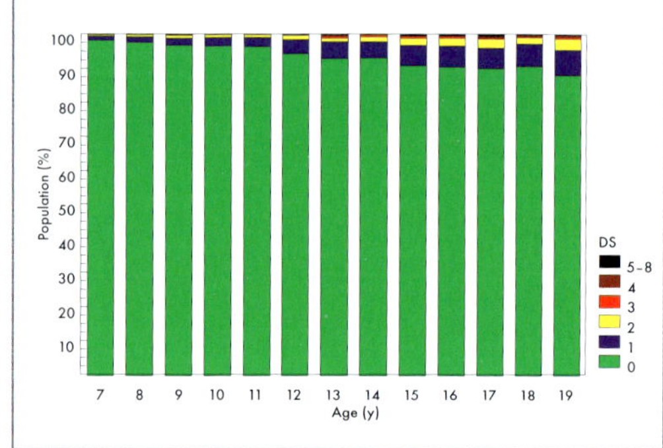

Fig. 2-26 Frequency distribution of new decayed surfaces (DS) in individuals aged 7 to 19 years in the county of Värmland, Sweden, in 1999. (from Axelsson et al. [2004][17] with permission.)

respectively, the caries incidence for all surfaces was reduced from 0.85, 1.15 and 2.0 new decayed surfaces per individual in 1979 to 0.02, 0.06 and 0.2 in 1999 (Fig. 2-25). In the same groups, caries incidence for the approximal surfaces declined from 0, 0.2 and 0.9 new decayed surfaces per individual in 1979 to 0, 0.03 and 0.2 in 1999. The frequency distribution of new decayed surfaces showed that 88–98% of the children in the different age groups did not develop any new decayed surfaces, in 1999 (Fig. 2-26). Among 7-year-old children, 98% did not develop any new decayed surfaces, 1% developed one new decayed surface and 0.4% developed two new decayed surfaces. The corresponding figures for 12-year-olds were 94%, 4% and 1%, respectively. Among 19-year-old individuals, 88% developed no new decayed surfaces; 8% had one new decayed surface; 3% had two new decayed surfaces; 1% had three or four new decayed surfaces, and 0.1% had five or six new decayed surfaces.

Treatment time and cost-effectiveness

According to data collected annually from all counties in Sweden by the Swedish Board of Health and Welfare, the mean treatment time by a dental clinician per child in 1979 was 1.75 h in the county of Värmland, and the national average was 1.7 h. However, one effect of our needs-related preventive program by preventive dental assistants and dental hygienists was a dramatic reduction, to only 20 min per child per year, by 1999 in the mean treatment time by a dental clinician, which was considerably lower than in any other Swedish county. Most of the dental clinician's time was spent on examinations, because the need for restorations was minimized.

The total costs per child per year (2001), including the needs-related preventive program by dental hygienists or preventive dental assistant, treatment by dental clinicians and orthodontic treatment by specialized orthodontists, was approximately 90 euros compared with 100 euros; as the average for all of Sweden. Because the average caries prevalence in children and young adults in this program is the lowest in Sweden, it must be concluded that this needs-related caries-preventive program is very cost-effective. The cost–benefit ratio of such a program is also very high because intact teeth and healthy gingivae are beautiful, functional and appealing, and this may positively influence our general health. As a contrast, unreasonable 'drilling, filling, killing the pulp and billing' should have gone out of fashion many decades ago.[17,71]

Summary

Nearly 100% of the goals of the needs-related caries-preventive program were achieved and currently we are still improving our results. Caries prevalence in those aged 19 years has been reduced from > 24 DFS in 1979 to only 2 DFS in 1999. Out of these, one DFS was occlusally. In Sweden, dental amalgam cannot be used in those 15 years of age or younger. Hence, only one of the two DFS in the 19 year olds was filled with amalgam. Therefore, very few occlusal amalgam fillings exist because of caries in the 19-year-old individuals, and in a few years there will be none. On average, there was only one approximal DFS in 1999 and < 0.5 was filled; this included non-cavitated dentin caries lesions diagnosed on bitewing radiographs, which should be arrested by 'prevention instead of extension' or at least 'prevention before extension.'

Needs-related self-care habits based on self-diagnosis were established as early as possible. In addition, PMTC and chemical plaque control was supplemented for at-risk individuals at needs-related intervals. As a consequence, approximal loss of periodontal attachment was prevented. It can be concluded that close to 100% of the goals in 1979 had been achieved by 1999. In addition, it seems reasonable that individuals who at 20 years of age have no lost teeth, only 2 DFS, no loss of periodontal attachment and well-established excellent self-care habits should maintain at least 25 healthy natural teeth for the rest of their lives.[17] This conclusion is supported by the results of the 30-year longitudinal study in adults. Subjects aged 51–65 and 66–80 in 2002, who had participated in a needs-related preventive and supportive care program performed by a dental hygienist from 1972 to 2002, on average lost only 0.4 and 0.7 teeth, respectively, did not loose periodontal attachment and developed only two new decayed surfaces per subject over the 30 years.[66]

It seems reasonable to believe that caries prevalence in children and young adults can be further reduced at very low cost by application of ongoing clinical research in new preventive materials and methods and in techniques to predict risk for oral diseases, and by new knowledge and continuing professional development of well-trained and highly motivated dental professionals. Finally, it is important to emphasize the importance of the evaluation of new methods, as well as the re-evaluation of established methods by means of clinical research prior to large-scale implementation. There are 'evergreen' methods, but preventive measures should be tailored to reflect trends in the pattern of dental disease in a population.

The effect of needs-related programs in adults

Experience gained from our 30-year longitudinal study is applied in the two-year training program for dental hygienists at the University of Karlstad, Sweden, and in preventive programs for adults at

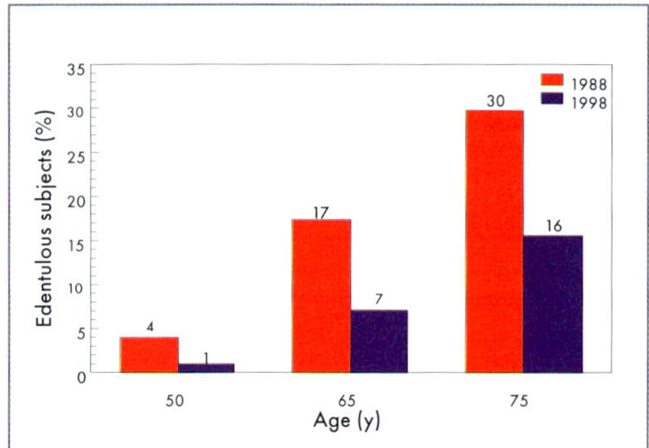

Fig. 2-27 The percentage of edentulous subjects aged 50, 65 and 75 years in the county of Värmland, Sweden in 1988 and 1998.
(Modified from Axelsson et al. [2000][72] with permission.)

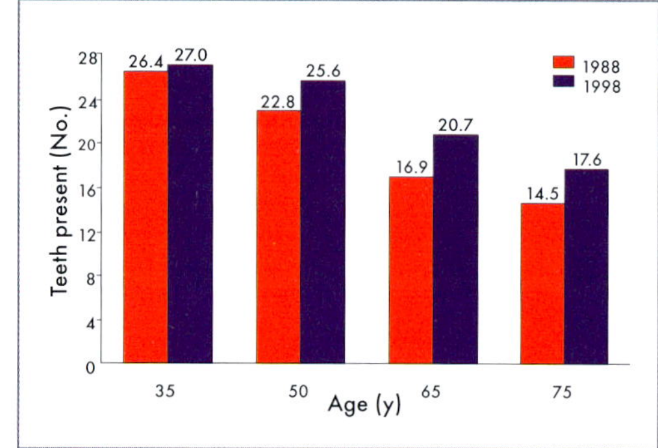

Fig. 2-28 Mean number of teeth in those aged 35, 50, 65 and 75 years in 1988 and 1998.
(Modified from Axelsson et al. [2000][72] with permission.)

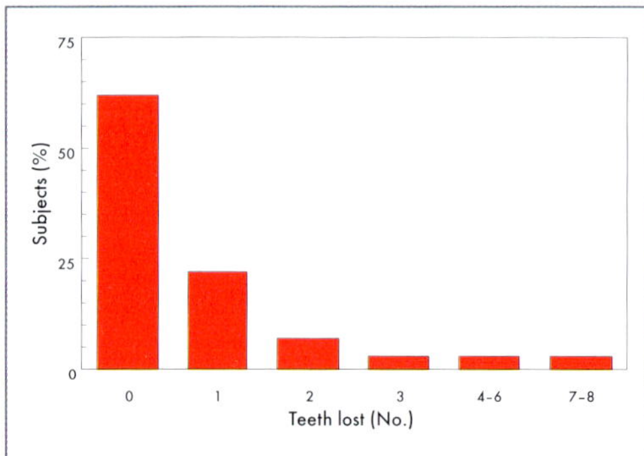

Fig. 2-29 Frequency distribution of tooth loss from the age of 50 years (1988) to the age of 60 years (1998) in a randomized sample of 313 subjects.
(From Axelsson et al. [2000][72] with permission.)

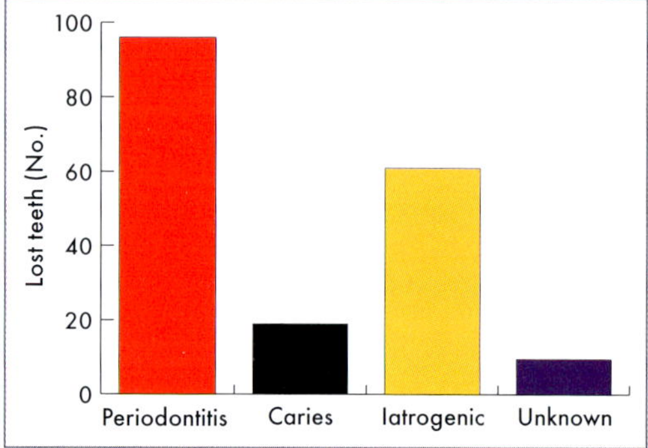

Fig. 2-30 Estimated frequency distribution of tooth loss from the age of 50 years (1988) to the age of 60 years (1998) in a randomized sample of 313 subjects, according to cause: periodontitis, caries, iatrogenic reasons (mainly root fractures in teeth with a post) and unknown.
(Modified from Axelsson et al. [2000][72] with permission.)

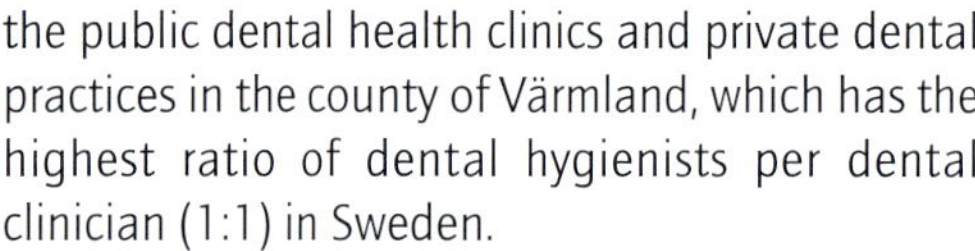

the public dental health clinics and private dental practices in the county of Värmland, which has the highest ratio of dental hygienists per dental clinician (1:1) in Sweden.

As a consequence, dental health status has improved considerably in the adult population, as shown in our analytical epidemiologic studies in randomized samples of 35-, 50-, 65- and 75-year-old adults in 1988 and 1998.[72] The percentage of edentulous individuals aged 50, 65 and 75 years decreased from 4, 17 and 30%, respectively, in 1988 to 1, 7 and 16%, respectively, in 1998 (Fig. 2-27). These data indicate that approximately 2% of those aged 65 years and < 10% of those aged 75 years will be edentulous in 2008. The number of teeth (third molars excluded) increased from 26.4, 22.8, 16.9 and 14.5 to 27.0, 25.6, 20.7 and 17.6 teeth in those aged 35, 50, 65 and 75 years, respectively (Fig. 2-28). It is estimated that the mean number of teeth will increase to 26, 24 and 20 in those aged 50, 65 and 75 years in 2008. The frequency distribution of lost teeth in a randomized sample of individuals from age 50 years (in 1988) to 60 years (in 1998) is shown in Fig. 2-29. The most common reason for lost teeth

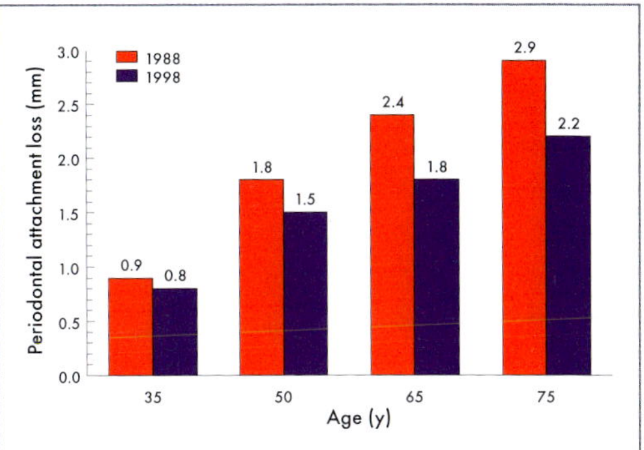

Fig. 2-31 Mean periodontal attachment loss (mm) in those aged 35, 50, 65 and 75 years in 1988 and 1998. (Modified from Axelsson et al. [2000][72] with permission.)

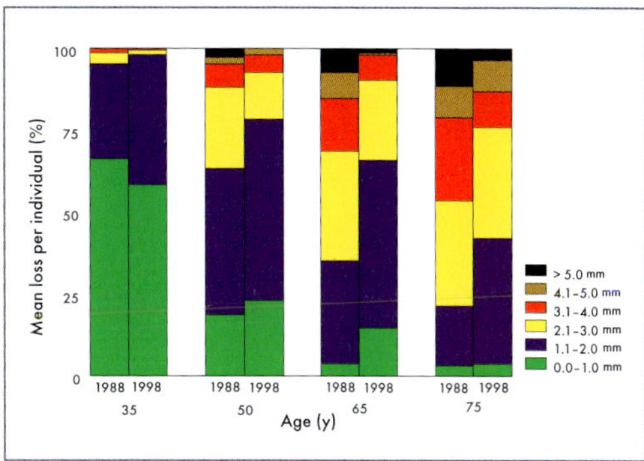

Fig. 2-32 Frequency distribution (%) of individuals with mean periodontal attachment loss at mesial sites of 0-1.0, 1.1-2.0, 2.1-3.0, 3.1-4.0, 4.1-5.0 and > 5 mm in 1988 and 1998. (Modified from Axelsson et al. [2000][72] with permission.)

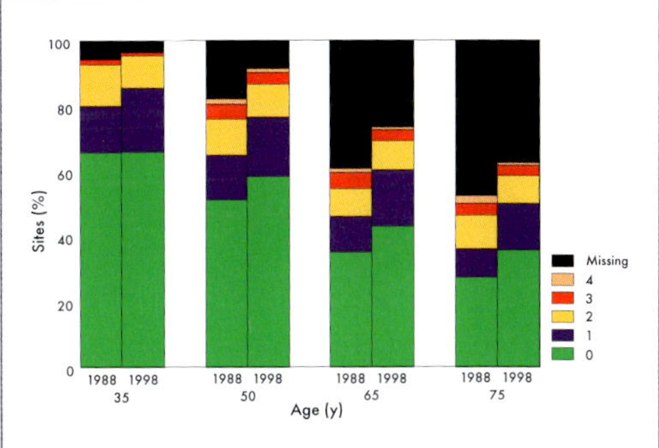

Fig. 2-33 Frequency distribution of missing sites and sites with Community Periodontal Index of Treatment Needs scores of 0, 1, 2, 3 and 4 in 1988 and 1998. (Modified from Axelsson et al. [2000][72] with permission.)

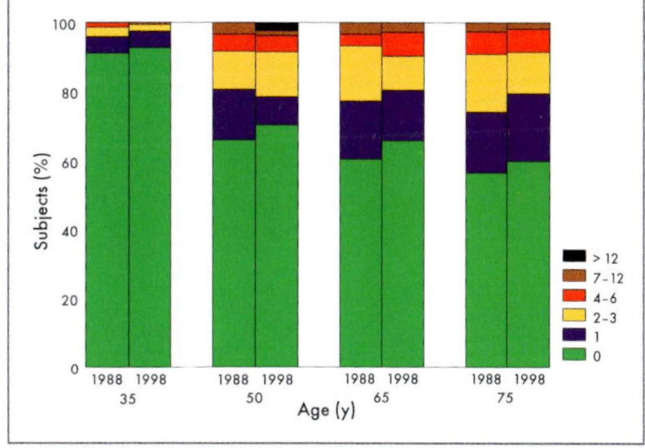

Fig. 2-34 Frequency distribution of individuals with 0, 1, 2-3, 4-6, 7-12 and > 12 sites with Community Periodontal Index of Treatment Needs score 4 in 1988 and 1998. (Modified from Axelsson et al. [2000][72] with permission.)

was periodontitis, followed by iatrogenic reasons (root fractures in teeth with post) (Fig. 2-30).

The mean periodontal attachment loss measured mesiobuccally, mesiolingually, buccally, distobuccally and lingually decreased from 0.9, 1.8, 2.4 and 2.9 mm to 0.8, 1.5, 1.8 and 2.2 mm in the individuals aged 35, 50, 65 and 75 years, respectively (Fig. 2-31). The frequency distribution of individuals with mean mesiobuccal and mesiolingual periodontal attachment loss of 0-1.0, 1.1-2.0, 2.1-3.0, 3.1-4.0, 4.1-5.0 and > 5 mm in the four age groups in 1988 and 1998 is shown in Fig. 2-32. The frequency distribution of all sites (mesial, buccal, distal and lingual) according to CPITN scores 0, 1, 2, 3 and 4, as well as missing sites, in 1988 and 1998 is shown in Fig. 2-33. The percentage of individuals with 0, 1, 2-3, 4-6, 7-12 and > 12 sites with CPITN score 4 (periodontal pocket depth > 5 mm) in the four age groups in 1988 and 1998, respectively, is shown in Fig. 2-34. From 1988 to 1998, notably in those aged 35 and 50 years, the mean number of intact teeth increased significantly. The number of missing teeth decreased most obviously in those aged 50, 65 and 75 years (Fig. 2-35).[72]

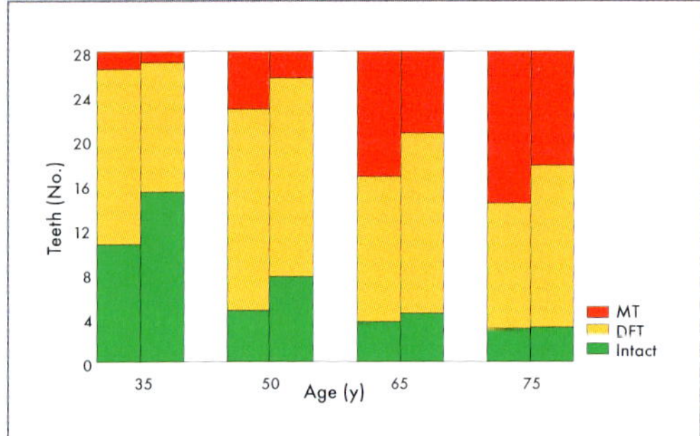

Fig. 2-35 Frequency distribution of the mean number of intact teeth, decayed and filled teeth (DFT) and missing teeth (MT) in randomized samples of subjects aged 35, 50, 65 and 75 years in 1988 compared with 1998.
(Modified from Axelsson et al. [2000][72] with permission.)

In conclusion, longitudinal clinical studies have shown that gingival plaque control by self-care and supportive care based on frequent PMTC and needs-related subgingival debridement in patients with periodontal disease will result in reduced probing depth, increased or maintained periodontal attachment, reduced quantities of subgingival microflora, reduced range of subgingival periopathogenic microflora and improved healing of periodontal soft tissues as well as of intrabony pockets after periodontal surgery and regenerative therapy. It also prevents recurrence of periodontal disease.

Longitudinal clinical studies have also shown that such supportive care performed by dental hygienists can prevent the recurrence of periodontitis as well as dental caries in adults because these strategies target the causes of the diseases. The range of effects reported in different clinical studies is strongly correlated with the materials and methods used, the sample size and the incidence of the disease in the population. If needs-related plaque-control habits for self-care are established and supplemented by needs-related intervals of PMTC, very significant preventive effects will be achieved, particularly in high-risk individuals, compared with a randomly matched control group.[17,63,73-77]

Global oral health personnel resources and trends

There has been a dramatic decrease in the previously high levels of dental caries among children in most industrialized countries since the mid 1970s.[78] In many developing countries, however, caries prevalence has increased from previous levels. In addition, the prevalence of moderate periodontal treatment needs (CPITN score 1–3) is much higher in developing countries than in industrial-

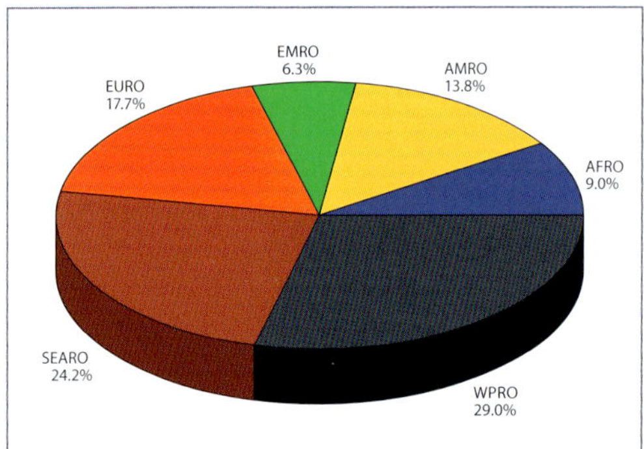

Fig. 2-36 World population by World Health Organization regions. EURO, Europe Regional Office; EMRO, Eastern Mediterranean Regional Office; AMRO, Americas Regional Office; AFRO, Africa Regional Office; WPRO, Western Pacific Regional Office; SEARO, Southeast Asia Regional Office. (Modified from World Health Organization [1994][79] with permission.)

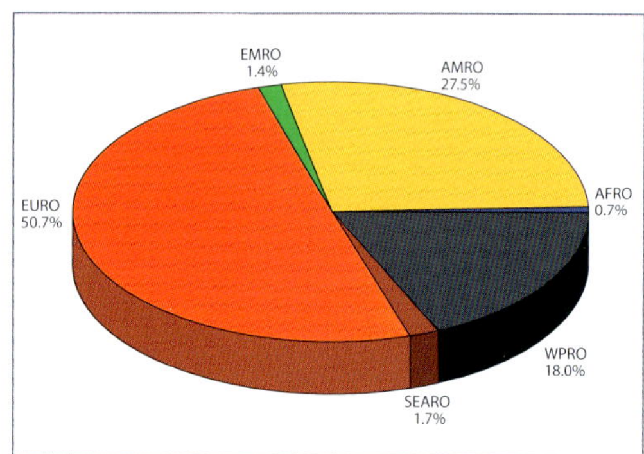

Fig. 2-37 Oral health personnel by World Health Organization regions. EURO, Europe Regional Office; EMRO, Eastern Mediterranean Regional Office; AMRO, Americas Regional Office; AFRO, Africa Regional Office; WPRO, Western Pacific Regional Office; SEARO, Southeast Asia Regional Office. (Modified from World Health Organization [1994][79] with permission.)

ized countries, despite a similar prevalence of advanced periodontal treatment needs (CPITN score 4). The dilemma is that the developing countries represent the majority of the world's population.

The percentage of the world's population by World Health Organization (WHO) regions in 1986 is shown in Fig. 2-36.[79] Asia alone (Southeast Asia Regional Office and Western Pacific Regional Office) contains more than 50% of the world's population. China and India have 2.5 billion inhabitants (40%).

According to WHO's Data Bank in 1986,[80] Europe has more than 50% of the world's oral health personnel resources - dental clinicians, dental therapists, hygienists, dental assistants, technicians, etc. (Fig. 2-37) - although it has only 17.7% of the world's population (Fig. 2-36). The extremes of the ratio of dental clinicians to inhabitants are found in Scandinavia (1:1000) and in China and India (1:120 000).[79,80]

Increasing the availability of oral health personnel

Overcoming this imbalance in the ratio of oral health personnel, particularly of dental clinicians, to the population in different countries is a major challenge. Many developing countries are experiencing either an actual increase in caries prevalence or an inability to reduce the existing level. Although the disease prevalence is, or threatens to be, only moderate, its impact is much more serious than would be the case in industrialized countries, because of the almost total lack of effective care.

These countries have responded to the problems by attempting to develop new dental schools with curricula adapted from those that were common, but are now changing, in industrialized countries. More serious still is the fact that, irrespective of which curricula these countries may have chosen, there is a crippling lack of qualified teaching staff. In practical terms, this shortfall results in failure to deliver, often by a wide margin, whatever curricula are offered in faculty handbooks.

This predicament is not limited to developing countries. There is a wide divergence of dental school performance across the range of industrialized countries, let alone within any country in which there are a number of dental schools. Even where schools may be judged to be similar in quality, strength and creativity may vary markedly from subject to subject. The profession is consequently facing a challenge to minimize undesirable variation in learning and teaching and to provide up-to-date and high-quality education for all.

In addition to the overwhelming need for dental treatment by dental clinicians, in particular in developing countries in Asia, Africa and Latin America, which are home to the majority of the world's population, there is a clear indication for training of dental hygienists who are committed exclusively to prevention and control of dental caries and periodontal diseases and periodontal treatment. In addition, initiating such work is very cost-effective, as discussed above.[65,66,73]

The role and supply of dental hygienists are of increasing interest worldwide, mainly because of a growing acknowledgment of the importance of oral health as a part of general health, renewed emphasis on setting and attaining health policy goals, and recognition of dental hygienists as a major resource for attaining those goals. Dental hygienists today constitute one of the largest and fastest growing groups in the oral health service. They practice, in collaboration with other health professionals, primarily as clinicians and health educators. Their work involves the use of preventive and therapeutic methods to promote good health and to prevent and control oral diseases.

According to Fédération Dentaire Internationale surveys in 1990, dental hygienists are now trained in more than 25 countries. The pioneers were the USA (1906) followed by Norway (1924), the UK (1943), Canada (1947), Japan (1949), Nigeria (1958) and Sweden and the Netherlands (1968). The USA has the highest ratio of dental hygienists per head of the population (1:2500), followed by Japan, Sweden and Canada (approximately 1:4000) (Fig. 2-38). The USA also has the highest

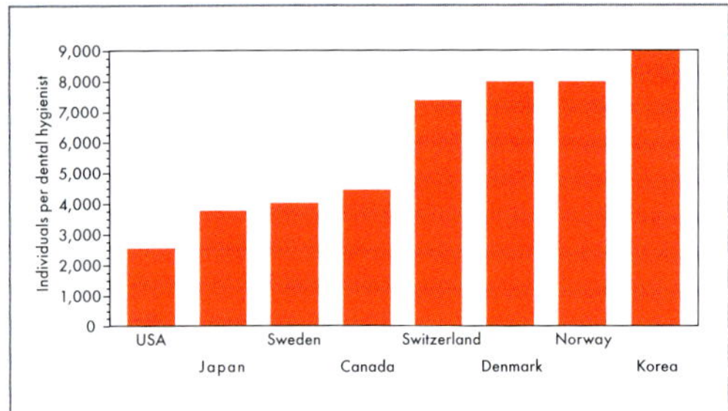

Fig. 2-38 Population per dental hygienist in 1990. (Modified from World Health Organization [1994][79] with permission.)

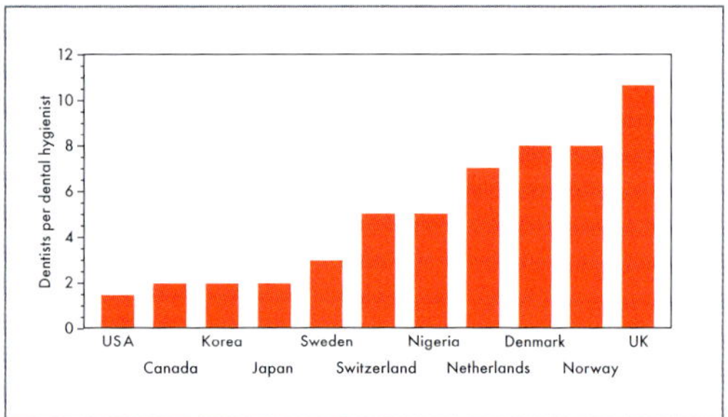

Fig. 2-39 Dentists per dental hygienist in 1990. (Modified from World Health Organization [1994][79] with permission.)

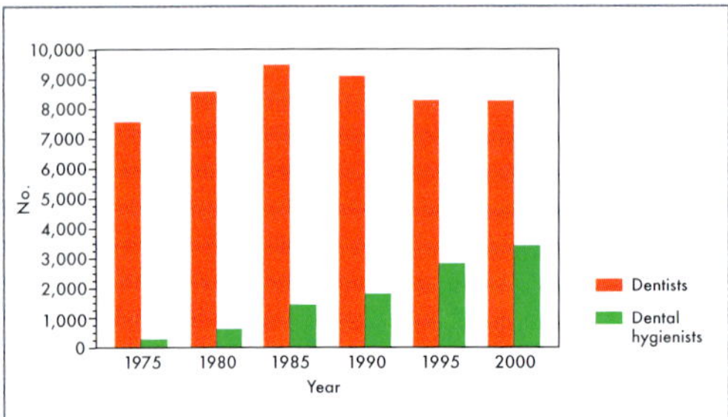

Fig. 2-40 Number of dentists and dental hygienists in Sweden from 1975 to 2000. (Modified from Axelsson et al. [1993][81] with permission.)

ratio of dental hygienists to dental clinicians (0.75:1), followed by Japan (0.5:1), South Korea (0.5:1), Canada (0.5:1) and Sweden (0.3:1) (Fig. 2-39). The ratio of dental hygienists to dental clinicians in Sweden retrospectively from 1975 to 2000 is shown in Fig. 2-40.[81] In some areas of Sweden, the ratio is especially high. For example, in the county of Värmland, there is one dental hygienist and one preventive dentistry assistant per dental clinician. In my private clinic, I have had the pleasure of having six to eight times more hours practiced by dental hygienists than dentists during the last 30 years.

In most countries, the length of the dental hygienist training program is two years, but it may range from one to four years. The entrance requirement is qualification as a dental assistant (nurse) or matriculation from high school. The occupation is held predominantly by women (more than 90%).

According to a Fédération Dentaire Internationale survey in 1990 of 13 countries (Australia, Canada, Denmark, Italy, Japan, Korea, the Netherlands, Nigeria, Norway, Sweden, Switzerland, UK and the USA), which covers most of the world's dental hygienists, the legal scope of their clinical practice is remarkably similar. It is characterized by a common set of procedures and activities, including treatment planning for the dental hygiene stages of care, history taking on general health, socioeconomic and oral health aspects, provision of optimized self-care for individuals and groups, scaling, root planing, debridement and professional mechanical tooth cleaning, topical application of fluoride gels and varnishes, use of fissure sealants, finishing of restorations and removal of overhangs, dietary evaluations and counselling, and administration of salivary and oral microbiology tests. In some countries, including Sweden, the training program also emphasizes behavioral science. Dental hygienists are also trained in local anesthesia (infiltration and regional block).

In Sweden, the training program for dental assistants also includes practical preventive dentistry. They are responsible for most of the preventive measures so successfully carried out in children and young adults, as discussed earlier in this chapter (Figs 2-23 to 2-26). Because the training program for preventive dentistry assistants is less than half the time required for the dental hygiene program, this category of dental personnel could be of value in other countries.

Needs-related preventive and supportive care programs based on risk prediction and risk profiles

In countries with high prevalence and incidence of dental caries and/or periodontal diseases and limited resources of dental clinicians, a so-called 'whole population strategy' for preventive programs performed by other oral health personnel such as dental hygienists and preventive dentistry assistants should still be cost-effective. For example, if all countries with non-fluoridated water, high or very high caries prevalence and incidence, little or no daily tooth cleaning and no use of fluoride dentifrice were to introduce water fluoridation and daily supervised tooth brushing with a fluoride dentifrice in schools, it would prove very cost-effective for caries prevention and control in children.

For successful prevention and control of dental caries in both children and adults, some basic principles must be adopted: for example, the higher the risk of developing caries (new caries surfaces) in the population, the greater the effect of one single preventive measure. This may be illustrated by the Swedish experience, where in the late 1950s, caries prevalence was extremely high. Almost every child developed several new lesions every year, mainly because of very poor oral hygiene. Regular tooth brushing was not an established habit, and no effective fluoride dentifrice was available. The introduction of well-organized, school-based fluoride mouthwash programs in which 0.2% NaF was provided once every one to two weeks resulted in caries reductions of 25–40%.[11,12] However, a 3-year randomized controlled double-blind study revealed no specific benefit from weekly rinsing with NaF compared with rinsing with distilled water, as discussed above.[11] There was a dramatic fall in both caries prevalence and caries incidence from 1964 to 1984, and especially after 1974, following the introduction of needs-related preventive programs (Fig. 2-41).[17] As an analogy, a raincoat is very cost-effective for a week in London in November but not for a visit to the Sahara Desert.

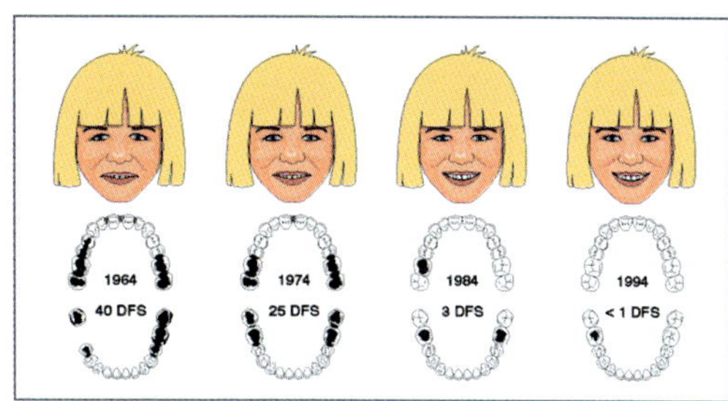

Fig. 2-41 Change in caries prevalence among 12-year-old residents of the county of Värmland, Sweden, 1964 to 1994. DFS, decayed or filled surface.
(From Axelsson [1998][73] with permission.)

In populations with poor oral hygiene standards and limited oral healthcare resources, most children have gingivitis and most adults have gingivitis and untreated chronic periodontitis. Under these conditions, and until the existing treatment needs are met, a whole-population strategy for general oral health promotion should be applied. School-based education in self-diagnosis and daily oral hygiene should be very cost-effective, as periodontitis always is preceded by gingivitis, as discussed above. In addition, such a program is rational as 'clean teeth never decay.'

At the population level, it is easy to find a positive correlation between one single risk factor and caries incidence in populations with high caries prevalence and incidence, where almost 100% of individuals develop new lesions of caries every year. In contrast, in populations with low or moderate caries incidence, well-established self-care habits and well-organized oral healthcare, administration of one single preventive measure to all subjects in the population, irrespective of predicted risk, will not be cost-effective; individual risk prediction and needs-related combinations of preventive measures are necessary. To ensure high sensitivity of risk prediction, several etiologic and modifying risk factors must be combined. For cost-effectiveness, the so-called high-risk strategy would be the method of choice.

There are several similarities between periodontal diseases and dental caries. Both are multifactorial infectious diseases. Besides etiologic, preventive and control factors, many other factors may modify the prevalence, onset and progression of the diseases. These modifiers may be divided into external (environmental) and internal (endogenous) factors, as discussed above.

Probability statements

For cost-effectiveness, the methods used to select and predict groups and individuals at 'true' risk for disease development should be as sensitive as possible. The optimal sensitivity for a diagnostic risk test is 100%, ie of 100 individuals selected as 'risk individuals,' all are true risk individuals. Similarly, for methods used to select true 'non risk' individuals, specificity should be as high as possible, ie of selected non-risk individuals, 100% are at no risk.

Usually, the higher the sensitivity is, the lower the specificity. Consequently, the clinician is usually forced to choose a test based on the consequences of making an error. A test method with high sensitivity and low specificity is likely to err in the direction of false positives. For a disease such as periodontitis, the implications are not usually serious when people are incorrectly identified as having active disease: they do not suffer extreme anxiety or undergo radical treatment. They may undergo intensified preventive treatment and incur increased treatment costs.

The consequence of a false-negative result, when a person with disease is incorrectly identified as healthy, is that the disease may progress further before it is diagnosed at a subsequent examination. This may be serious in the case of aggressive disease and of major consequence when there are prolonged intervals between examinations. For periodontal disease, as well as dental caries, the consequences of a false-positive diagnosis are less serious than those of a false-negative diagnosis. To avoid this impasse, several tests, one highly sensitive and one highly specific, may be combined.

The probability of developing dental caries or periodontitis given the result of a test method is known as the predictive value. The positive predictive value is the probability that a patient with a positive test result actually has active caries or periodontitis. Similarly, the negative predictive value is the probability that a patient with a negative test result actually has inactive dental caries or periodontal disease.

Risk categories

For the clinician, accurate prediction of patients or sites at high risk of developing caries or periodontitis is of fundamental importance. Because of the particular nature of dental caries and periodontal diseases, prediction of disease progression is important. Diagnostic tests differentiate whether or not a person has a specific disease at the time.

A risk indicator is a factor that has proved to be significantly associated with the occurrence of a specific disease, but only in cross-sectional studies. A risk factor, by comparison, is a factor that significantly increases the likelihood that people without disease, if exposed to this factor, will succumb to the disease within a specified time interval. Although diagnostic tests and risk factors can be evaluated by cross-sectional research design, longitudinal studies are necessary to confirm risk factors. The term risk factor is rather loosely used and can refer to an attribute or exposure associated with increased probability of disease (not necessarily causal): any type of determinant (cause), or a determinant that can be modified. This loose terminology may cause confusion when multivariate aspects of diseases are considered. Use of the term should be restricted as follows: risk factors are characteristics of the person or environment that, when present, directly result in an increased likelihood that a person will get a disease and, when absent, directly result in a decreased likelihood.

Exposure to a risk factor means that a person has been exposed to or manifested the factor prior to the onset of the disease. There may be continuous exposure, an isolated episode or multiple exposures over a period of time. Clinicians must recognize that risk factors, like etiologic factors (the periopathogens and the cariogenic microflora), are based on the current state of knowledge about a direct relationship: in light of further knowledge, a current risk factor for a specific disease may in the future be excluded. Because dental caries and periodontal diseases are the result of multiple etiologic factors (different species of the cariogenic microflora and periopathogens) and modifying factors, removal of a risk factor, such as the cessation of smoking in periodontal diseases and reduced sugar intake in dental caries, does not necessarily cure the disease. It should reduce the likelihood of disease development, but, once a person has the disease, removal of the risk factor may or may not result in cure.

Prognostic risk factors are factors which increase the risk that an already existing disease will progress. For example, in patients with existing periodontal disease, smoking will increase the risk for progression of the disease. Therefore, for adults we should speak about prognostic risk factors instead of risk factors.[82]

Risk markers and risk predictors (eg advanced attachment loss and deep diseased pockets in periodontal disease and DFS in dental caries) are usually biologic markers that indicate either disease or disease progression but currently are thought not to be causal or represent historical evidence of the disease: for example, the number of missing teeth, DFS or past evidence of periodontal disease. If a risk predictor is more strongly associated with the disease than a risk factor, and the risk predictor and risk factor are also associated with each other, then the risk predictor will appear in the multivariate model instead of the risk factor. For example, baseline periodontal status and number of decayed/missing/filled surfaces are usually strongly associated with the occurrence of new disease because these are measures of past disease and thus risk predictors.

Microorganisms are etiologic risk factors associated with new disease. They are also associated with baseline periodontal status and caries prevalence (prognostic risk) because they are partially responsible for this status.

Dental caries and periodontal diseases have multiple levels of measurement: person, tooth, and surface or site. A person can have disease, although many teeth and even more tooth sites may be disease free. Thus, the same person can have sites with disease onset as well as established sites of disease exhibiting progression. If the risk factor for disease onset differs from the prognostic factors for disease outcome, established sites should be evaluated under prognosis and not under risk prediction. Currently, however, both types of site tend to be considered together when risk factors are delineated. In the future, it may be useful to consider the two as separate entities.

In addition to etiological and preventive factors, many other factors may modify the prevalence, onset and progression (incidence) of dental caries and periodontal diseases, as discussed above. Such factors are divided into external (environmental) and internal (endogenous) factors.

External modifiers

External modifying risk indicators, risk factors and prognostic risk factors include

- for dental caries: frequent intake of sticky sugar-containing products (prolonged sugar clearance time), poor oral hygiene, irregular dental care habits, regular intake of medicines with salivary depressive side-effects and low socioeconomic (particularly low education) level
- for periodontal diseases: smoking, poor oral hygiene and irregular dental care are most important; others are use of smokeless tobacco, low socioeconomic (particularly low education) level, infectious and other acquired diseases, side-effects of medication and poor dietary habits.

It can be seen that poor oral hygiene habits, irregular dental care habits and low educational level are external risk factors and prognostic risk factors for both dental caries and periodontal diseases.

Internal modifiers

The most important internal modifying risk indicators, risk factors and prognostic risk factors are:

- for dental caries: reduced salivary flow, buffer capacity and antimicrobial effects; impaired host response, atypical plaque-retaining features of tooth crowns (particularly the fissures of the molars); low quality of the tooth enamel

- for periodontal disease: genetic factors, impaired host factors, chronic diseases, reduced salivary flow and quality.

Most studies of genetic factors in periodontal disease have concerned the aggressive forms of disease. Family studies suggest that susceptibility to the aggressive forms of disease, in particular in prepubertal and adolescent children, is at least in part influenced by host genotype. Inherited phagocytic cell deficiencies appear to confer risk for aggressive periodontitis in prepubertal children. The prevalence and distribution of aggressive periodontitis in affected families are most consistent with an autosomal recessive mode of inheritance. Comparisons between adult monozygous twins reared together and reared apart indicate that early family environment has no appreciable influence on probing depth and attachment loss in adults.[83] A number of apparently genetically determined syndromes or diseases appear to carry an associated increased risk for periodontal destruction. Defects of phagocytic cell function, especially polymorphonuclear leukoytes but also mononuclear phagocytes, are common in patients with aggressive periodontitis.

Genetic polymorphism of proinflammatory cytokines, particularly interleukin-1, has been shown to be a risk factor and prognostic risk factor for periodontal diseases.[84] It has also been shown that genetic polymorphism of interleukin-1 together with smoking has a synergistic negative effect.[85,86] It is estimated that approximately 50–80% of the most severe forms of periodontital disease could be explained by the combined effect of these two factors. Of the chronic diseases, poorly controlled diabetes mellitus, both type 1 and type 2, is the most important risk factor and prognostic risk factor for periodontal disease.[87]

Individual caries risk selection

By combining etiologic factors, caries prevalence (experience), caries incidence (increment), external and internal modifying risk indicators, risk factors and prognostic risk factors, as well as preventive factors, caries risk may be evaluated at the individual level, as no risk (C0), low risk (C1), risk (C2) and high risk (C3). These conditions may vary in different age groups. Therefore, the criteria for C0, C1, C2 and C3 should be defined for at least the following general groups: pre-schoolchildren (primary teeth), schoolchildren (permanent teeth), adults and the elderly.

Caries prevalence and caries incidence as well as socioeconomic conditions may vary considerably among different populations and countries. The individual risk selection is recommended to start with etiologic factors, followed by caries prevalence; caries incidence; external modifying risk indicators, risk factors and prognostic risk factors; internal modifying risk indicators, risk factors and prognostic risk factors; and preventive factors. The more factors that can be identified in the individual subject, the greater the validity of the predicted risk evaluation.[17,88]

Individual periodontitis risk selection

The relative risk for developing periodontal disease can be evaluated by combining clinical examination, preventive factors, etiologic factors, the absence or presence of environmental (external) and host-related (internal) risk indicators, risk factors, prognostic risk factors, risk markers and risk predictors. Periodontal risk increases in accordance with the severity and number of these factors to which the individual is exposed.[17,89]

Since the 1970s, almost 100% of the children and young adults (1–20 years of age) in Värmland, Sweden have been categorized into C0, C1, C2 and C3 groups for our needs-related caries-preventive program. In addition, nearly 100% of the adult patients at the public dental health clinics, representing approximately 50% of the adult population in Värmland, and the majority of the adult patients in private clinics have been categorized into four classes – general risk, periodontal risk, caries risk and iatrogenic risk – since the mid 1980s. This was to improve our needs-related preventive program for adults, which was initiated in 1985.[74]

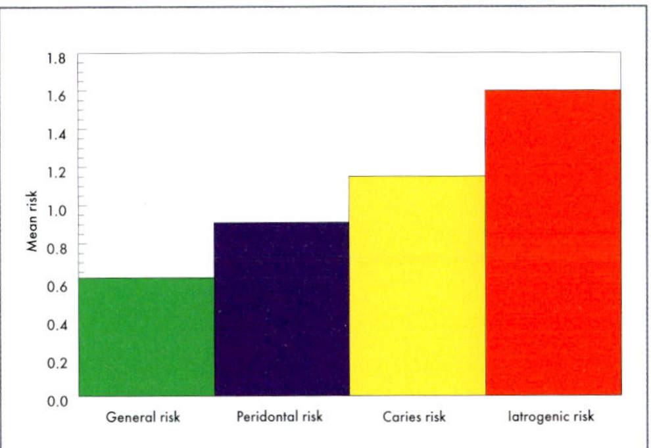

Fig. 2-42 Mean risk scores for general risk, periodontal risk, caries risk and iatrogenic risk in the adult population, county of Värmland, Sweden. Risk was assessed with the following scale: 0, no risk; 1, low risk; 2, risk; 3, high risk. (Modified from Axelsson et al. [2004][17] with permission.)

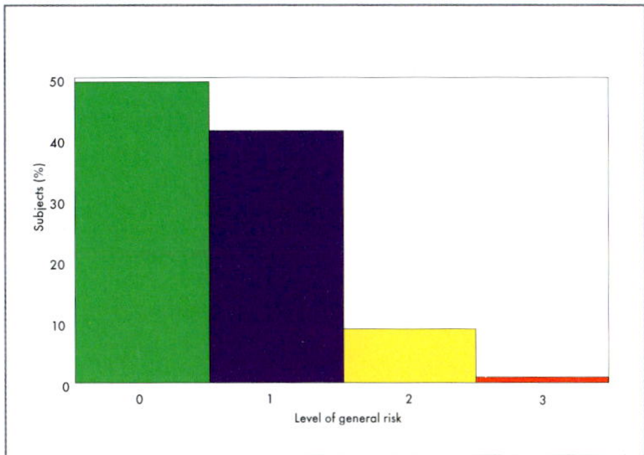

Fig. 2-43 Frequency distribution of general risk scores (0, no risk; 1, low risk; 2, risk; 3, high risk) in adult patients aged 20 to 80 years in the county of Värmland, Sweden. (Modified from Axelsson et al. [2004][17] with permission.)

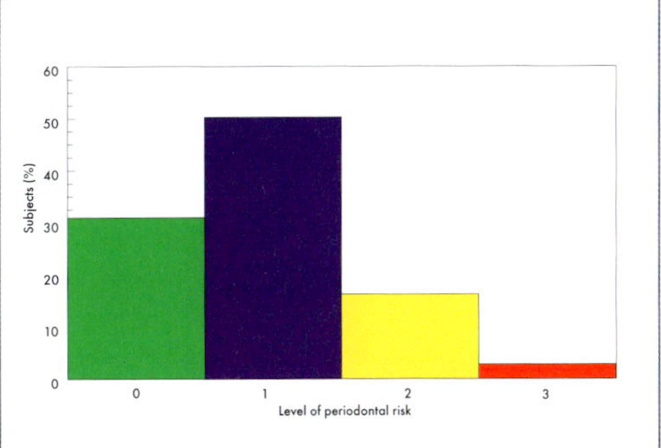

Fig. 2-44 Frequency distribution of periodontal risk scores in adult patients, aged 20 to 80 years, in the county of Värmland, Sweden. Results indicated that 32% had no periodontal risk (P0); 50% had low periodontal risk (P1); 16% had periodontal risk (P2), and 2% had high periodontal risk (P3). (Modified from Axelsson et al. [2000][72] with permission.)

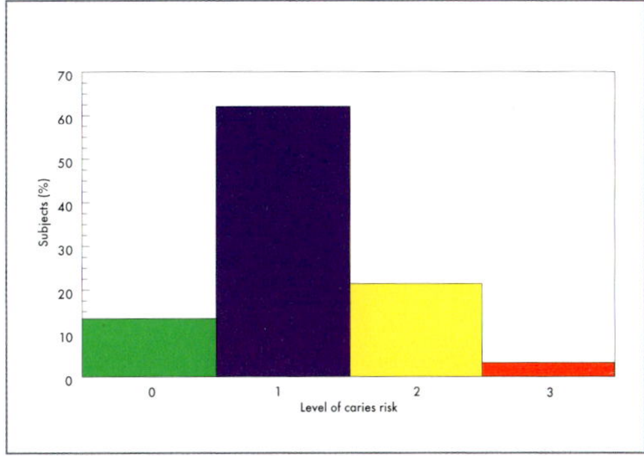

Fig. 2-45 Frequency distribution of caries risk scores (0, no risk; 1, low risk; 2, risk; 3, high risk) in adult patients aged 20 to 80 years in the county of Värmland, Sweden. (Modified from Axelsson et al. [2004][17] with permission.)

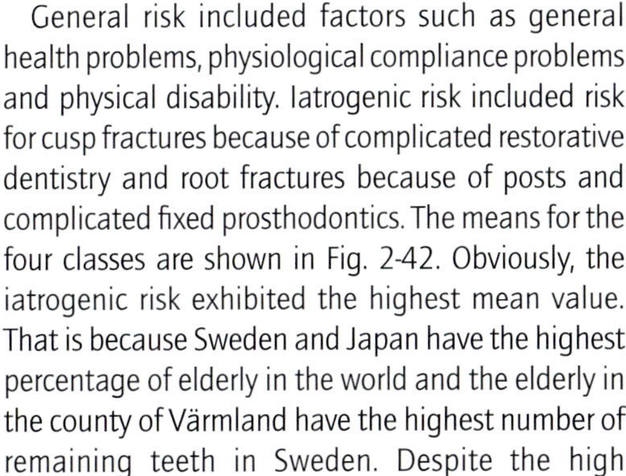

General risk included factors such as general health problems, physiological compliance problems and physical disability. Iatrogenic risk included risk for cusp fractures because of complicated restorative dentistry and root fractures because of posts and complicated fixed prosthodontics. The means for the four classes are shown in Fig. 2-42. Obviously, the iatrogenic risk exhibited the highest mean value. That is because Sweden and Japan have the highest percentage of elderly in the world and the elderly in the county of Värmland have the highest number of remaining teeth in Sweden. Despite the high percentage of elderly, the general risk exhibited the lowest mean value. The frequency distribution of general risk scores is shown in Fig. 2-43. The frequency distribution of the four classes of periodontal risk (P0, no risk; P1, low risk; P2, risk; P3, high risk) in the 20–80-year-olds is shown in Fig. 2-44.

The frequency distributions of P0, P1, P2 and P3 were 61, 36, 2 and 1%, respectively, in those aged 20 years; 24, 59, 15 and 2%, respectively, in those aged 40 years; 11, 58, 27 and 4%, respectively, in those aged 60 years; and 12, 55, 28 and 4%, respectively, in those aged 80 years. Notably, the

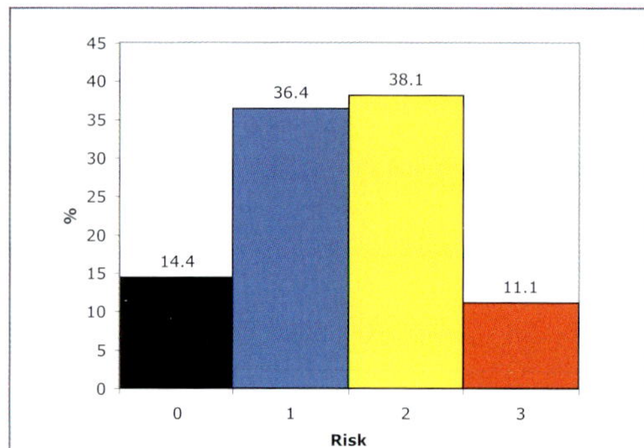

Fig. 2-46 Frequency distribution of iatrogenic risk scores (0, no risk; 1, low risk; 2, risk; 3, high risk) in adult patients aged 20 to 80 years in the county of Värmland, Sweden. (Modified from Axelsson et al. [2004][17] with permission.)

frequency distribution of high-risk patients even in the 80-year-old group is < 5%. In developing countries with limited dental care resources as well as in industrialized countries, the prevalence of the more severe (aggressive) forms of periodontitis is estimated to be between 5 and 15%.

The frequency distribution of the four classes of caries risk in the adult population is shown in Fig. 2-45. Only 3–4% of patients were classified as high risk. In those aged 60–80 years, the percentage is higher than in those aged 20–30 years because of reduced stimulated salivary flow, exposed root surfaces (increased risk for root caries), higher frequency of physical and mental disability and other general health problems. The frequency distribution of the four classes of iatrogenic risk is shown in Fig. 2-46. Because approximately 50% of our adult population are more than 50 years old, they exhibit a high prevalence of restored tooth surfaces and teeth with posts. When they became adult, Sweden had among the highest caries prevalence in the world. That is the main reason why more than 40% are classified with iatrogenic risk and almost 15% at high iatrogenic risk. By comparison, the majority of those aged 20–30 years has no iatrogenic risk.

The fee per year required for needs-related preventive programs and so-called supportive care is based on the sum of the scores in the risk classes: general risk, periodontal risk, caries risk and iatrogenic risk.

Risk profiles

Risk profiles are a tool for individualized preventive programs and communication with the patient. Risk profiles for tooth loss, dental caries and periodontal diseases can be presented graphically by combining symptoms (risk markers) of disease (eg prevalence, incidence, treatment needs); etiologic factors; external modifying risk indicators, risk factors and prognostic risk factors; internal modifying risk indicators, risk factors and prognostic risk factors; and preventive factors. This can be done manually or by computer. Degrees of risk (0, 1, 2 or 3) are displayed in green, blue, yellow or red, respectively (Figs 2-47 to 2-49). The graphs are very useful tools for communication with the patient when discussing the oral health status, etiology, modifying factors, prevention, possibilities, responsibilities and re-evaluations.[17,73,88,89] Tables 2-1, 2-2 and 2-3 show the abbreviations used for the most important variables related to tooth loss, caries risk and periodontal risk, respectively.

- *Risk profiles for tooth loss.* As illustrated in Fig. 2-47, a profile of risk for future tooth loss can be compiled by combining several risk indicators, risk factors and prognostic risk factors. Among these are age, estimated risk for periodontal diseases (P0 to P3), and dental caries (C0 to C3), poor socioeconomic conditions, chronic diseases, iatrogenic root fractures, trauma, genetics and impaired host response, medication and irregular dental care habits. In many industrialized countries, elderly people have heavily restored dentitions because of high caries incidence 30 to 50 years previously, when dental treatment comprised 'drilling, filling, killing (the pulp) and billing.' In such populations, the most frequent reason for tooth loss would be iatrogenic root fractures caused by posts in endodontically treated teeth. In developing countries with very limited oral healthcare resources, the main reasons for tooth loss would be untreated periodontal disease and dental caries among elderly people, and untreated dental caries and trauma among young people.
- *Detailed risk profiles for dental caries.* If a patient is at high risk predominantly for either caries or

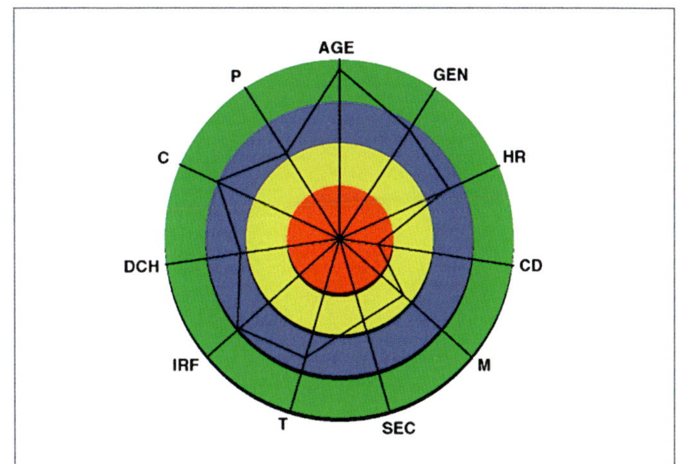

Fig. 2-47 Risk profile for tooth loss. Degrees of risk (0, 1, 2 or 3) are displayed in green, blue, yellow or red, respectively. For explanation of abbreviations, see Table 2-1. (Modified from Axelsson et al. [2004][17] with permission.)

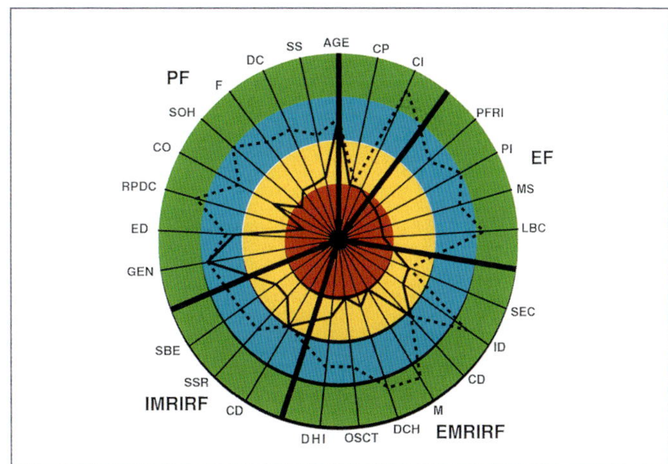

Fig. 2-48 Risk profile for dental caries: initial presentation, C3 (solid line); 1-year re-call, C1 (dotted line). For explanation of abbreviations, see Table 2-2. (Modified from Axelsson et al. [2004][17] with permission.)

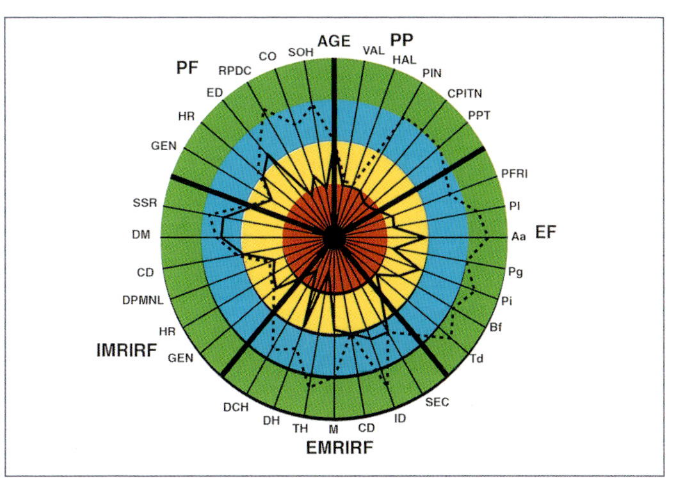

Fig. 2-49 Risk profile for periodontal diseases: baseline, P3 (solid line); 2 years later, P1 (dotted line). For explanation of abbreviations, see Table 2-3. (Modified from Axelsson et al. [2004][17] with permission.)

Table 2-1 Abbreviations related to tooth-loss

Term	Abbreviation
Age	AGE
Genetic factors	GEN
Host response	HR
Chronic diseases	CD
Medication	M
Socioeconomic conditions	SEC
Trauma	T
Iatrogenic root fracture	IRF
Dental care habits	DCH
Dental caries	C
Periodontal disease	P

Table 2-2 Abbreviations for caries-risk variables

Term	Abbreviation
Caries risk	
No risk	C0
Low risk	C1
Risk	C2
High risk	C3
Symptoms of dental caries	
Caries prevalence	CP
Caries incidence	CI
Etiologic factors	EF
Plaque Formation Rate Index	PFRI
Plaque Index	PI
Salivary mutans streptococci count	MS
Salivary lactobacilli count	LBC
External modifying risk indicators, risk factors and prognostic risk factors	EMRIRF
Infectious diseases	ID
Medication	M
Dental care habits	DCH
Oral sugar clearance time	OSCT
Dietary habit index	DHI
Internal modifying risk indicators, risk factors and prognostic risk factors	IMRIRF
Age	
Chronic diseases	CD
Stimulated salivary secretion rate	SSR
Salivary buffering effect	SBE
Genetic factors	GEN
Preventive factors	PF
Educational level	ED
Regular preventive dental care habits	RPDC
Compliance	CO
Standard of oral hygiene	SOH
Use of fluorides	F
Dietary control	DC
Salivary stimulation	SS

periodontal disease, a more detailed risk profile is available for the specific disease. How a high-risk patient (C3) has been transformed to a low-risk patient (C1) by improved self-care supplemented by professional preventive measures is illustrated in Fig. 2-48. The greater the difference between the solid line (baseline) and the dotted line, the greater the improvement. The absence of any change suggests that this particular factor cannot be influenced (eg genetic factors, age and some chronic diseases).[17,88]

- *Detailed risk profiles for periodontal disease.* A detailed risk profile for patients at high risk predominantly for periodontal disease is shown in Fig. 2-49. The risk profile illustrates graphically how high periodontal risk has been reduced to low risk (from P3 to P1) by improved needs-related plaque-control measures via self-care and supplementary professional treatment. The greater the difference between the solid line (baseline) and the dotted line, the greater the improvement. The absence of any change suggests that this particular factor cannot be influenced (eg genetic factors, host response and some chronic diseases).[17,88]

Table 2-3 Abbreviations related to periodontal risk

Term	Abbreviation
Periodontal risk	
No risk	P0
Low risk	P1
Risk	P2
High risk	P3
Clinical periodontal diagnosis	
Periodontitis prevalence (experience)	PP
Vertical attachment loss	VAL
Horizontal attachment loss (furcation involvement)	HAL
Periodontitis incidence (activity)	PIN
Periodontal pocket temperature	PPT
Etiologic factors	EF
Plaque Formation Rate Index	PFRI
Plaque Index (scores and pattern)	PI
Aggregatibacter actinomycetemcomitans	Aa
Porphyromonas gingivalis	Pg
Prevotella intermedia	Pi
Bacteroides forsythus	Bf
Treponema denticola	Td
Term	**Abbreviation**
External modifying risk indicators, risk factors and prognostic risk factors	EMRIRF
Socioeconomic conditions	SEC
Infectious diseases	ID
Chronic diseases	CD
Medication	M
Tobacco habits	TH
Dietary habits	DH
Dental care habits	DCH
Term	**Abbrev'n**
Internal modifying risk indicators, risk factors and prognostic risk factors	IMRIRF
Genetic factors	GEN
Host response	HR
Defective polymorphonuclear leukoyte function	DPMNL
Chronic diseases	CD
Diabetes mellitus	DM
Stimulated salivary secretion rate	SSR
Preventive factors	PF
Host response	HR
Educational level	ED
Regular preventive dental care habits	RPDC
Compliance	CO
Standard of oral hygiene	SOH

In the USA, the computer-aided risk calculator by Previsor has been frequently used for prediction of periodontal diseases.[90] Lang and Tonetti[91] have also presented a graphic model for risk prediction of periodontal diseases.

Schedules for needs-related preventive programs based on risk prediction

In countries with ample oral health personnel, oral health resources and relatively high standards of living and oral health, by far the most cost-effective strategy for improvement of oral health status is needs-related self-care based on self-diagnosis, supplemented with PMTC and topical application of fluoride agents at needs-related intervals. A schedule for needs-related preventive and maintenance (supportive) care for new and maintenance patients is outlined in Fig. 2-50.

According to current thinking, all new patients should be introduced to a needs-related preventive program in the following order.

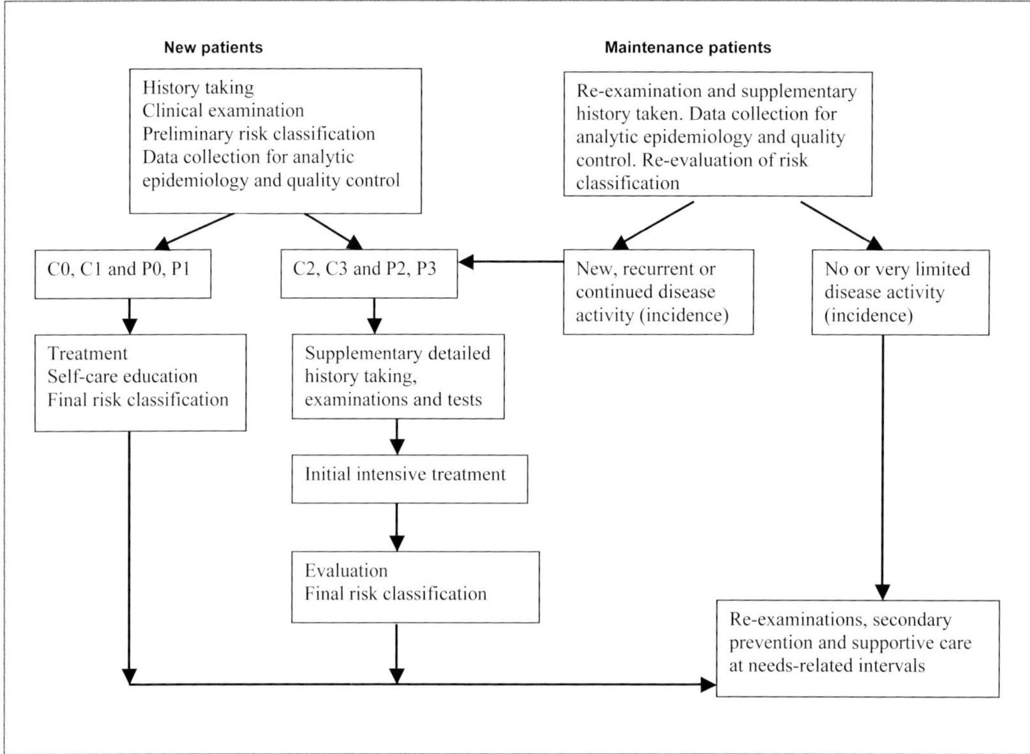

Fig. 2-50 Schedule for needs-related preventive and maintenance (supportive) care.

Screening and history taking

At the very first appointment, the goals are:

- to obtain a brief overview of oral health status by screening diagnosis, supplemented with clinically indicated radiographic examinations
- to gain an impression of the owner of the oral cavity by taking an oral and a general history.

In oral history evaluation, dental care, oral hygiene, fluoride, dietary and smoking habits and attitudes to oral health are of great importance. The most important variables for general history evaluations are level of education, occupation, lifestyle, general diseases, use of medicines, attitudes to general health and body mass index.

It is important to remember that the diagnosis reveals only the present oral status, while the history discloses the reasons for that status. On the basis of the results of screening and history taking, appropriate detailed supplementary examinations and tests are selected.

Examinations and tests

The goals of supplementary examinations and tests are:

- to obtain detailed information on oral health status
- to obtain detailed information on etiologic and modifying factors related to the patient's oral health status.

The most important clinical variables related to periodontal diseases are vertical periodontal attachment loss (mm), horizontal attachment loss (furcation involvement score 0–3), gingival index, pocket depth, alveolar bone level, shape and structure based on full-mouth radiographs (conventional or computer-aided digital images), bleeding on probing, purulent exudate, periodontal pocket temperature, gingival crevicular fluid (amount and content), subgingival plaque-retention factors (eg calculus, rough root surfaces, overhangs of restorations). If retrospective data are available, the incidence of periodontal attachment loss can be estimated.

From an etiological point of view, the PFRI, PI, occurrence of subgingival plaque biofilms and specific periopathogens such as *Aggregatibacter* (formerly *Actinobacillus*) *actinomycetemcomitans*, *Porphyromonas gingivalis*, *Bacteroides forsythus*, *Treponema denticola* and *Prevotella intermedia* (formerly *Bacteroides intermedius*) (diagnosed using the DNA-DNA checkerboard technique) are of great importance. The most important external and internal modifying factors for periodontal disease are the pattern of oral and dental care, smoking habits, educational level, systemic disease (especially diabetes types 1 and 2) and genetic susceptibility.

For the diagnosis of dental caries, the most important clinical variables are caries prevalence expressed in prognostic risk, the location and size of non-cavitated and cavitated enamel and dentin lesions, the color and texture (active or inactive) of non-cavitated and cavitated root lesions and the location and size of lesions diagnosed in radiographs (conventional bitewing or computer-aided digital images). If retrospective data are available, the rate of caries progression (incidence) can be evaluated.

The most important etiological factors related to dental caries are PFRI and specific cariogenic bacteria, in particular the salivary counts of mutans streptococci and Lactobacillae.

Important modifying factors related to dental caries are dietary habits (particularly estimated sugar clearance time), oral hygiene, fluoride and dental care habits, educational level, stimulated and unstimulated salivary flow (mL/min), buffer capacity of the saliva, use of medicines with negative effects on salivary flow, general diseases and the shape and morphology of the teeth. In the near future, antimicrobial and genetic tests of saliva should also be available.

Risk classification

Based on all data from the diagnosis and history taking, the patient is classified according to risk for dental caries and periodontal diseases – no risk (C0 and P0, respectively), low risk (C1 and P1), risk (C2 and P2), or high risk (C3 and P3) – and the individual risk profile is established as a tool for case presentation and communication with the patient, as discussed and illustrated earlier in this chapter.

Initial intensive treatment

The number of visits and the materials and methods used are strictly related to the patient's classification and predicted risk. The main goals of the initial intensive treatment are:

- to establish needs-related self-care habits based on self-diagnosis and education
- to heal diseased periodontal tissues as soon as possible, resulting in a dramatic reduction in plaque formation rate (PFRI)[92]
- to achieve remineralization and arrest of caries lesions without cavitation
- to eliminate plaque-retentive factors, such as restoration overhangs, unpolished restorations, calculus, rough root surfaces and cavitated caries lesions.

For patients at no risk (C0 and P0) or at low risk (C1 and P1) without any treatment need, the initial preventive treatment may be limited to one or two visits. For patients at risk (C2 and P2) and at high risk (C3 and P3), the initial intensive treatment may range from three to six visits. These visits will be concentrated to as short period as possible (seven to ten days) and at about two-day intervals. However, the first two should be at close to a 24 h interval for evaluation of PFRI and establishment of needs-related oral hygiene habits based on PFRI and education in self-diagnosis.

In order to facilitate mechanical plaque control by self-care as well as PMTC, plaque-retentive factors will be eliminated as early as possible. The outstanding most severe plaque-retention factors are remaining roots untreatable because of caries and untreatable teeth because of advanced periodontal disease. Such teeth should be extracted as soon as possible. Overhangs and undercut of restorations (fillings and crowns) will be eliminated. Rough surfaces of restorations will be finished and polished. Cavitated caries are excavated and restored at least semipermanently with glass-ionomer cement or acrylic resin-modified glass-ionomer cement, which should be of extra benefit in caries-risk patients as the glass-ionomer cement may act as a slow-release fluoride agent; this can be recharged with fluoride by the daily use of fluoride dentifrice and the professional use of fluoride varnishes and gels.

Subgingival as well as supragingival calculus will be eliminated and rough root surfaces planed with 'non-aggressive' techniques without exposal of the root dentin tubules. During these procedures, subgingival biofilms should be removed as well. By re-contouring, the plaque retention in root grooves and furcation involved teeth can be reduced.

The so-called 'full mouth disinfection' method should be implemented in those with caries risk (C2 and C3) as well as periodontal risk (P2 and P3) during this initial intensive treatment period. For C2 and C3 patients, this means mechanical cleaning of all tooth surfaces and the dorsum of the tongue and rinsing afterwards with 0.1% or 0.2% chlorhexidine solution twice a day. At every visit PMTC and tongue scraping is performed, followed with chlorhexidine mouthrinsing and interproximal placement of chlorhexidine gel or the use of chlorhexidine varnish on the key risk tooth surfaces. In P2 and P3 patients, the 'full mouth disinfection' also includes subgingival mechanical removal of the biofilm in combination with irrigation with iodine solution (bacteriocidic). Depending on the outcome of the analyses of the subgingival microflora, topical use of doxycyclin gels or systemic use of antibiotics (amoxicillin and/or metronidazole) may be indicated in susceptible patients with impaired general health (eg severe cardiovascular problems, poorly controlled diabetes type 1 and 2).

This intensive combination of mechanical and chemical plaque control by self-care and professional (dentist or dental hygienist) care will enable the periodontal tissues, in particular the free gingivae, to heal. In addition the PFRI will be dramatically reduced and this will facilitate the daily oral hygiene procedure. In C2 and C3 patients, non-cavitated enamel and dentin caries may be arrested and active root caries transformed to inactive lesions if patients chew fluoride-containing gum for 20 min after every meal and fluoride varnish is used on the key-risk surfaces at every clinic visit.

Re-evaluation

The goals of the re-evaluation are:

- to evaluate the results of the initial intensive treatment
- to assess patient compliance
- to evaluate supplementary need for regenerative therapy because of lost periodontal support and restorative treatment
- to determine the materials and methods needed for the maintenance period and the optimal recall intervals.

Patients evaluated as C2–C3 and P2–P3 should be recalled within three to six months after the initial intensive treatment for evaluation of the effects of treatment on the symptoms of active caries lesions, gingivitis and periodontitis that were exhibited at the baseline examination.

Non-cavitated caries may have been arrested and active root caries should be inactive in C2 and C3 patients. Inflamed gingival sites should be healed and pocket depth significantly reduced in the P2 and P3 patients.

Repeated oral microbiology tests may be indicated in C2 and C3 patients with very high counts of salivary mutans streptococci and Lactobacillae and P2 and P3 patients with high levels of periopathogens in deep diseased pockets at baseline.

At this re-evaluation, the dental clinician decides whether supplementary restorative dentistry or regenerative periodontal therapy is indicated. By interview and questionnaires, patient's knowledge, attitude and compliance are evaluated. The quality of the patient's self-performed oral hygiene is evaluated by plaque disclosing. It is of great importance to activate the patient to participate in the evaluation by self-diagnosis at every visit. Based on the outcome of the initial intensive treatment and the risk classification, the material and methods needed for the maintenance period (supportive care) and the optimal recall intervals are determined.

Maintenance period (supportive care)

Intervals, materials and methods of the maintenance program are strictly related to the patient's classification and predicted risk. The optimal goals of the maintenance program are:

- to ensure that healthy individuals with no experience of oral diseases remain healthy (primary prevention)
- to prevent recurrence of oral disease (secondary prevention) after initial successful symptomatic treatment (tertiary prevention), ie, to ensure no new caries lesions and no further loss of periodontal attachment
- to encourage continuous improvement in self-care habits to prolong the intervals and reduce the need for professional preventive measures.

All the above goals have been shown to be successfully achieved over a period of 30 years in adults by a dental hygienist[66] and by dental hygienists and preventive dentistry assistants from birth to 20 years of age in large-scale preventive programs.[17]

If the effect of the maintenance (supportive) care is failing and the patient develops new caries or exhibits new or further loss of periodontal attachment, new detailed history, tests and diagnosis are undertaken to evaluate the reasons for new continued disease activity (incidence). Based on the outcome of these detailed analyses, another needs-related intensive treatment will be carried out according to Fig. 2-50.

Recall examination

Intervals, diagnosis and supplementary history taking are strictly related to the patient's classification and predicted risk. The goals of the re-examination are:

- to evaluate the effect of the supportive care program
- to prolong the intervals of the supportive program and the recall re-examinations, provided that the patient's self-care has improved and there is no oral disease activity
- to evaluate whether new treatment needs have occurred
- to repeat an intensive treatment period and introduce a more comprehensive supportive care program if the previous program has proved unsuccessful.

The recall examination should always be carried out by a dental clinician and in patients classified as P2 or P3. An alternative might be a dentist specializing in periodontal diseases.

Implementation

These principles for needs-related preventive programs are based on an ideal ratio of dental professionals, well-developed oral healthcare systems, high economic and educational standards among the population and recent knowledge about diagnosis and preventive materials and methods. Local conditions may limit full implementation of this state of the art program.

For example, in Sweden, almost all children and young adults and 80–90% of the adults are so-called recall patients; they receive some kind of regular maintenance program, but only a minority of the adults receive a strictly needs-related preventive program. In many other countries, however, maintenance programs are still non-existent, at least for adults.

Quality control of preventive programs

Analytical computerized oral epidemiology can be used for quality control of preventive programs and treatment (at surface, tooth, individual, clinic and regional levels). A great deal of time, effort and money are spent on oral healthcare each year, so it is reasonable that the government agency responsible for healthcare has an audit system that regularly evaluates the total effect of the national oral care and dental insurance systems on the oral health status and treatment needs of the population. At the same time, it encourages and motivates dental clinicians to evaluate continuously the efficiency of their own preventive program at surface, tooth and individual levels, as well as for their total patient population. In addition, a national dental insurance scheme should promote preventive dentistry and analytical epidemiology for quality control.[17,72,93]

According to Swedish Medical Terminology,[94] the definition of epidemiology is 'the medical science of the spread, etiology, and prevention of the epidemic (infectious) diseases.' Because certain species of transmissible microorganism that colonize tooth surfaces are implicated in the etiology of both caries and periodontal diseases, these diseases are regarded as epidemic diseases.

In contrast to other medical disciplines, dentistry has well-established and measurable variables for evaluation of health. These variables should be stratified according to their importance. The main reasons for loss of teeth are dental caries and periodontal diseases. Variables associated with these conditions should be given priority in oral health epidemiology. The masticatory efficiency of the dentition and the condition of the oral mucosa should also be included.

The WHO, in collaboration with the Fédération Dentaire Internationale, international dental associations and ministries of health, established goals for the level of oral health to be attained by the year 2000 for selected indicator age groups in children and adults. One goal recommended that computer-based epidemiologic systems be established to monitor whether these goals were being attained. Epidemiologic surveys in randomized samples of the population were recommended to be repeated at five-year intervals.

Very powerful personal computers are now available and portable computers are suitable for field surveys. As a consequence, large volumes of epidemiologic data may be collected, and direct statistical evaluation and graphic presentation of the results are readily accomplished.

Tooth loss

The final outcome of untreated caries and periodontal disease is edentulousness. According to WHO's goals, edentulousness in those aged 35–44 years and 65 years should have been reduced from the levels in 1969 by 50% and 25%, respectively, by the year 2000.

In field surveys, retrospective determination of the reason for missing teeth is frequently difficult and uncertain. Information with respect to which teeth are most frequently missing and the reason for extraction is important for planning appropriate preventive measures. A number of important questions arise.

1. Why are the maxillary molars the teeth most frequently missing?
2. Why are maxillary premolars missing more frequently than mandibular premolars?
3. Why are the mandibular canines the most resistant of all the teeth?

Loss of occlusal contacts

Mastication is the primary function of the teeth. Masticatory efficiency (ie chewing capacity) may be expressed in terms of the Eichner Index, based on the number of occlusal contacts in the molar and premolar areas.[95,96]

Dental caries and periodontal disease

There is a strong correlation between oral health status and the occurrence of dental caries and periodontal disease. The prevalence of these diseases is, therefore, the most important dental health variable. Many parallels may be drawn between these two diseases. The etiologies are known for both diseases; pathogenic microorganisms that colonize the tooth surfaces are implicated. Both diseases are site-related: not evenly distributed among the teeth and tooth surfaces.

For example, the difference in prevalence of both caries and marginal periodontitis between the distal surfaces of the maxillary first molars and the mandibular canines is usually more significant than the difference in total prevalence between individuals: there are specific, highly susceptible, key-risk teeth and surfaces.

If the standard of oral health is to be improved by preventive measures, such facts must be acknowledged and the mechanisms explained. The prevalence of both caries and periodontal disease should be presented at the individual level as well as at tooth surface levels.

The prevalence of both diseases represents the end result of all incidences and does not progress linearly. In other words, prevalence represents the results of unpredictable site-specific exacerbations and periods of disease quiescence.

Apical periodontitis

In most countries, the prevalence of apical periodontitis has not been determined because complete-mouth intraoral radiographs or orthopantomograms are required for diagnosis.

Endodontic treatment

Data on the prevalence of endodontic treatment should also be collected. In an adult population, the number of root fractures is strongly correlated with the number of endodontically treated teeth restored with the aid of posts. Most coronal fractures also occur in root-filled teeth.

Mucosal diseases

From the oral health aspect, diagnosis of and collection of data on diseases of the oral mucosa are very important. In many countries, the prevalence of serious diseases, such as precancerous and cancerous lesions and human immunodeficiency virus-associated lesions, is increasing.

Treatment needs

To plan and organize the resources necessary to meet the need for oral treatment, an estimate must be made of treatment needs, not only for marginal periodontal diseases but also for caries, apical periodontitis, malocclusion, oral mucosal diseases and bone diseases. Some indices for treatment needs of caries (Community Caries Index of Treatment Needs [CCITN])[97] and apical periodontitis (Apical Periodontal Index of Treatment Needs [APITN])[98] have, therefore, been designed, analogous to the well-established CPITN.[99]

Etiological and modifying factors

In addition to epidemiologic data on prevalence and treatment needs, epidemiologic studies should also include causal and modifying factors, in terms of the previous definition of epidemiology. This is also confirmed by the definition of epidemiology in the *Encyclopaedia Britannica* (1963): 'The medical science concerned with the description of factors and conditions that are significantly associated with the occurrence of an infectious process, disease or abnormal physiological state in a human community with elucidation of the manner in which these factors and conditions operate in the causative complex.'

The variables to be included in an analytic oral epidemiology system are set out in rank order in Table 2-4.[17,71,93]

Questionnaire

Prior to the clinical examination, participants should answer a questionnaire about their dental care habits, oral hygiene habits, dietary and smoking habits, systemic diseases and use of medicines, socioeconomic background, lifestyle, and knowledge of causes and prevention of oral diseases. In addition, full-mouth radiographs should be taken where indicated clinically.

Some results of our preventive and supportive care programs for adults have been presented earlier in this chapter (Figs 2-27 to 2-35).[17,72]

Vision 2020

Improvement of personal qualifications in oral health

Communication skills, which are so essential in keeping information at hand and in offering opportunities for interaction with undergraduates and

Table 2-4 Variables included in the analytic computer-based oral epidemiology system

Code	Variable
1. Oral epidemiology	
1.1	Percentage edentulous
1.2	Number of teeth
1.3	Function of teeth: modified Eichner's Index
2. Prevalence	
2.1	Dental caries: decayed/missing/filled teeth (DMFT), decayed/filled teeth (DFT), decayed/missing/filled surfaces (DMFS), decayed/filled surfaces (DFS)
2.2	Marginal periodontitis
2.2.1	Vertical loss of attachment (mm)
2.2.2	Horizontal loss of attachment; furcation involvement score 0–3
2.3	Apical periodontitis[17,93]
2.4	Oral mucosal lesions and bone diseases
2.5	Malocclusion
3. Treatment needs	
3.1	Dental caries: Community Caries Index of Treatment Needs (CCITN)[17,97]
3.2	Marginal periodontitis: Community Periodontal Index of Treatment Needs (CPITN)97
3.3	Apical periodontitis: Apical Periodontal Index of Treatment Needs (APITN)[17,98]
3.4	Oral mucosal and bone diseases
3.5	Malocclusion
4. Etiologic factors	
4.1	Non-specific oral microflora: Plaque Index (PI) and Plaque Formation Rate Index (PFRI)[8,17]
4.2	Specific microflora
5. Modifying factors	
5.1	External modifying risk indicators, risk factors and prognostic risk factors: poor oral hygiene and dietary habits, smoking and snuffing habits (other unhealthy lifestyle habits), socioeconomic background (particularly low educational level), use of medicines, infectious and other acquired diseases
5.2	Internal modifying risk indicators, risk factors and prognostic risk factors: chronic diseases (eg diabetes mellitus, cardiovascular diseases, Sjögren's syndrome), impaired host response (particularly reduced polymorphonuclear leukoyte function), genetic susceptibility for periodontal disease, reduced salivary secretion rate

graduates as well as teaching staff, should be enhanced. An obvious outcome will be the development of a new type of student as well as new types of teacher. Major elements of this initiative would include:

- much greater ease in pooling intellectual resources
- speedy exchange of information, especially in relation to effective new methodologies and materials
- development of common assessment methods
- access to a wide variety of databanks
- greater opportunity to remodel careers over extended period of time according to the speed of change in society and the job market.

Preparation of a broad set of modules serving the oral health stream within a health sciences structure will demonstrate what might be achieved and thus initiate a 'snowballing' effect toward the ultimate objective of a complete computer-assisted curriculum. Already there are several centers of excellence around the globe producing the type of interactive materials needed for computer-assisted training. Such programs are steadily increasing and are available on CD-ROM and the Internet. There is a need to direct that excellence toward the overall objective. This is what the WHO hopes to do in collaboration with the International Federation of Dental Education Associations, which is enthusiastic about this approach.[79]

Succinctly, empowerment of the learner is the principal aim of this concept, in both a variation on the theme of universities without walls and an attempt to make excellence available whatever the constraints of quantity and quality in teaching staff. It will benefit dental schools where the resources needed to deliver an adequate and appropriate curriculum are very scarce. Every school will need a certain core of staff to administer, coordinate, guide, evaluate and conduct practical exercises. The specific teaching and learning, however, would come largely from the student, the graduate and the teachers interacting with the computer programs at their disposal. The excellence of those programs would depend on having a 'braintrust' group of the very best experts responsible for devising the programs. In this way, the best available courses would be offered to all students everywhere, rather than the wide range of messages, often contradictory or outdated, that students currently receive.

Whatever the approach chosen, an initiative of this type will streamline the training of health personnel, with sufficient flexibility to ensure that such training will keep pace with the leading edge of science to a much greater extent than is the case today.

For too long, the oral cavity has been separated from the rest of the body and 'donated' to dental clinicians, a profession more or less independent from the medical profession. At the beginning of the last century, dentistry centered around extraction of teeth and making complete and partial dentures, with the assistance of technicians. Then in most industrialized countries came an era of 'drilling, filling and billing,' and 'aggressive' exploration of the tooth crown in the management of dental caries. During the second half of the twentieth century, in many industrialized countries, the roots of the teeth have also been exploited by specialists in periodontology and endodontics, and teeth have been moved around for functional and esthetic reasons by specialists in orthodontics.

Recently, successful reconstructions using implant technology have been achieved through teamwork by oral surgeons, periodontists, prosthodontists and dental technicians. Specialists in periodontology now offer regeneration of periodontal support.

According to the *lege artis* principles, modern knowledge and experience obliges dental professionals to focus on prevention and the control of dental caries, periodontal diseases and other oral conditions, while eliminating existing treatment needs.

Increasing numbers of individuals worldwide will have intact tooth crowns and no loss of periodontal support. Therefore, the crowns and roots of teeth have to be reunited in considerations of the oral cavity, and the oral cavity must be returned to its rightful place in the body. This requires a holistic approach, centered on the owner of the oral cavity. Preventive dentistry and oral health promotion have to be integrated with general health promotion, in collaboration with general health personnel. Dental education has to be reoriented to serve the changing needs of oral health, linked more closely to the requirements of the health sector.

As an alternative to existing schools, many of which are specific to medicine, dentistry, nursing and pharmacy, the aim should be to create an integrated system for educating all health personnel within a health sciences school structure. Elimination of separate training of auxiliary and professional personnel is also desirable. A 'ladder' system of education is envisaged, in which, for the oral health team, the 'oral physician,' instead of today's dental clinician, is seen as the leader, at parity with colleagues in the other medical specialties. Other oral health personnel, such as dental assistants, preventive dentistry assistants and dental hygienists, would leave this ladder at various levels, corresponding to defined lists of duties, as would be the case for personnel focusing on any other health areas. A number of dental schools, predominantly but not exclusively in Europe, have already begun to move toward this type of structure.

Integrated health teams

At the community and city levels, integrated local health teams should be established to improve oral health as well as general health among the population. Such a team should consist of well-trained professionals, highly experienced in prevention and health promotion rather than treatment and each donating specific skills.

- *General physician*. The general physician should be the leader of the team. Therefore, he or she should be the most highly qualified and experienced in leadership and communication, general medicine, general health promotion and epidemiology.
- *Psychologist*. The psychologist should be highly qualified and experienced in behavioral science, with special reference to establishing good health lifestyle habits and eliminating bad habits, such as smoking.
- *Nutritionalist*. The nutritionalist should be highly qualified and experienced in the concept of 'input and output' related to eating at the cellular level as well as the individual level. Emphasis should be placed on the consequences of healthy versus unhealthy dietary habits.
- *Sociologist*. The sociologist should be well educated and experienced in the influence of socioeconomic conditions on health status.
- *Physiotherapist*. The physiotherapist should be well educated and experienced in how to prevent the development (primary prevention) and the recurrence (secondary prevention) of musculoskeletal orthopedic problems (eg back pain), as well as diagnosis and early rehabilitation of such problems.
- *Physical education teacher*. The physical education teacher should be well educated and experienced in the consequences of physical training and activity versus physical inactivity for general health and how to activate all members of the population.
- *Engineer*. The engineer should be well educated and experienced in the effects of the external and internal environment on health and how to diagnose and eliminate unhealthy environments.
- *Oral physician*. The oral physician will be the leader of the oral health personnel team and highly qualified and experienced in preventive dentistry and oral health promotion as an integrated part of general health promotion.
- *General health nurse*. The general health nurse will be responsible for education of the population in self-diagnosis and self-care, with special reference to prevention and control of diseases.
- *Dental hygienist*. The dental hygienist should be well educated and experienced in optimizing oral self-diagnosis and self-care for prevention and control of dental caries, periodontal diseases and other oral diseases, supplemented by needs-related professional preventive measures.

The local health team should be backed up, at the area/county level, by a central resource team with a great variety of specialists and subspecialists. Most should have a scientific background at the doctorate (PhD) level:

- physicians, all specialties
- psychologists
- sociologists
- nutritionalists
- oral physicians
- epidemiologists
- statisticians
- economists.

The remainder should have extensive research experience:

- physiotherapists
- sports professionals
- engineers
- general nurses
- dental hygienists
- public relations officers: art directors and copywriters.

The effects of such teams on the health status of the population and the costs should be repeatedly evaluated in terms of the following:

- absence from work because of disease
- internationally accepted (WHO) disease-specific variables
- cost-effectiveness and cost-benefit ratio.

Oral health goals

Governments and communities should recognize the need to develop and maintain preventive programs for oral diseases, and communities should be responsible for these activities. All communities should be able to afford and manage basic health-promoting oral care so that adult teeth will be retained throughout life. Realistic goals for the effects of all preventive dental care programs should be set up at global as well as national, county, district and clinic levels. Such goals should also be updated in accordance with improved oral health status at certain intervals. As shown earlier in this chapter, for those who had followed our needs-related program from birth to the age of 20 years, the goals we set in the county of Värmland, Sweden, in 1979 were essentially achieved in 1999.

Oral health for life should be approaching reality for all. To promote improved oral health worldwide, the WHO's Oral Health Unit drew up international oral health goals to be achieved by the year 2000 for severity of oral disease involvement at various key ages: 12, 35–44 and 65 years and older. These goals included the following.

1. The WHO databases for oral health will be further developed. Coordinated national database systems will be established. A WHO personal computer card for oral health recordings will be defined and produced.
2. Of those aged five to six years, 50% will be caries free.
3. Children will have no more than three decayed, missing or filled teeth at 12 years.
4. 85% of the population will have all their teeth left at 18 years.
5. A 50% reduction in edentulousness at ages 35 to 44 years will be achieved compared with the level in 1969.
6. A 25% reduction in levels of edentulousness at age 65 years and older will be achieved compared with the level in 1969.

In 1988, the first International Conference on Preventive Dentistry and Epidemiology was held in Karlstad, Sweden, in collaboration with WHO, Fédération Dentaire Internationale, and the Swedish Board of Health and Welfare. Among other topics discussed at the workshops were realistic goals for the years 2010 and 2020 to follow the WHO's goals for 2000, what was known about existing preventive measures, and the future potential of large-scale implementation of recent clinical research.[73] The goals for the years 2010 and 2020 were set:

1. Creation and subsequent refinement of well-developed computerized analytic epidemiologic systems for quality control of oral as well as general health programs and cost-effectiveness.
2. A focus on education of all the population in self-diagnosis and self-care as the most cost-effective oral healthcare.
3. Prevention and control of caries and periodontitis in the vast majority of the adult population (secondary prevention) parallel with efficient primary prevention in children, resulting in about 90% caries-free young children.

The following goals for the year 2010 should be achieved:

1. A complete electronic global, nation-based WHO database for oral health and a coordinated general health database will be established.
2. 90% of five year olds will be caries free.
3. Children will have no more that two decayed, missing or filled teeth at 12 years of age.
4. 75% of 20 year olds will be caries inactive.
5. 75% of 20 year olds will not develop destructive periodontal disease.
6. More than 75% of all children and young adults will have sufficient knowledge of etiology and prevention of oral diseases to motivate self-diagnosis and self-care.

The goals for the year 2020 should be:

1. A global electronic database for automatic oral and general health evaluation, including possibilities for health economy analysis, will be established.
2. 90% of five year olds will be caries free.
3. Children will have no more than one decayed, missing or filled tooth at 12 years of age.
4. 90% of 20 year olds will be caries inactive.
5. 90% of the whole population will not develop destructive periodontal disease.
6. More than 75% of the total population will have sufficient knowledge of etiology and prevention of oral diseases to motivate self-diagnosis and self-care.

Of course more detailed and tougher goals can be set up at national, county, city and clinic levels, depending on the actual oral health status and dental care resources.

The importance of changing the attitudes toward oral health

If the goal of oral healthcare is to maintain a natural dentition throughout life, the loss of all teeth is the ultimate failure, closely followed by a high percentage of people with only 20 or fewer remaining teeth. The relevant question is why such a high failure rate has been accepted by the public and the dental profession. Intact teeth and healthy gingivae are simply beautiful, attractive functional parts of the body and should be much more highly regarded by the population. Carious teeth, swollen, red, bleeding gingivae and bad-smelling breath are most unattractive.

Individuals would never accept destruction of other parts of the body: an ugly false nose or other parts of the body normally covered by clothes. Why should they accept false teeth? Patients would not accept having even 1% of the nose replaced by amalgam or gold. Imagine having to amputate a finger once every five years and accept a gold replacement despite regular checkups once or twice a year, in particular when the cause of the disease is well known and prevention can be successful.

It is the duty of dental professionals to educate and motivate the public, health personnel and politicians to regard intact teeth and healthy gingivae as highly as, for example, a healthy nose, eyes or ears and a justifiable external mode of dress. It is all a matter of changing attitudes and priorities. Famous clothing designers change fashion annually, and people accept the extra costs without hesitation.

A healthy and well-cared mouth facilitates communication and human relationships. In addition, the boost in health, well-being and self-confidence is very important for quality of life and contributes at a very basic biologic level to protection from systemic infection and other general health problems. For example, analytical studies have disclosed a clear relationship between periodontal disease and cardiovascular diseases,[100,101] as well as preterm low birth weight deliveries,[102,103] diabetes mellitus[87] and other general health problems. Therefore, when oral health is compromised, overall health and quality of life are also compromised.

Patient responsibility

Motivation is defined as readiness to act or the driving force behind our actions. Responsibility has been identified as the motivating factor of longest duration. Optimized responsibility may result in lifelong motivation, in contrast to the limited duration of encouragement provided by, for example, commendation or a salary increase.

Adults should believe that 'no dentist or dental hygienist should accept more responsibility for my oral status than I do myself, because it is my mouth.' However, in many industrialized countries with well-organized social health and welfare systems, the population is more or less passive; patients regard the dental clinician and dental hygienist as responsible for their oral health, the physician as responsible for their general health and the politicians as responsible for their social welfare.

With the current level of knowledge about the etiology, prevention and control of dental caries and periodontal diseases, it has been shown that patients who are well motivated and well educated in self-diagnosis and self-care can prevent and control these diseases by themselves. Of much greater importance to general health, quality of life and costs for health and welfare are the following examples: It is estimated that, among external (environmental) carcinogenic factors, an unhealthy diet accounts for approximately 30% of cancers, smoking for approximately 20% and viruses for approximately 10%. The simple message on diet is reduction of animal fat and increased intake of fiber-rich vegetables and fruits, which are the cheapest and most accessible food products in tropical and subtropical climates where most of the world population lives. For cardiovascular diseases, unhealthy diet and smoking, along with physical inactivity and chronic infectious diseases such as periodontal disease, are also highly ranked as external (environmental) risk factors. Physical inactivity may also result in skeletal disasters, in particular back pain. The important question is, 'Who is responsible for what you eat, whether you smoke, whether you exercise, and whether you clean your teeth?' Health maintained and controlled by self-diagnosis and self-care not only is cost-effective but also is an important factor in quality of life and maintaining independence and health.

Practitioner responsibility

The *lege artis* principles require clinicians to practice dentistry according to modern science and established evidence-based methods: that is, the latest or 'state of the art' techniques. From experimental and well-controlled longitudinal clinical studies in humans, the following conclusions may be drawn.

- Dental caries and periodontal diseases can successfully be prevented and controlled by self-care supplemented by needs-related professional preventive measures.
- Non-cavitated caries affecting enamel, root and even dentin can be remineralized or at least arrested successfully.
- Regeneration of periodontal attachment is a reality.

To realize these clinical outcomes, the profession must concentrate on prevention, control and arrest of dental caries and periodontal diseases. For dental caries, 'prevention instead of extension' or at least 'prevention before extension,' should be given priority. By the same token, aggressive treatment of dental caries with extractions and 'drilling, filling, killing the pulp and billing,' and of periodontal diseases with aggressive scaling, extensive flap surgery, extractions and replacement of teeth with very expensive implant therapy must be regarded as outdated and lacking justification.

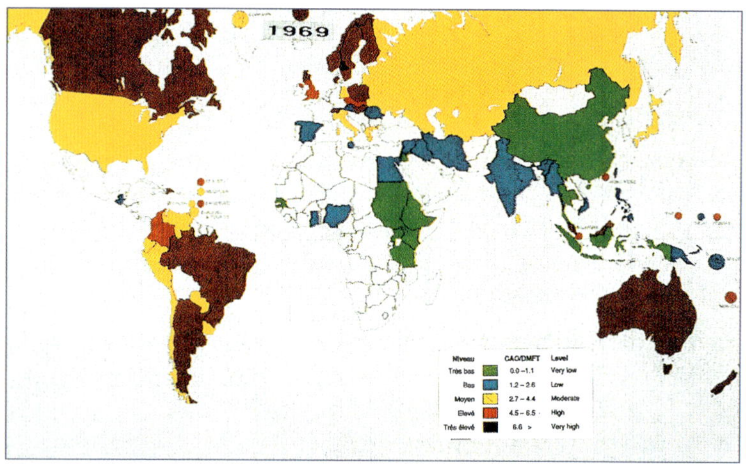

Fig. 2-51 Worldwide caries prevalence among 12-year-old children in 1969. In Sweden, County of Värmland (the black area) had the highest caries prevalence. DMFT, decayed, missing or filled teeth. (From World Health Organization [1994][79] with permission.)

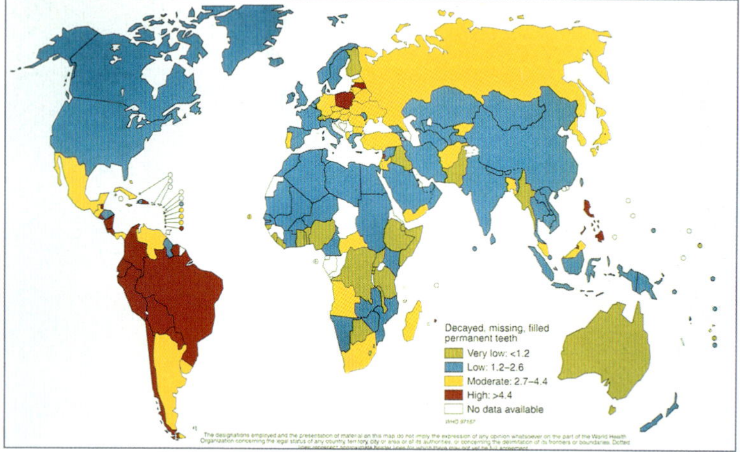

Fig. 2-52 Worldwide caries prevalence in 1997 among 12-year-old children. (From World Health Organization [1997][78] with permission.)

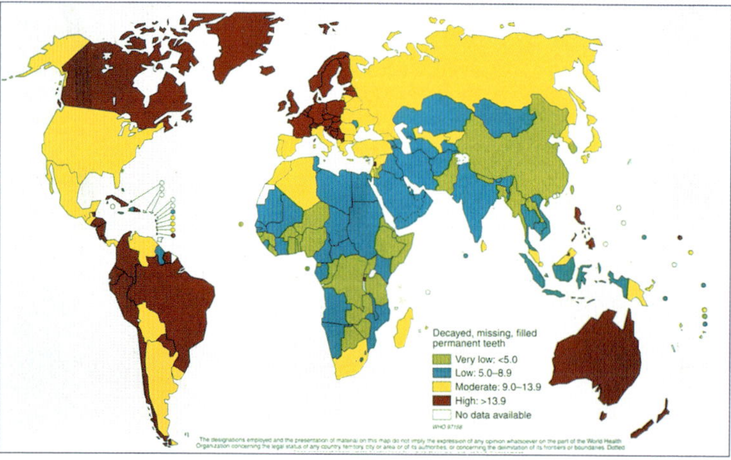

Fig. 2-53 Worldwide caries prevalence among those aged 35–44 years in 1997. (From WHO [1997][78] with permission.)

Oral and general health is strongly correlated with the level of education. Worldwide, the level of education is improving. Eventually, increasingly well-educated patients will learn the implications of high-quality dentistry according to *lege artis* principles and will request more preventive dentistry, instead of 'drilling, filling and billing.' Dentists who are not willing to comply with their patients' requests will find that their practices decline.

Improving access to oral care

Traditional systems for oral care are based on various combinations of public-salaried services and private practice. The public services are usually responsible for prevention and the care of schoolchildren and disadvantaged groups. Private practitioners provide a wide range of treatment to the general public. All the systems are oriented in such a way that the dental clinician provides most of the care.

As discussed above, the level of dental caries in developing countries has rarely been as high as in industrialized countries, except for Latin America (Figs 2-51 to 2-53). In some developing countries, successful preventive programs have been implemented. In many countries, however, there is still a threat of increasing caries, related to changing diet and lifestyles in combination with poor oral hygiene and a failure to use fluoride dentifrice. In many communities, the oral care systems do not meet even the basic needs of the public. Most public services have very low coverage; communities in low-income rural and urban areas cannot afford private oral care. Furthermore, developing countries cannot afford to establish, staff and run education facilities for dental clinicians or hope to provide adequate employment opportunities for dental clinicians trained abroad.

In all countries, economic restraints, changes in demand for oral healthcare, political pressures to extend services to underprivileged groups and concerns about quality, costs and effectiveness of care demand that alternative ways of organizing oral healthcare be examined and implemented. Cost and lack of access for underprivileged and low-income groups constrain all oral healthcare systems.

What actions can be taken to combat this neglect, breakdown the barriers of costs and improve access to oral healthcare? Alternative systems must be developed so that many more people can have access to and can afford oral healthcare. Several recent advances give great scope for the transformation of the delivery and quality of oral care:

- new educational technologies make the acquisition of new knowledge and skills, simpler and faster for all types of personnel
- simplified and logical design of oral healthcare clinics improves the workplace and substantially reduces the capital cost of equipment and the need for maintenance
- better materials that are easier and simpler to use.

Based on these technological advances, three types of care can be defined.

1. Simple low technology: very cost-effective
2. Moderate level of technology: rather expensive
3. High technology: often extremely expensive.

The first level of oral care includes education of the population in self-diagnosis and self-care on an individual and group basis, PMTC, use of fluoride varnish and fissure sealants, scaling, root planing and debridement, plus low-technology treatment of single-surface caries cavities with the so-called atraumatic restorative technique, which has the potential to revolutionize the type of care that can be given in developing countries with a low ratio of dental clinicians.

For small caries cavities, hand instruments can be used to remove the diseased tissue. The damaged area can then be repaired with glass-ionomer cement, which also has a preventive effect as it functions as a slow-releasing fluoride agent that can be recharged with fluoride from other agents, such as fluoride dentifrice.

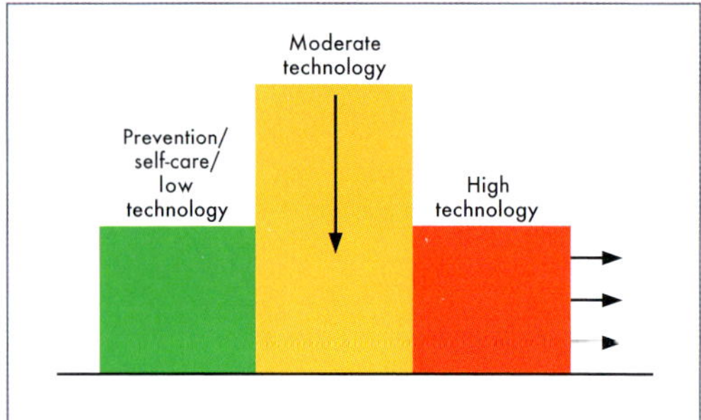

Fig. 2-54 Changes in distribution of tasks in oral healthcare from past to present in highly industrialized countries. (Modified from WHO [1994][79] with permission.)

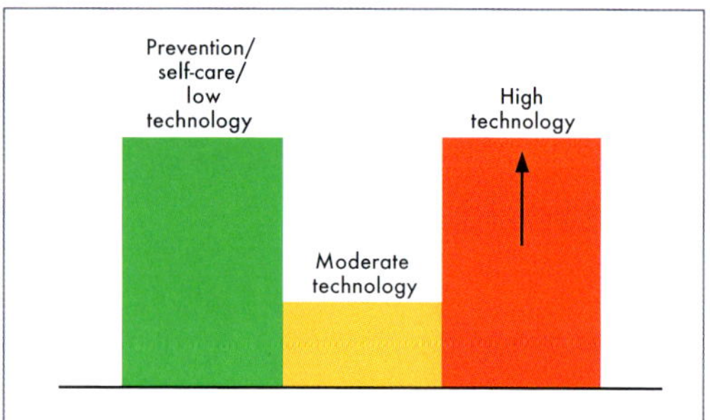

Fig. 2-55 Distribution of tasks in oral healthcare in highly industrialized countries. (Modified from WHO [1994][79] with permission.)

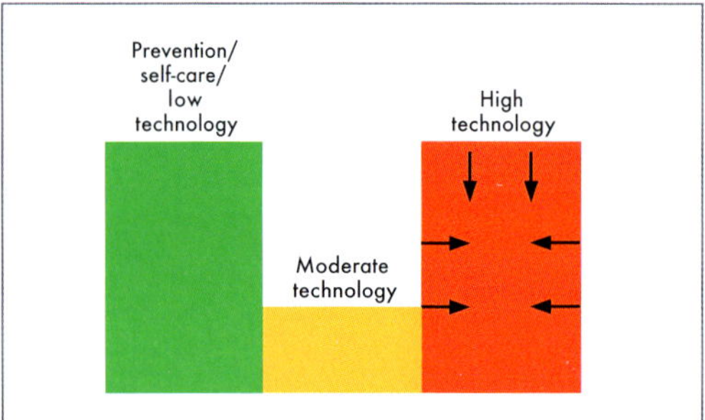

Fig. 2-56 Future distribution of tasks in oral healthcare in highly industrialized countries. (Modified from WHO [1994][79] with permission.)

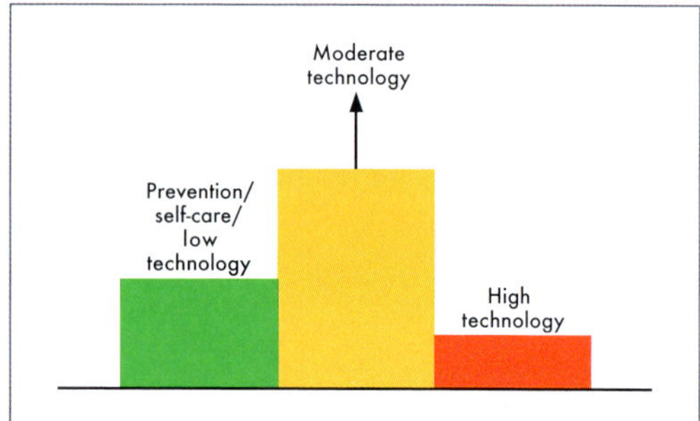

Fig. 2-57 Typical distribution of tasks in oral healthcare in developing countries. (Modified from WHO [1994][79] with permission.)

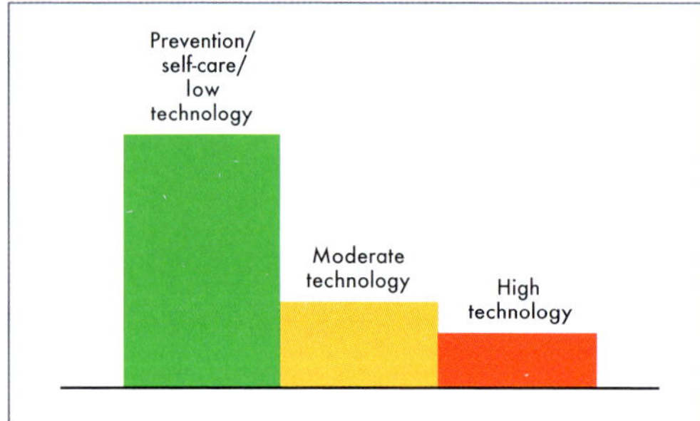

Fig. 2-58 Eventual future distribution of tasks in oral healthcare in all countries. (Modified from WHO [1994][79] with permission.)

The aim of the first level (low technology) of oral care is to prevent the need for more traditional and costly invasive (moderate technology) oral care.

The second level (moderate technology) includes multiple-surface restorations, extractions, simple periodontal surgery, removable prostheses and traditional invasive oral care, practiced by most dental clinicians worldwide.

The third and most complex high-technology level of oral care includes precision prosthetics, implants, laminates and ceramic inlays and onlays, orthodontics, regenerative periodontal treatment and complex oral surgery and medicine: in other words, the costly and complex procedures that require highly qualified specialists or 'oral physicians.' In any society, the availability of high-technology oral care will remain limited.

A rational, health-promoting, affordable mix of oral care should be planned and implemented in all countries. Emphasis on prevention and control of oral diseases will minimize the need for intervention at the moderate- and high-technology levels. As a consequence of improving oral health in most industrialized countries, the need for moderately complex care is decreasing. With further emphasis on prevention, the need and demand for first-level interventions will increase slightly, while the need for high-technology care will probably increase for the foreseeable future, because of the desire to preserve natural teeth and the increasing numbers of elderly people who retain some natural teeth and edentulous people who will want implant treatment.

In developing countries, the first (low-technology, non-invasive) level of oral care will continue to be the major need. In those developing countries in which the prevalence of caries is increasing, a rising demand for the moderate level of technology will continue for some time to come. High-technology oral care will remain limited.

The proportion of the population taking advantage of oral healthcare services varies from country to country, but in only a few might it be considered optimum. For example, in Sweden, almost 100% of those aged 1–19 years receive well-organized and regular oral care, predominantly preventive dentistry, free of charge.[17,71] In the county of Värmland, Sweden, 90% of the adult population visits oral healthcare clinics regularly for care, including prevention.[17,72] In most countries, total coverage is an unrealistic goal, but steps should be taken to ensure that oral care is available to all those who need it.

The pattern of oral healthcare levels in highly industrialized countries, from the past to the future, is shown in Figs 2-54 to 2-56, modified from the WHO data.[102] The typical distribution and trends of different oral healthcare levels in developing countries are shown in Fig. 2-57. The eventual future distribution of oral healthcare levels in all countries is illustrated in Fig. 2-58.

The influence of dental insurance systems on oral health status

There is no doubt that different financing and insurance systems will significantly influence oral health status. Some of the different approaches to financing oral care include quality control guidelines, fixed fee agreements, capitations schemes, health maintenance organizations, rewarding increased preventive care and public health funding.

Quality control guidelines

Using information about the duration of treatment methods and acceptable care products, quality control guidelines are being prepared, indicating the average number of years each type of care should last. If care procedures do not last the specified time, the clinician is then obliged to provide retreatment free of charge. Such guidelines are intended to reduce unnecessary treatment that results in progressive destruction of tooth substance and periodontal support and higher costs for oral care.

Fixed fees

In some countries, dental clinicians may charge only fixed fees for most procedures that are agreed between the health authorities and the professionals. These fees may be exceeded only for special treatment and after a review of the diagnosis and proposed procedure. In countries using this system, the costs of oral care are not rising, but possibly even decreasing.

Dental insurance systems based on fixed fees for different specified treatment procedures, such as one anterior acrylic resin composite restoration versus complicated multisurface restorations, crowns or endodontic treatment, are not a guarantee for improved oral health status among the population. For example, in Germany and Japan, the dental insurance systems are heavily concentrated on restorative dentistry: so-called tertiary prevention.

For items such as crowns and restorations, the dental clinicians are relatively well reimbursed, but there is virtually no reimbursement for preventive dentistry according to the schedules issued by the national dental insurance scheme. As a consequence, dental practices concentrate on 'drilling, filling and billing' to survive.

This may explain why, in contrast to other industrialized countries such as the Scandinavian countries, Canada and Australia, Germany and Japan maintain a moderate to high caries prevalence (Figs 2-51 and 2-52).[78]

This is possibly surprising, on the one hand, given that Germany and Japan have well-educated dental clinicians, very high scientific standards and a well-educated population with a high standard of living. On the other hand, it indicates the very powerful influence the prevailing dental insurance system has on the oral health status of the population.

Capitation schemes

Capitation schemes pay the dental clinician a fixed sum for each person enrolled as a patient in the practice. For this fixed annual fee, a dental clinician contracts to maintain the oral health of the enrolled patient. Patients must, however, undertake to attend for checkups on a regular basis or they lose their rights and have to pay for treatment needed to restore their oral health. It is anticipated that costs will be reduced and the oral health status improved by this type of program.

Health maintenance organizations

Health maintenance organizations contract with a group of oral care professionals to provide care to a group of communities or individuals at agreed fees. Health maintenance organizations are usually organized and managed by companies that specialize in health insurance. This has proved an effective way to limit the costs of providing comprehensive oral care.

Rewarding increased preventive care

In some countries, projects to encourage preventive care give dental care managers a financial reward if disease levels are reduced in the patients in their catchment area.

Public health funding

In most Scandinavian countries, oral healthcare programs for children and young adults, including school-based preventive programs, have been organized free of charge by the departments of health. This is one reason for the vast improvement in caries prevalence in Scandinavian children from 1969 to 1997 (Figs 2-51 and 2-52).

For example, the Swedish Public Dental Health Service has been granted a fixed annual allowance by the Department of Health to carry out needs-related dental care for all individuals up to 20 years of age. This has encouraged and motivated the service to focus on preventive dentistry and to delegate preventive treatment to dental hygienists and preventive dentistry assistants, to minimize costly restorative dentistry by dentists. Notably, in the county of Värmland, Sweden, needs-related programs practiced by dental hygienists and preventive dentistry assistants have been successfully implemented under capitation arrangements.[17,71]

Oral health insurance system

In 1973, a national dental insurance was introduced for all adults in Sweden, irrespective of whether they chose the public Dental Health Service (40%) or private practice (60%). Approximately 80–90% of the Swedish adult population visit dental clinics regularly for maintenance programs. Up until 1999, restorative dentistry, including crown and fixed partial denture, was based on an itemized fee schedule, while preventive dentistry and periodontal treatment was based on an hourly fee, with different rates for specialized periodontists, general dental practitioners, dental hygienists and preventive dental assistants. In 1999, the insurance system was reviewed. A capitation system based on the individual's predicted risk (Figs 2-42 to 2-46) combined with analytical epidemiology for quality control was introduced parallel to a modified version of the earlier system.

As discussed in this chapter, the oral health professionals must practice according to modern scientific principles and established methods. The cause of both dental caries and peridontal diseases are known as are efficient preventive measures, which have been confirmed over a 30-year period irrespective of age. Therefore, high-quality oral healthcare must focus on prevention and control of dental caries and periodontal diseases and other oral diseases: primary and secondary prevention. Existing treatment needs (tertiary prevention) must also be addressed.

In this context, it seems that all national dental health insurance schemes and finance systems should promote prevention and control of oral diseases, combined with analytic epidemiology for quality control, and cost-effectiveness analyses by the government in accordance with national and global oral health goals. In other words, the dental professionals should expect to be well paid for successful prevention and control of oral diseases. An increasingly well-educated and well-motivated population will undoubtedly prefer an oral healthcare program giving priority to prevention and control of oral diseases compared with extractions, big flaps, drilling, filling, billing, killing the pulp and costly implant therapy, and as a consequence maybe impaired general health and reduced 'quality of life.'

Ancient Chinese doctors were said to be very well paid as long as they were able to keep their patients healthy. If they failed, they received no reimbursement at all.

The following proposal for an oral health insurance system is based on 'state of the art' knowledge and understanding. The system would involve a capitation system based on the predicted risk, including needs-related primary, secondary and tertiary prevention. The individual annual fee would be combined with a negative fee based on the effect of the needs-related maintenance program on disease progression.

For example, if the patient developed a new caries lesion, the patient's annual fee would be increased by US$60 and the dental clinician's reimbursement would be reduced by US$60. Likewise the annual fee would be increased by a certain amount for the patient and reduced by the same amount for the dental clinician if the patient exhibited further loss of periodontal support.

For quality control of such an oral health insurance system, a computer-aided analytical oral epidemiologic system should be introduced. The dental clinician could present graphs in the waiting room to show the success of the practice in improving oral health status and eliminating treatment need among the patients. It would significantly increase the dental clinician's reputation and create good will. The patients would feel privileged to belong to the practice and pleased with the effects of their own efforts in self-care; they would be willing to pay a reasonable fee for the high quality of oral healthcare they were being offered. Non-participating colleagues focused on 'drilling, filling and billing' would lose patients and fear that they are cutting off the branch they are sitting on by not practicing preventive dentistry. The more treatment needs are reduced, the more successful the practice.

Undoubtedly, no single preventive measure or combination of preventive measures would have the impact on the improvement of oral health status as the proposed scheme. Patients would be motivated to learn and improve self-diagnosis and self-care to improve their oral health status and prevent increased annual fees for oral healthcare. Dentists would have opportunity to practice state-of-the-art dentistry and, as a consequence, their annual reimbursement would be secure.[17]

References

1. Orland F, Blayney J, Wendell-Harrison R. Use of the germ-free animal technique in the study of experimental dental caries. J Dent Res 1954;33:147–174.
2. Fitzgerald RJ, Keyes PH. Demonstration of the etiologic role of streptococci in experimental caries in the hamster. J Am Dent Assoc 1960;61:9–19.
3. Gustafsson B, Quensel C, Lanke L, Lundqvist C, Grahnen H, Bonow B et al. The Vipeholm dental caries study. The effect of different levels of carbohydrate intake on caries activity in 436 individuals observed for 5 years. Acta Odontol Scand 1954;11:232.
4. von der Fehr F, Löe J, Theilade E. Experimental caries in man. Caries Res 1970;4:131.
5. Löe H, von der Fehr F, Schiött C. Inhibition of experimental caries by plaque prevention. The effect of chlorhexidine mouthrinses. Scand J Dent 1972;80:1–9.
6. Scheinin A, Mäkinen K. Turku sugar studies I-XXI. Acta Odontol Scand 1975;33:307–320.
7. Imfeld T. Apples, salted peanuts and plaque pH. A telemetric in vivo re-examination. Br Dent J 1978;145:303–305.

8. Axelsson P. A four-point scale for selection of caries risk patients, based on salivary *S. mutans* levels and Plaque Formation Rate Index. In: Johnson NW (ed). Risk Markers for Oral Diseases Caries, vol 1. Cambridge, UK: Cambridge University Press, 1991:158–170.
9. Dean HT, Arnold FA Jr, Elvove E. Domestic water and dental caries. V. Additional studies of the relation of fluoride domestic waters to dental caries experience in 4425 white children aged 12–14 years of 13 cities in 4 states. Public Health Rep 1942;57:1155–1179.
10. Murray JJ, Rugg-Gunn AJ, Jenkins GN. Fluorides in caries prevention, 3rd edn. London: Wright, 1992.
11. Forsman B. Effect of mouthrinses with sodium fluoride in schools at Växjö, Sweden. Sved Tandlakforb Tidn 1965; 57:705–709.
12. Torell P, Ericsson Y. A 2-year test with different methods of local caries-preventive fluoride application in Swedish schoolchildren. Acta Odontol Scand 1965;23:287–322.
13. Axelsson P, Paulander J, Nordqvist K, Karlsson R. The effect of fluoride containing dentfrice, rinsing and varnish on interproximal dental caries. A 3-year clinical trial. Community Dent Oral Epidemiol 1987;15:177–180.
14. Knutson J. Sodium fluoride solution: technique for applications to the teeth. J Am Dent Assoc 1948;36:37–39.
15. Buonocore MG. A simple method of increasing the adhesion of acrylic filling materials to enamel surfaces. J Dent Res 1955;34:849–853.
16. Feigal RJ. Sealant and preventive restorations: review of effectiveness and clinical changes for improvement. Pediatr Dent 1998;20:85–92.
17. Axelsson P. A Clinical Textbook on Preventive Materials, Methods and Programmes. Hanover Park, IL: Quintessence, 2004.
18. Carvalho J, Ekstrand K, Thylstrup A. Dental plaque and caries on occlusal surfaces of first permanent molar in relation to stage eruption. J Dent Res 1989;68: 773–779.
19. Carvalho J, Thylstrup A, Ekstrand K. Results after 3 years of non-operative occlusal caries treatment of erupting first permanent molars. Community Dent Oral Epidemiol 1992;20: 187–192.
20. Thylstrup A, Vinther D, Christiansen J. Promoting changes in clinical practice. Treatment time and outcome studies in a Danish public child dental health clinic. Community Dent Oral Epidemiol 1997;25:126–134.
21. Wright G, Banting D, Feasby W. The Dorchester dental flossing study: final report. Clin Prev Dent 1979;1:23–26.
22. Weinstein P, Getz I. Changing Human Behaviour: Strategies for Preventive Dentistry. Chicago,IL: Science Research Associates, 1978.
23. Axelsson P, Buischi Y, Barbosa MFZ, Karlsson R, Pradi MCB. The effect of a new oral hygiene training programme on approximal caries in 12–15-year-old Brazilian children: results after 3 years. Adv Dent Res 1994;8:278–284.
24. Albandar JM, Axelsson P, Buischi Y, Mayer M. Long-term effect of two preventive programmes on the incidence of plaque and gingivitis in adolescents. J Periodontol 1994;65:605–610.
25. Nyvad B, Fejerskov O. Active root surface caries converted into inactive caries as a response to oral hygiene. Scand J Dent Res 1986;94:281–284.
26. Löe H, Theilade E, Jensen S. Experimental gingivitis in man. J Periodontol 1965;36:177–187.
27. Lang NP, Cumming BR, Löe H. Toothbrushing frequency as it relates to plaque development and gingival health. J Periodontol 1973;44:396–405.
28. Bosman CW, Powell RN. The reversal of localized experimental gingivitis. J Clin Periodontol 1977;4:161–172.
29. Lindhe J, Hamp SE, Löe H. Experimental periodontitis in the beagle dog. J Periodontol Res 1973;8:1–10.
30. Saxe SR, Greene JC, Bohannan HM, Vermillion JR. Oral debris, calculus and periodontal disease in the beagle dog. Periodontics 1967;5:217.
31. Lang NP, Karring T. Proceedings of the 1st European Workshop on Periodontology. Hanover Park, IL: Quintessence, 1994.
32. Lövdal A, Arno A, Schei O, Werhaug J. Combined effect of subgingival scaling and controlled oral hygiene on the incidence of gingivitis. Acta Odontol Scand 1961;19:537–555.
33. Suomi JD, Greene JC, Vermillion JR, Doyle Chang JJ, Leatherwood EC. The effect of controlled oral hygiene procedures on the progression of periodontal disease in adults: results after third and final year. J Periodontol 1971;42:152–160.
34. Rosling B, Nyman S, Lindhe J, Jern B. The healing potential of the periodontal tissues following different techniques of periodontal surgery in plaque-free dentitions. A 2-year clinical study. J Clin Periodontol 1976;3:233–250.
35. Nyman S, Lindhe J, Rosling B. Periodontal surgery in plaque-infected dentitions. J Clin Periodontol 1977;4: 240–249.
36. Nyman S, Lindhe J. A longitudinal study of combined periodontal and prosthetic treatment of patients with advanced periodontal disease. J Periodontol 1979;50: 163–169.
37. Lindhe J, Westfelt E, Nyman S, Socransky SS, Haffajee AD. Long-term effect of surgical/non-surgical treatment of periodontal disease. J Clin Periodontol 1984;1:448–458.
38. Wennström A, Wennström J, Lindhe J. Healing following surgical and non-surgical treatment of juvenile periodontitis. A 5-year longitudinal study. J Clin Periodontol 1986;13:869–882.
39. Ramfjord SP, Nissle RR, Schick RA, Cooper H. Subgingival curettage versus surgical elimination of periodontal pockets. J Periodontol 1968;39:167–175.
40. Ramfjord SP, Knowles JW, Nissle RR, Schick RA, Burgett FG. Results following three modalities of periodontal therapy. J Periodontol 1975;46:522–526.

41. Ramfjord SP, Morrison EC, Burgett FG, Nissle RR, Schick RA, Zann GJ, et al. Oral hygiene and maintenance of periodontal support. J Periodontol 1982;53:26-30.
42. Ramfjord SP, Caffesse RG, Morrison EC, Hill R, Kerry GJ, Appleberry E, et al. Four modalities of periodontal treatment compared over 5 years. J Clin Periodontol 1987;14:445-452.
43. Knowles JW, Burgett FG, Nissle RR, Schick RA, Morrison EC, Ramfjord SP. Results of periodontal treatment related to pocket depth and attachment level. Eight years. J Periodontol 1979;50:225-233.
44. Knowles JW, Burgett FG, Morrison EC, Nissle RR, Ramfjord SP. Comparison of results following three modalities of periodontal therapy related to tooth type and initial pocket depth. J Clin Periodontol 1980;6:32-47.
45. Renvert S, Wikström M, Dahlen G, Slots J, Egelberg J. Effect of root debridement on the elimentation of *Actinobacillus actinomycetemcomitans* and *Bacterioides gingivalis* from periodontal pockets. J Clin Periodont 1990;17:345-350.
46. Mousqués T, Listgarten MA, Phillips RW. Effect of scaling and root-planing on the composition of the human subgingival microbial flora. J Periodontol Res 1980;15:144-151.
47. Magnusson I, Lindhe J, Yoneyama T, Liljenberg B. Recolonization of subgingival microbiota following scaling in deep pockets. J Clin Periodontol 1984;11:193-207.
48. Sbordone L, Ramaglia L, Gullettta E, Iacono V. Recolonization of the subgingival microflora after scaling and root planing in human periodontitis. J Periodontol 1990;61:579-584.
49. Axelsson P, Lindhe J. The significance of maintenance care in the treatment of periodontal disease. J Clin Periodontol 1981;8:281-294.
50. Cortellini P, Pino Prato G, Tonetti M. Long term stability of clinical attachment following guided tissue regeneration and conventional therapy. J Clin Periodontol 1996;23: 106-111.
51. Gottlow J, Nyman S, Karring T. Maintenance of new attachment gained through guided tissue regeneration. J Clin Periodontol 1992;19:315-317.
52. Lindhe J, Nyman S. Long-term maintenance of patients treated for advanced periodontal disease. J Clin Periodontol 1984;11:504-514.
53. Rosling B, Serino G, Hellström M, Socransky SS, Lindhe J. Longitudinal periodontal tissue alterations during supportive therapy. Findings from subjects with normal and high susceptibility to periodontal disease. J Clin Periodontol 2001;28:241-249.
54. Listgarten MA, Schifter C. Differential dark field microscopy of subgingival bacteria as an aid in selecting oral intervals: results after 18 months. J Clin Periodontol 1982;9:305-316.
55. Listgarten MA, Levin S, Schifter CC, Sullivan P, Evian CI, Rosenberg ES, Laster L. Comparative longitudinal study of 2 methods of scheduling maintenance visits;2-year data. J Clin Periodontol 1986;13:692-700.
56. Axelsson P, Lindhe J. The effect of a plaque control programme on gingivitis and dental caries in schoolchildren. J Dent Res 1977;56(special issue):142-148.
57. Axelsson P, Lindhe J. The effect of a preventive programme on dental plaque, gingivitis and caries in schoolchildren. Results after one and two years. J Clin Periodontol 1974;1: 126-138.
58. Klock B. Long-term effect of intensive caries prophylaxis. Comm Dent Oral Epidemiol 1984;12:69-71.
59. Axelsson P, Lindhe J. The effect of fluoride on gingivitis and dental caries in a preventive programme based on plaque control. Community Dent Oral Epidemiol 1975;3:156-160.
60. Axelsson P, Lindhe J, Wäseby J. The effect of various plaque control measures on gingivitis and careis in schoolchildren. Community Dent Oral Epidemiol 1976;4:232-239.
61. Axelsson P, Lindhe J. Effect of oral hygiene and professional tooth cleaning on gingivitis and dental caries. Community Dent Oral Epidemiol 1981;6:251-255.
62. Axelsson P. Concept and practice of plaque control. Pediatr Dent 1981;3:101-113.
63. Hotz P. Role of dental plaque control in the prevention of caries. In: Lang NP, Attström R, Löe H (ed). Proceedings of the European Workshop on Mechanical Plaque Control. Berlin: Quintessence, 1998:35-49.
64. Axelsson P, Lindhe J. Effect of controlled oral hygiene procedures on caries and periodontal disease in adults. Results after 6 years. J Clin Periodontol 1981;8:239-248.
65. Axelsson P, Lindhe J, Nyström B. On the prevention of caries and periodontal disease. Results of a 15-year longitudinal study in adults. J Clin Periodontol 1991;13:182-189.
66. Axelsson P, Nyström B, Lindhe J. The long-term effect of a plaque control programme on tooth mortality, caries and periodontal disease in adults. Results after 30 years of maintenance. J Clin Periodontol 2004;31:749-757.
67. Håkansson R. Dental care habits and dental status in 1974-1985 among adults in Sweden. Comparative cross-sectional and longitudinal investigations. Thesis, Lund University, Sweden, 1991.
68. Jansson L, Lavstedt S, Zimmerman M. Marginal bone loss and tooth loss in a sample from the county of Stockholm: a longitudinal study over 20 years. Swed Dent J 2002;26: 21-29.
69. Fure S. 10-year incidence of tooth loss and dental caries in elderly Swedish individuals. J Caries Res 2003;37:462-469.
70. Hugoson A, Laurell L. A prospective study on periodontal bone height changes in a Swedish population. J Clin Periodontol 2000;27:665-674.
71. Axelsson P, Paulander J, Svärdström G, Tollskog G, Nordensten S. Integrate caries prevention. The effect of a needs-related preventive programme on dental caries in children: County of Värmland, Sweden - results after 12 years. Caries Res 1993;27(suppl 1):83-84.
72. Axelsson P, Paulander J, Svärdström G, Kaijser H. Effects of population based preventive programmes on oral health conditions. J Parodontol Implantol Oral 2000;19(300): 255-269.

73. Axelsson P. Needs-related plaque control measures based on risk prediction. In: Lang NP, Attström R, Löe H (eds). Proceedings of the European Workshop on Mechanical Plaque Control. Berlin: Quintessence, 1998:190–247.
74. Baehni PC, Tessier JF. Supportive periodontal care. In: Proceedings of the 1st European Workshop on Periodontology. Berlin: Quintessence, 1994:274–288.
75. Garmyn P, van Steenberghe D, Quirynen M. Efficacy of plaque control in the maintenance of gingival health: plaque control in primary and secondary prevention. In: Lang NP, Attström R, Löe H (ed). Proceedings of the European Workshop on Mechanical Plaque Control. Berlin: Quintessence, 1998:107–120.
76. Lang NP, Brügger U, Salvi G, Tonetti M. Supportive periodontal therapy (SPT). In: Lindhe J, Lang NP, Karring T (ed). Clinical Periodontology and Implant Dentistry. Copenhagen: Blackwell-Munksgaard, 2003:781–805.
77. Renvert S, Persson GR. Supportive periodontal therapy. Periodontology 2000;36:179–195.
78. World Health Organization. Global Oral Data Bank. Geneva: World Health Organization, 1997.
79. World Health Organization. WHO Oral Health Country Profile Programme. Geneva: World Health Organization, 1994.
80. World Health Organization. Oral Health Surveys: Basic Methods, 3rd edn. Geneva: World Health Organization, 1987.
81. Axelsson P, Rolandsson M, Bjerner B. How Swedish dental hygienists apply their training programme in the field. Community Dent Oral Epidemiol 1993;21:297–302.
82. Machtei EE, Dunford R, Hausmann E, Grossi SG, Powell J, Cummins D, et al. Longitudinal study of prognostic factors in established periodontitis patients. J Clin Periodontol 1997;24:102–109.
83. Michalowicz BS, Aeppli DP, Kuba RK. A twin study of genetic variation in proportional radiographs alveolar bone height. J Dent Res 1991;70:1431–1435.
84. Kornman KS, Crane A, Wang HY, di Giovine FS, Newman MG, Pirk FW, et al. The interleukin 1 genotype as a severity factor in adult periodontal disease. J Clin Periodontol 1997;24:72–77.
85. Axelsson P, Paulander J, Nordström L, Jonsson AS, Appel B. The role of genetic interleukin-1 polymorphism on tooth loss and periodontal support loss in 50–60-year-old smokers and non-smokers. Presented at the Scientific Congress of the Department of Periodontology, University of Gothenburg, Sweden, 2001.
86. McGuire MK, Nunn ME. Prognosis versus actual outcome. IV. The effectiveness of clinical parameters and IL-1 genotype in accurately predicting prognoses and tooth survival. J Periodontol 1999;70:49–56.
87. Grossi S, Genco R. Periodontal disease and diabetes mellitus: a two-way relationship. Ann Periodontol 1998;3:51–61.
88. Axelsson P. A Clinical Textbook on Diagnosis and Risk Prediction of Dental Caries. Hanover Park, IL: Qu ntessence, 2000.
89. Axelsson P. A Clinical Textbook on Diagnosis and Risk Prediction of Periodontal Diseases. Hanover Park, IL: Quintessence, 2002.
90. Page RC, Martin J, Krall EA, Mancl LA, Garcia R. Longitudinal validation of a risk calculator for pericdontal disease. J Clin Periodontol 2003;30:819–827.
91. Lang NP, Tonetti MS. Periodontal risk assessment for patients in supportive periodontal therapy (SPT). Oral Health Prevent Dent 2003;1:7–16.
92. Ramberg P, Axelsson P, Lindhe J. Plaque fo·mation at healthy and inflamed gingival sites in young individuals. J Clin Periodontol 1995;22:85–88.
93. Axelsson P, Paulander J, Tollskog G. A new computer-based oral epidemiology system. Presented at the 1st International Conference on Preventive Dentistry and Epidemiology, Karlstad, Sweden, 1988.
94. The National Board of Health and Welfare. Swedish Medical Terminology. Sweden: Stockholm, 1975.
95. Eichner K. Über eine Gruppeneinteiling des Lückengebisses für die Prothetik. Dtsch Zahnärztl Z 1955;10: 1831–1834.
96. Österberg T, Landt H. Index for occlusal status. Tandlakartidn 1976;68:1216–1223.
97. Axelsson P. The Community Caries Index of Treatment Needs (CCITN). Presented at the 1st Internaticnal Conference on Preventive Dentistry and Epidemiology, Karlstad, Sweden, 1988.
98. Axelsson P. The Apical Periodontal Index of Treatment Needs (APITN). Presented at the 1st Internaticnal Conference on Preventive Dentistry and Epidemiology, Karlstad, Sweden, 1988.
99. Ainamo J, Barmes D, Beagrie G, Cutress T, Martin J, Sardo-Infirri J. Development of the WHO community periodontal index of treatment needs (CPITN). Int Dent J 1982;32: 281–291.
100. Beck J, Garcia R, Heiss G. Periodontal disease and cardiovascular disease. J Periodontol 1996;67(suppl):1123–1137.
101. Kolltveit KM, Eriksen HM. Is the observed association between periodontitis and atherosclerosis causal? Eur J Oral Sci 2001;109:2–7.
102. Offenbacher S, Katz V, Fertik G. Periodontal infection as a risk factor for preterm low birth weight. J Periodontol 1996;67(10 suppl):1103–1113.
103. Offenbacher S, Jared HL, O'Reilly PG Wells SR, Salvi GE, Lawrence HP et al. Potential pathogenic mechanisms of periodontitis-associated pregnancy complications. Ann Periodontol 1998;3:233–250.

CHAPTER 3

Dental radiology and imaging

Keith Horner

Definition

Dental radiology and imaging encompasses those techniques that can be used to create images of the dental and maxillofacial region for clinical purposes. The purpose is principally diagnosis, but imaging during treatment and the assessment of treatment outcome are also important. When discussing imaging, emphasis is often placed upon the technology of acquiring the image. In itself, however, an image is useless without effective interpretation. Finally, the two steps of image acquisition and interpretation must be complemented by considering the impact of the imaging investigation upon treatment.

Medical imaging is a vast subject, including an increasingly varied array of techniques. To generalize, all medical imaging can be seen to involve the receipt of data from the body that reflect its nature: structural or physiological. Using this all-embracing definition, therefore, medical imaging may even include such investigations as electroencephalography and electrocardiography. In a dental context, this would mean that such tools as apex locators and electric pulp testers may be considered a form of 'imaging.' Most people would agree, however, that an essential element in medical radiology is the acquisition of data for the purpose of constructing an image rather than to collect a mass of data. This chapter has been written from this more generally accepted perspective.

To manufacture an image, it is necessary to input some kind of energy to the body. Subsequently, an output of energy from the body must be detected and transformed into an image. This process for some of the main imaging techniques used in dental and maxillofacial radiology is illustrated in Table 3-1. In the majority of cases, the notable exception being ultrasound, the energy imparted to the patient is in the form of radiation from the electromagnetic spectrum.

Despite the experience in medicine, where a range of techniques is widely used, dental imaging has traditionally been about the use of X-rays. Today, while X-ray imaging remains overwhelmingly dominant, we are beginning to see the emergence of newer techniques that may begin to challenge this monopoly. Furthermore, while inter-

Table 3-1 The input and output of energy used in the imaging techniques most applicable to dental and maxillofacial radiology. CT, computerized tomography; CBCT, cone beam computerized tomography; CCD, charge-coupled device; CMOS, complementary metal oxide semiconductors.

Input energy	Output energy	Detector system
X-rays (radiography, CT and CBCT)	Attenuated X-rays	Film
		Film + intensifying screen combinations
		Phosphor plates
		Solid state (CCD, CMOS, selenium)
		Scintillation detectors (CT)
		Others
Ultrasound (diagnostic ultrasonography)	Reflected ultrasound	Piezoelectric transducer
Radiofrequency and magnetic field (magnetic resonance imaging)	Emitted radiofrequency and magnetic field changes	Radiofrequency transmitter coils
Visible light (quantitative light-induced fluorescence)	Light fluorescence	CCD camera

pretation remains ultimately a clinical skill that is dependent upon the subjective judgement of the observer, computer-aided diagnosis has already appeared in a few areas. For the future, there is a developing prospect of automated diagnosis from clinical images. In this chapter, the past and present will be reviewed and a window opened on the likely future of dental radiology and imaging.

Historical milestones

While dental imaging may involve other forms of radiation, its history stems directly from the discovery of X-rays by Wilhelm Conrad Röntgen in 1895. Röntgen was a 50-year-old Professor of Physics (Ordentlicher Professor und Rektor) at the University of Würzburg in Germany. The story of his discovery has joined the ranks of those landmarks in the history of science when serendipity and inspired thinking combine in a momentous way. On 8 November 1895, Röntgen was working late in his laboratory studying the effect of passing electrical currents through Hittorf–Crookes vacuum tubes, following some earlier observations that fluorescence of a barium platinocyanide screen occurred when it was placed close to the apparatus. At this stage, Röntgen thought that this effect was caused by 'cathode rays' (electrons), but on this dark November evening, with the room lights dimmed, he noticed that fluorescence was occurring on a piece of screen on a bench a good meter away. Realizing that electrons cannot travel such a distance in air, he postulated that he had produced an hitherto unrecognized form of radiation, which he called 'X-rays' using the usual notation for an unknown quantity.

Apparently, Röntgen worked almost continuously for days on his discovery. One of his earliest experiments was to investigate the penetrative ability of the rays by placing different materials in the path of the radiation. He discovered that materials of similar thickness attenuated the X-rays to different degrees. It is also said that at one point in this experiment, his fingers entered the radiation beam and he briefly saw an image of his bones on the fluorescent screen. He had thereby produced the first X-ray image of the body, albeit a transitory one. Röntgen soon found, however, that he could produce a permanent record of the effect of exposing objects to X-rays using photographic materials instead of the barium platinocyanide screen. It is following this discovery that he famously recorded X-ray images of the hands of both his colleague Albert von Kölliker, the Professor of Physiology and Anatomy at Würzburg, and of his wife Anna Bertha (Fig. 3-1). It is tempting to wonder whether the conversation between Röntgen and von Kölliker might have touched on the potential medical uses of X-rays. As far as Anna Bertha Röntgen was concerned, however, she is said to have announced 'I have seen my death' when she saw the bones of her hand.

Röntgen published his paper 'Über eine neue Art von Strahlen' ('On a new kind of rays') shortly before the end of the year.[1] Within the month of January 1896 alone, commentaries upon and translations of his discovery appeared in highly influential scientific journals, including Nature, and news appeared in the popular press. Röntgen went on to publish other papers on X-rays and was rewarded by receiving several honours, including the Nobel Prize for Physics in 1901. He never profited financially from his work because he did not attempt to patent his discovery. He died of cancer in 1923 in impoverished circumstances. Whether his final illness was related to his X-ray work is impossible to establish. It was for others to take forward his work into medical use, but he must have been proud to be considered the father of medical imaging.

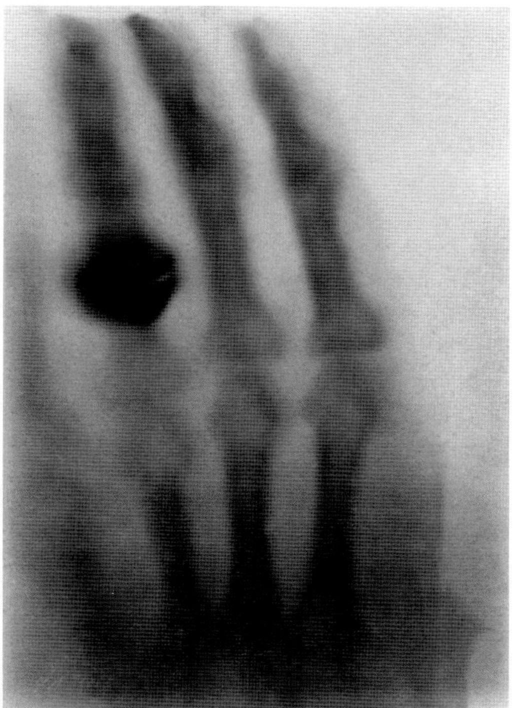

Fig. 3-1 One of the first X-ray images produced by Röntgen.

The birth of dental imaging

Röntgen's discovery of X-rays hit the news stands as well as the scientific literature. Apart from scientists eager to reproduce his findings, clinicians were stimulated to experiment with X-rays, helped by the relative simplicity of the equipment needed. Excellent and detailed descriptions of the history of the early years of dental radiography are available,[2,3] so only some key points will be addressed here.

Scientists interested in imaging teeth, and dental clinicians themselves, first made radiographs of patients in the early months of 1896, within weeks of the publication of Röntgen's discovery of X-rays. No one person can be confidently nominated as having taken the first dental radiograph, but at least four individuals were independently experimenting with X-rays in the oral cavity: Walkhoff and Koenig in Germany, Kells in the USA and Harrison in the UK. Walkhoff was a dental clinician in Braunsweig, Germany. He used a photographic glass plate, wrapped in rubber dam, placed between his tongue and his teeth and exposed himself to X-rays for 25 min while lying on the ground to avoid movement (Fig. 3-2). Harrison is notable because he care-

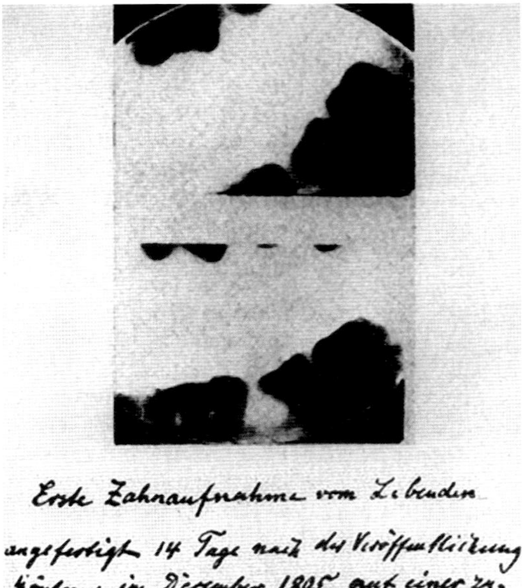

Fig. 3-2 One of the first radiographs of teeth, taken by Otto Walkhoff in the early months of 1896.

fully recorded and published his work in June of 1896.[4] His radiographs were remarkable because of their acceptable clinical quality (Fig. 3-3).

As Harrison's records show, these pioneers used battery power in the absence of a mains electrical supply, to which was added a transformer (home-made) to produce a high voltage. Hand-crafted glass X-ray tubes were used (Fig. 3-4), the same as those described by Röntgen. As far as recording the image was concerned, the Walkhoff method of wrapping carefully trimmed photographic glass plates was used by all the early dental radiographers. Interestingly, however, Harrison switched to the more convenient 'Eastman's Kodac' [sic] film, avoiding the hazards of cutting glass in a darkroom.

With extremely long exposure times, it is not surprising that radiation injuries were reported. Harrison was amongst the earliest to do this, recording the dramatic events that followed the

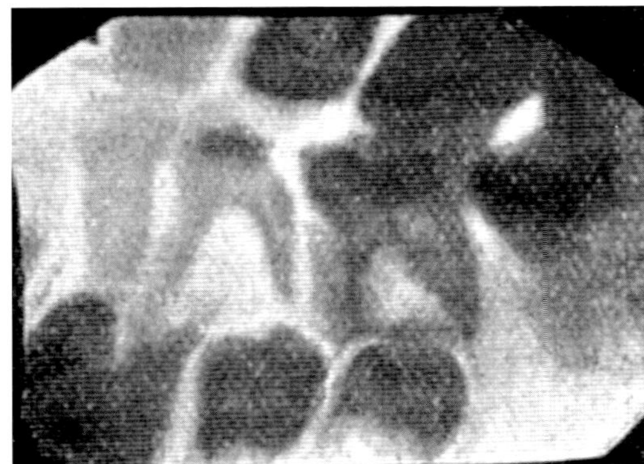

Fig. 3-3 Radiograph of a 7-year-old girl taken by Harrison in 1896.[4] The exposure was of several minutes duration.

exposure of his male assistant, acting as a patient, over a four-week period in 1896:[4]

> *On June 4 the patient complained of an itching and burning sensation, with slight redness over the area subjected to the X-rays; shaving had to be discontinued on account of pain ... On the 6(th) the hair follicles of the beard and right side of the moustache appeared to pustulate. On June 8 ... the skin commenced to desquamate; on the next day the hair over the affected region began to fall. The hair has continued to fall up to the date of writing (June 24), and the skin of the face is quite bald, and the glossy skin in slight wrinkles.*

The American dental clinician William Morton identified that this kind of skin injury was the result of a very close positioning of the X-ray source against the skin. He recommended that injuries could be avoided by using an 18 inch source-to-skin distance and a more powerful X-ray source,[5] thus preempting the advent of the 'long cone' X-ray set by many years.

The collective experience of early pioneers of dental radiography was of unpredictable, home-assembled X-ray-generating equipment, adapted photographic materials and sporadic radiation-induced injuries. It was a poor start to radiographic imaging in dentistry. It is unsurprising that Harrison's conclusions about X-ray use in dentistry were

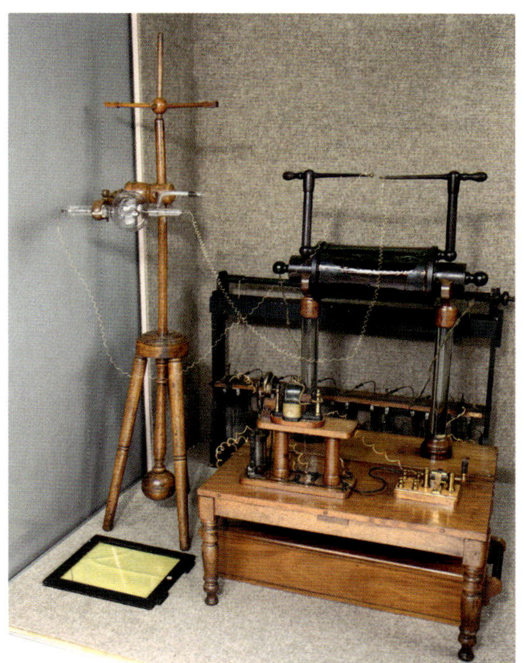

Fig. 3-4 An X-ray installation from 1896–7. On the left is the X-ray tube and on the right is the electrical apparatus required to produce the required voltage. (Courtesy of the Science Museum, London.)

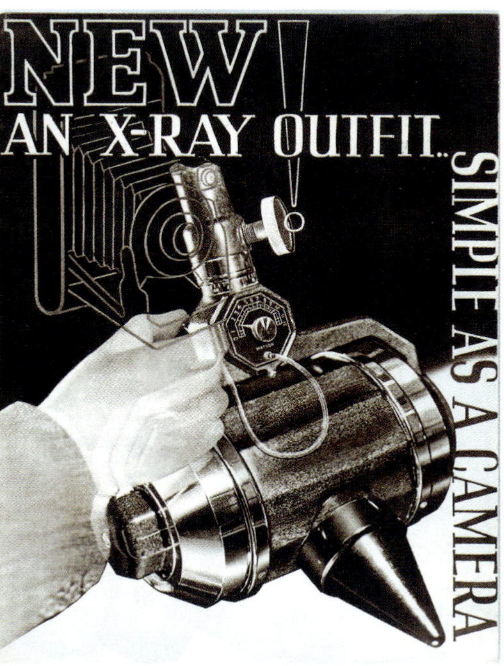

Fig. 3-5 An advertisement for a state-of-the-art dental X-ray set from the 1930s. Note the pointed cone used to aid positioning. (Courtesy of the Science Museum, London.)

that 'the work is altogether too complicated and too expensive to be added to the dental outfit.'

The first twenty years

Until equipment was more robust and predictable in its performance, Harrison's pessimism was entirely justified. It would take almost 20 years for dental radiography to be feasible for any dental clinician to consider. Two developments were key to this change: first, the increased prevalence of a mains electrical supply and transformers and, second, the development of reliable X-ray tubes. While the former reflects the general advance in technology of the early twentieth century, the latter represents a real drive to make radiology a clinically acceptable specialty.

Within months of Röntgen's discovery, several scientists had independently developed a 'focus tube,' in which the anode was moved from a position perpendicular to the electron beam to one in which it was set at an angle, leading to a smaller source of X-rays and giving sharper 'focused' images and improving tube life. This form of tube is presumably the improved form of X-ray tube reported by Morton in 1897 as being safer to use on patients.[5] Unlike modern X-ray tubes, which require a very good vacuum to function properly, early X-ray tubes actually required the inclusion of air to act as the electron source. The air content needed to be adjusted by the operator using a small valve to maintain the correct X-ray output. This element of subjectivity to the exposure was far from ideal and led to the practice of 'setting the tube', whereby the user had to test the exposure, usually using his own, or assistant's, hand as a test object, by assessing the brightness of the image on a fluorescent screen. This stored up much trouble for the future in the form of delayed radiation injuries and cancer induction.

The first commercially manufactured dental X-ray set was produced in 1905 in Germany. This was followed in 1912–13 by equipment from two US manufacturers. The milestone development, however, came in 1913 with the patenting of the 'hot cathode' X-ray tube by Coolidge. This changed the method of X-ray production from the old 'gas' tubes to vacuum tubes and used a heated tungsten filament as the electron source. Essentially, this is the basis of the X-ray technology used through to today, albeit that vast improvements in performance have been achieved over the intervening years.

Early dental X-ray sets were hazardous not only because of the X-ray risks but also because of exposed high-voltage wires; the risk of electrocution during use was serious. In 1918, the first 'shock-proof' dental X-ray set, the Victor CDX, was introduced in which the X-ray tube and electrical elements were housed in an oil-filled container. Nonetheless, other manufacturers continued to manufacture equipment with exposed high-voltage wires for some years. By the 1930s, however, dental X-ray equipment was being produced that was truly recognizable as an ancestor of today's intraoral X-ray sets, with a streamlined outer casing and a position-indicating device to improve accuracy in techniques (Fig. 3-5). Such equipment had sufficient robustness to remain in clinical use well into the lifetime of some older dental clinicians still working today.

While good equipment is obviously essential, excellence in radiographic technique is a prerequisite of a useful diagnostic image. The challenges of intraoral radiography were recognized in the very first year of dental radiography by both Kells and Harrison. Kells advocated placing the film parallel with the tooth in 1896, although this was more widely recognized in 1904 following Price's publications. Harrison described a customized stent to support the film, manufactured from dental composition to facilitate the technique. For most dental clinicians, however, the individualized manufacture of film holders was an additional problem, and the advent of the bisecting angle technique by Cieszynski in 1907 was a major advance. He used the principle of isometry to cast accurate 'shadows' of the teeth on to a film positioned at a different angle, allowing patients to support the film with their finger. Although one of the first dental radiographs taken by Walkhoff in 1896 can be thought of as the first bitewing image, this technique was only formally described and recommended for clinical use by Kells in 1925. The bitewing technique has stood the test of time and remains the single most useful X-ray image in the clinical practice of dentistry.

Imaging: a clinical essential

The period following the First World War can be seen as one of steady improvements and maturity in dental X-ray imaging. As we have seen, the equipment used for X-ray production could now be purchased by dental clinicians and had reasonable reliability. Dental radiology began to be seen as an integral part of dentistry, with the production of textbooks on techniques and interpretation of images.

While the bisecting angle technique became dominant in everyday dental practice, others persisted in advocating parallelism and accurate geometrical images. Franklin McCormick recommended a long X-ray source-to-skin distance as early as 1910. This became a family mission, with first his son and then his son-in-law, Gordon Fitzgerald, going on to develop the 'long cone' technique in 1947. This was accompanied by the introduction of film-holding beam-aiming devices to permit the technique to be feasible in everyday clinical practice. The short, pointed-cone, positioning device began to be seen as a problem in the 1970s. While it certainly simplified the technique, the cone itself added to scattered radiation; this problem could be addressed by using an open-ended positioning device. At the same time, the short focus-to-skin distance, addressed over 50 years previously by McCormick, was finally recognized by the equipment manufacturers with the widespread introduction of 'long cones' – correctly long cylinders. Despite the overwhelming superiority of the 'long cone' paralleling technique for intraoral radiography, it is

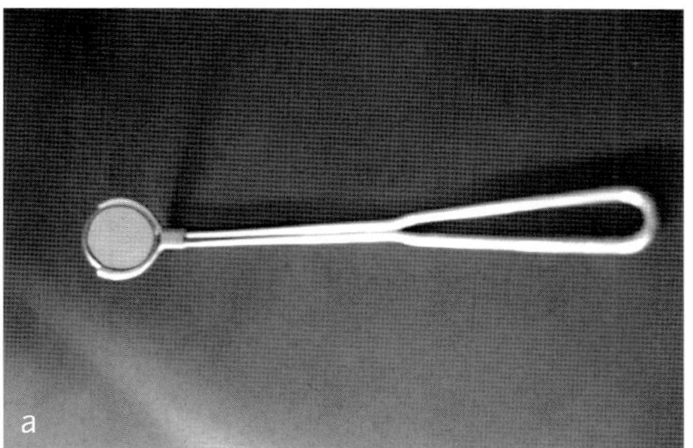

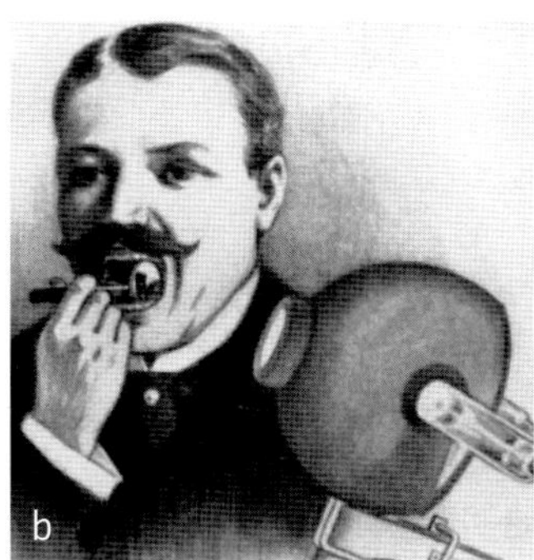

Fig. 3-6 Intraoral fluoroscopy. (a) A small fluorescent screen is fitted to a mouth mirror handle; (b) early drawing of this instrument in use.

salutary to note that short focus-to-skin distances and the bisecting angle technique have only recently become redundant in many dental practices.

Although the revolutions in X-ray set design and construction were complete by the 1930s, certain refinements, notably the introduction of electronic rather than clockwork timers, had to wait several decades for the technology to become available. This development was needed as the advances in film speed paved the way for increasingly shorter exposure times. This steady improvement in the speed of the image receptor really began in 1919, when the first machine-wrapped dental X-ray film was manufactured (Kodak Regular film). Up to this point, roll photographic film had been used with film 'packets' being made by the dental clinician for each patient examination.

Although film was always the main means of capturing an image, there was a vogue for intraoral fluoroscopy using a special instrument, resembling a large mouth mirror with the mirrored glass replaced by a fluorescent screen (Fig. 3-6). By holding this device in the mouth during an exposure, an instant but non-permanent image was produced on the screen. Although this had some advantages, the temptation for repeated exposures and for the dental clinician to hold the instrument for the patient meant that excessive X-ray doses were received by both patient and operator. Thankfully, this technique has been redundant, and in most countries illegal, for many years.

A double-sided emulsion for X-ray film was introduced by Kodak in 1924. This 'radiatized' film halved the exposures required. After this, improvements were related to increasing film speed. Kodak Ultraspeed was manufactured in 1940, further reducing exposure times by half, and the 1950s saw Ultraspeed improved, with several speed advances having been achieved. In the 1960s, the film base was switched from cellulose acetate to polyester, improving the archival quality of radiographs. By 1980, Ektaspeed (E-speed) film was introduced, giving approximately half the exposure of the latest Ultraspeed emulsion. In probably the final refinement of intraoral dental film, F-speed film, giving a 20% reduction in exposures compared with Ektaspeed, was marketed in 2000.[6]

Panoramic radiography

Taking multiple intraoral radiographs can be a tedious business, requiring time and skill from the operator and tolerance by the patient. The idea of using a single exposure to produce a complete image of the dentition is, therefore, an attractive one and had been in the minds of dental clinicians at an early stage in the development of radiology. The challenge was to overcome the curved shape of the jaws. Although one proposal for imaging curved surfaces such as the jaws was patented as early as 1922, the easiest approach was to use the oblique lateral view of the jaws. Two exposures, one

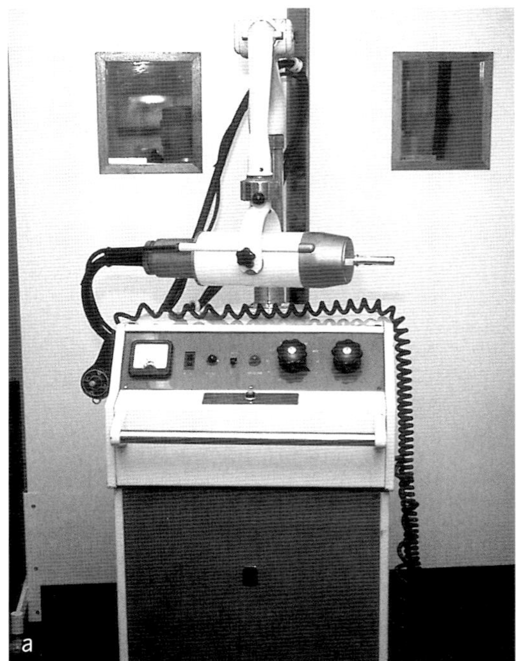

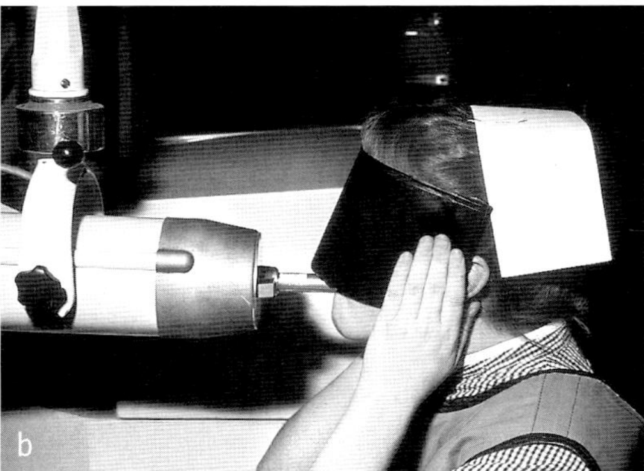

Fig. 3-7 Panograph intraoral panoramic unit. (a) The apparatus, showing the slender X-ray source; (b) the equipment in use. (From Rushton [2006][7] with permission.)

for each side of the face, using a radiographic cassette and a dental X-ray set, can produce a highly satisfactory image without recourse to the additional expense of specialized equipment.

One approach for obtaining a panoramic image was to employ an intraoral source of radiation and extraoral film applied closely to the face, patented by Koch und Sterzel Aktiengesellschaft in 1943 and by Ott in 1951. These principles were used in the manufacture and clinical use of the Panograph by Watson and Sons Ltd (Fig. 3-7). The anode – the source of X-rays – was located at the end of a rod that was placed in the patient's mouth. These units delivered a very high local dose of radiation to the mouth. The image quality, however, was poor, given geometric distortion. Despite some commercial success, the unacceptable radiation dose levels were mainly responsible for the withdrawal of the Panograph from clinical use.

While the intraoral X-ray tube method was a dead end, parallel developments would eventually lead to great success. In 1922, Zulauf patented 'Panoramic X-ray apparatus' in the USA. His patent shows that he devised a system using a narrow collimated X-ray source that was rotated around the patient's face on a track. A long film packet was placed intraorally and the maxilla and mandible were exposed individually. It is uncertain whether this design was ever developed subsequently. Early in the following decade, a Japanese researcher, Numata, produced a similar design, presumably without knowledge of Zulauf's patent.

In 1946, the Finnish dental researcher Paatero began his program of work, which would ultimately lead to the modern panoramic X-ray unit. Initially, he followed the earlier path of using an intraoral film, although in his design the patient was rotated while the X-ray source was fixed. In 1949, however, a major step forward was made when Paatero developed a system with a curved film cassette positioned extraorally, avoiding the need for the difficult and uncomfortable intraoral placement of a film. This again, however, involved the rotation of the patient and used a single axis of rotation, which led to poor image quality.

Two scientists in the USA, Nelson and Kumpula, were also working in this field and, in the 1950s, after some collaboration with Paatero, developed a machine that used a double eccentric axis rotation around a stationary patient. This was to develop into the commercially successful Panorex

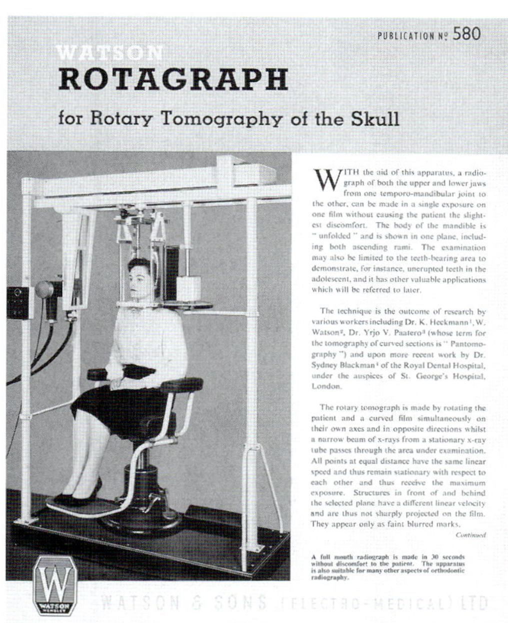

Fig. 3-8 The Rotagraph panoramic X-ray unit; an advertisement from the 1950s. (From Rushton [2006][7] with permission.)

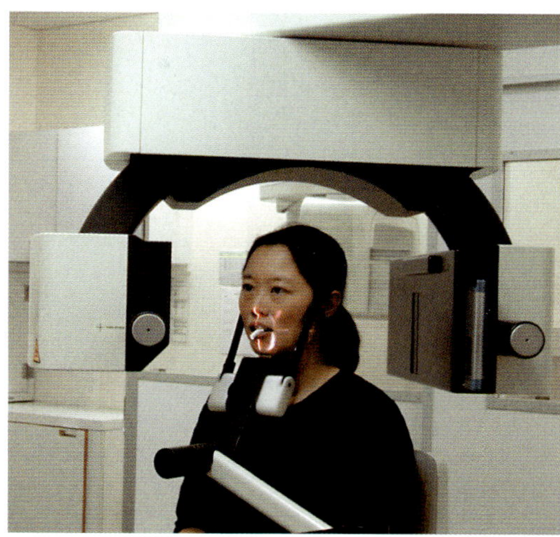

Fig. 3-9 The Scanora multifunctional tomographic unit.

unit. Meanwhile, Paatero continued his previous work using rotation of the patient and film in collaboration with Blackman, a dental radiologist from London, and Watson and Sons Ltd., producing the Rotagraph (Fig. 3-8). While these two systems worked in a satisfactory way, Paatero embarked on a new program of research that would lead, by the mid-1950s, to the development of the far superior 'orthopantography'.

Orthopantography was radically different in that it used three rotational axes, reducing considerably the troublesome overlap of teeth on the film. The 'ortho' element of its name reflected that the projection approximated more closely to one. That has at right angles to the line of the dental arch. With this development, Paatero had set the standard for panoramic radiography that made it a staple part of dental and maxillofacial radiology for over 50 years. Subsequent advances have been incremental refinements of the movement path taken during panoramic radiography, in particular the shift from three centers of rotation to a continuously moving, elliptical, one. We have, however, seen the incorporation of movement programs that allow the production of cross-sectional tomographic images at specified points along the dental arches.[8] This development, in the form of the Scanora (Soredex, Tuusula, Finland) was aimed principally at the needs of dental implantology.

It was subsequently followed by other manufacturers of panoramic equipment, with varying degrees of success (Fig. 3-9).

Those interested in exploring this aspect of dental imaging history are referred to definitive histories of panoramic radiography.[7,9]

The digital age begins

In dentistry, film remained the staple means of recording the attenuated X-ray beam through to the end of the twentieth century. Indeed, in many countries this remains the case today. In developed countries, however, dental film sales are steadily falling as digital imaging becomes predominant. The term digital radiography refers to X-ray imaging techniques which at some stage utilize a digital data format in acquiring, processing, displaying or managing a medical X-ray image.[10]

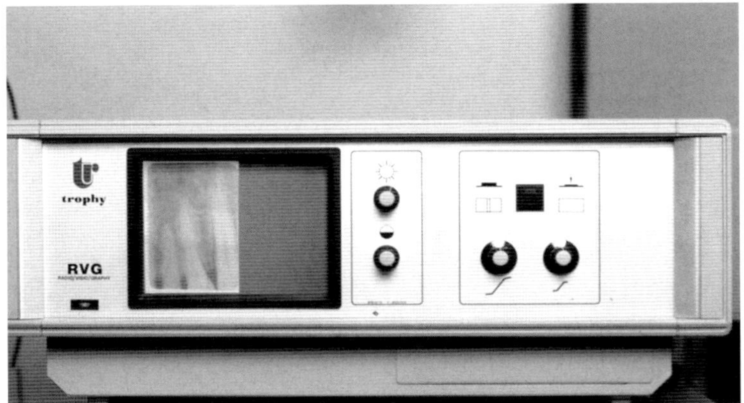

Fig. 3-10 RadioVisioGraphy, the first digital dental radiography system.[12]

Where did digital imaging originate?

Paradoxically, the oldest branch of medical imaging, radiography, has been the slowest to utilize new technologies. In the 1960s, nuclear medicine used computers to generate time-activity curves from a set of dynamic images. In the late 1960s and early 1970s, digital subtraction angiography and computerized tomography (CT) were developed and introduced. Digital subtraction angiography was developed to remove background data from images following the administration of intravenous contrast medium to patients. Both nuclear medicine and digital subtraction angiography originally involved an external computer to process data obtained in an analogue form. Both could be performed without the computed element. In contrast, CT was the first form of medical imaging in which the computer element was an essential component. CT is based upon the computer performing back projection of multiple X-ray projections. The first clinical CT scanner was installed at the Atkinson Morley Hospital in London in 1972 by Hounsfield.[11]

In dentistry, however, when we talk about digital imaging we are really considering image acquisition for conventional radiographic procedures. Medical digital image receptors can be divided into the following types:[10]

- digitization of conventional film
- image-intensifier-based digital fluorography
- photostimulable phosphor computerized radiography
- amorphous selenium technology
- flat-panel detectors.

Digitizing conventional film has developed along with flatbed scanners and digital photography. In terms of true digital imaging in dentistry, however, the first development in digital radiology employed the principles of image-intensifier-based digital fluorography, considerably simplified anc reduced in size, to produce dental digital images.

In 1989, a French dental clinician, Francis Mouyen, developed RadioVisioGraphy[12] using a combination of a fluorescent screen and charge-coupled device (CCD) camera technology (Fig. 3-10). A fragment of intensifying screen, such as used traditionally in radiographic cassettes, was adapted to a CDD chip using an optical fiber coupling into an intraoral sensor, connected by a cable to a small image-display unit. Images were instantaneously displayed after exposure.

This clever and simple idea, although not without its practical problems,[13] revolutionized dental radiography, bringing a backwater of medical imaging into the modern age. Subsequently, numerous manufacturers adopted this technology, including applications for panoramic radiography using a modified CCD chip to accommodate the long, thin collimated beam.

More recently, some manufacturers have introduced complementary metal oxide semiconductors as an alternative to CCDs.

Photostimulable phosphor computerized radiography was introduced in 1981,[10] but was first used for dental imaging in the mid-1990s, with the introduction of the Digora system (Soredex, Tuusula, Finland) for intraoral radiology. An imaging plate was exposed in the mouth and then scanned in a dedicated processing unit attached to a personal computer. Phosphor plate technology was found to offer the advantage over the then available CCD systems of wide exposure latitude and acceptable image quality compared with film.[14] Phosphor plate technology was subsequently used for some panoramic systems and, unlike CCD systems, occlusal-sized imaging plates were developed by some manufacturers.

Digital imaging technology is further discussed below, but the reader is also referred to the recent publication by Horner and co-workers[15] for a more extensive contemporary review.

Current 'state-of-the-art' techniques

Intraoral radiography

Radiography in which a small image receptor is positioned within the mouth and exposed using a simple X-ray set positioned outside the mouth is the commonest form of radiography performed worldwide. The X-ray sets used for this purpose, commonly referred to as intraoral X-ray sets (Fig. 3-11), are simple in construction, work from a mains electricity supply and are inexpensive to purchase. This uncomplicated nature is accompanied by robustness, with many sets being in daily use for 20 or more years.

Indeed, the replacement of intraoral X-ray sets has been often dictated by changing requirements of radiation protection regulations rather than

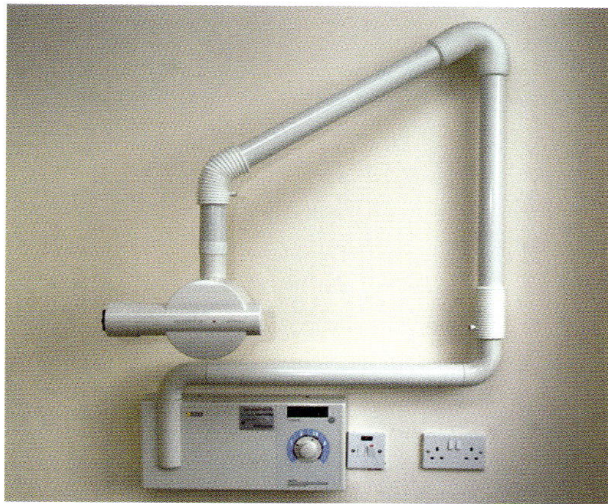

Fig. 3-11 A modern dental X-ray set.

functional failure. It is this need to reduce radiation doses for intraoral X-ray equipment that has driven the changes that have brought us to the state-of-the-art equipment available today.

The intraoral X-ray set is best considered systematically, according to function:

- kilovoltage and X-ray generation characteristics
- filtration methods
- collimation and irradiated volume limitation
- other factors.

The first two dictate the spectrum of X-radiation that is used on the patient. The X-rays generated in a simple X-ray tube are produced by interactions between the electrons emitted at the tungsten filament and the atomic nuclei of the tungsten target on the anode. The electrons are attracted to the anode by the potential difference (kilovoltage) between filament and anode. Such interactions vary in their intimacy, from minimal perturbation of each negatively charged electron's path by a positively charged tungsten nucleus through to a 'direct hit.' On each occasion that an interaction occurs between one electron and a nucleus, a single X-ray photon is emitted. The greater the interaction, the larger the energy of the X-ray photon created. A 'direct hit' by an electron on the nucleus results in a photon of maximum energy for that kilovoltage, where every last bit of energy from the electron is transferred to the X-ray photon. The consequence of this method of X-ray production is to produce X-rays that form a spectrum of energy, in which low-energy X-rays predominate and maximum energy X-rays are extremely rare. Consider, then, what may happen if X-rays with such a spectrum were used on a patient. The weakest X-rays would quickly be attenuated and only the stronger X-rays would succeed in reaching the image receptor in the mouth. Indeed, the energy imparted to the superficial skin – the 'dose' of radiation – would be very high.

It has long been recognized that the X-ray spectrum can be shaped to remove the weakest X-rays and largely preserve those with a useful energy. There are several ways of achieving this transformation. First, the potential difference across the X-ray tube and the method of X-ray generation can be optimized to provide an 'ideal' spectrum for penetration of the patient's jaws, while matching the spectral sensitivity of the image receptor. Second, the addition of filters to the exit port of the X-ray set allows weak X-rays to be preferentially attenuated.

Mains electrical supply has an alternating potential at 50 or 60 Hz providing, in turn, an alternating current at the same frequency. A transformer is used to 'step up' the mains potential to a higher level: many thousands of volts (kilovoltage). In the negative half of each cycle, there is no X-ray production, as electrons can only cross the X-ray tube in the filament-to-anode direction. Furthermore, the stated potential (kilovoltage) would only be achieved at the peak of the cycle, with a lower average potential difference being the reality. If this were used for X-ray production, the process would be inefficient, with X-rays being emitted in pulses and their mean energy being low. This would result in higher radiation doses to patients than are desirable. This was addressed many years ago by the incorporation of rectification circuits whereby the negative half of the voltage cycle is made positive (full-wave rectification) and the pulses smoothed to a ripple (three-phase rectification). 'State-of-the-art' intraoral X-ray sets incorporate capacitors into the circuitry that effective y remove any rippling at all, leaving a constant voltage for use in X-ray production. Such constant potential, or direct current equipment, produces proportionally fewer low-energy X-rays and hence gives reductions in skin dosage to patients. There are other consequences. The complete absence of pulsation in X-ray production means that exposure times are shorter, reducing the risk of movement artefact and facilitating the use of rapid digital imaging. A negative effect is that radiographic contrast is lower, all other factors being equal.[16]

Increasing the voltage acting across the X-ray tube, regardless of the method of generation used, also has significant effects. As voltage is increased, the maximum and mean X-ray energy is increased and the quantity of X-rays produced per unit time also increases. This allows greater penetration by the X-rays, shortens exposure times and reduces radiation dose to the patient. There is, however, a reduction in radiographic contrast associated with increasing voltage. Consequently, it can be seen that a 'high' kilovoltage and constant potential X-ray generation act similarly upon the X-ray spectrum. A reasonable question may be to ask why we do not continue increasing the voltage to ever higher levels. An important consideration in selecting the voltage in intraoral X-ray equipment is the spectral sensitivity of the image receptor and the image quality. Increasing the voltage much beyond 70 kV would result in a spectrum ill-matched to the optimal for dental image receptors, so the exposure would be less efficient. Higher voltage also gives greater scatter of X-rays, producing more random 'noise' in images and increasing radiation dose at depth in the patient. As such, a voltage of 60–70 kV has been recommended for intraoral radiography as being a reasonable compromise between diagnostic efficacy and dose limitation.[17] Increasing voltage and constant potential generation result in broadly similar effects and it has been shown that, for a constant potential set, a setting 5–8 kV lower is needed for the same radiographic contrast. Therefore, it has been recommended that 60 kV is used in constant potential X-ray units.

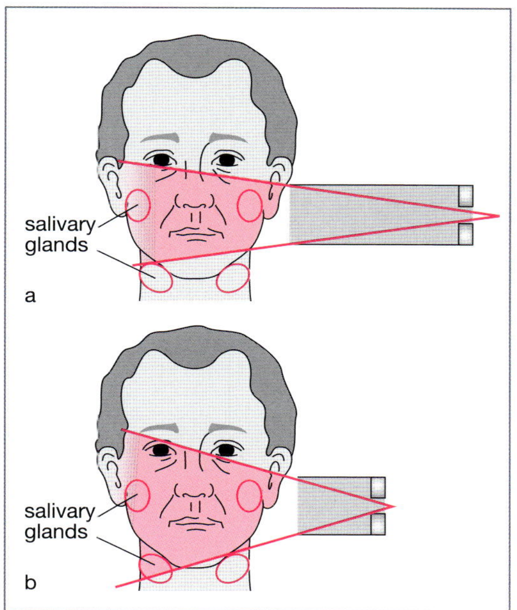

Fig. 3-12 Increasing the X-ray source-to-skin distance reduces the volume of the patient that is irradiated: (a) long distance; (b) short distance. Note the inclusion of more radiosensitive salivary gland tissue in the latter. (From Horner et al. [2007][15] with permission.)

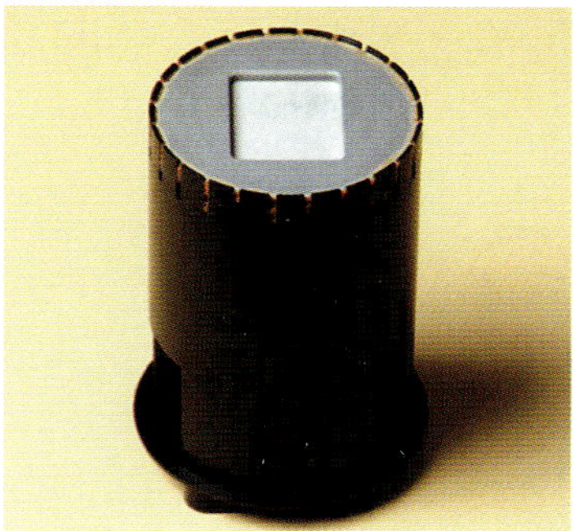

Fig. 3-13 An example of a rectangular collimator that may be fitted into the circular position-indicating device of a dental X-ray set.

Filtration was one of the earliest methods of radiation protection, which served to remove the very weakest X-rays, which contribute nothing to image production but substantially to radiation dose. The filter material is usually aluminum. As for voltage and constant potential generation, adding filtration alters the resulting X-ray spectrum in a beneficial way, but excessive filtration thickness leads to fewer X-rays being produced per unit time as well as reducing image contrast. Aluminum filtration of suitable thickness remains a standard on X-ray equipment, with manufacturers incorporating the filter material at the time of equipment assembly in line with nationally set standards. The use of additional filtration (K-edge filters) with materials other than aluminum, such as rare earth materials, was subject to substantial research in the 1980s and 1990s; however, while offering some advantages in specific situations, this approach appears to have faded into obscurity. To the author's knowledge, no 'state-of-the-art' X-ray set includes such filtration as standard.

The volume of patient that is in the X-ray beam is, obviously, proportional to the radiation dose received by the patient. This volume is determined by the area of the X-ray beam at the skin surface and the divergence of the beam. The former is controlled by the collimation incorporated into the X-ray set; the latter is dictated by the X-ray source–object–image receptor relationship, with the distance between the X-ray source and the skin being the only variable that can be significantly altered. By increasing this distance, the effective beam divergence is reduced and the volume of patient irradiated is less (Fig. 3-12). Therefore, for optimal dose reduction, the ideal situation is to reduce the area of the beam at the skin surface and lengthen the X-ray source-to-skin distance. Reducing irradiated volume also reduces the amount of scattered radiation arising in the patient. As scattered X-rays cause image noise, an added benefit is improved contrast on radiographs.

State-of-the-art intraoral X-ray sets match the beam area and shape at the skin surface to be slightly greater than the dimensions of the Size 2 (3 cm by 4 cm) dental film packet. This rectangular collimation (Fig. 3-13) alone reduces radiation doses to patients by 50–60% compared with a 6 cm round beam.[17] Despite the exact match in size between image receptor and beam area, so long as film

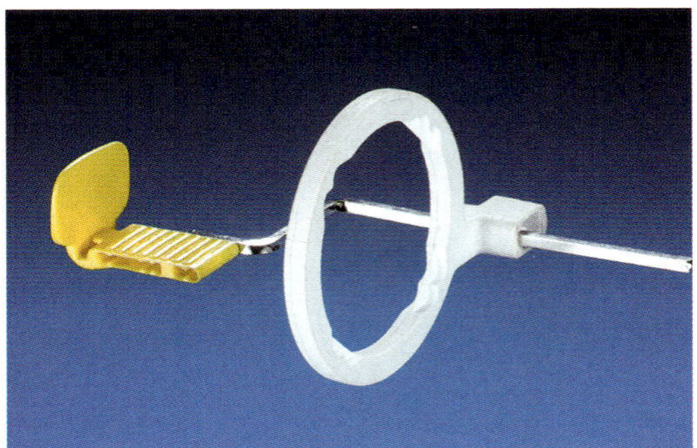

Fig. 3-14 Modern film holding/beam-aiming device for intraoral radiography.

holders with a beam-aiming device are used, reject rates do not appear to be a significant problem. Occlusal radiography is also easily performed using rectangular collimation. Many older X-ray sets without rectangular collimation can be readily upgraded by adding a suitable adapter.

Increasing the X-ray source-to-skin distance also has image-quality benefits by giving sharper images. It does this by reducing the penumbra around objects on radiographic images. The source-to-skin distance (indicated by the position-indicating device) does have an upper practical size limit. Increasing the distance reduces the intensity of the X-ray beam by the inverse square law; consequently, all other factors being equal, exposure times (but not radiation dose) will rise as X-ray source-to-skin distance is increased. While this can be compensated for by increasing voltage, extremely long X-ray source-to-skin distances are impractical owing to the increased risk of movement artefacts and the challenges of accommodating the length of the position-indicating device in a dental office. Most manufacturers of intraoral X-ray equipment currently set a distance of 20 cm from the X-ray source to the end of the position-indicating device, with a few providing a 30 cm option.

While the above are the main features of a modern X-ray set, there are other factors worth consideration. With modern digital imaging systems, there is a need for an ability to make precise, short exposures. Older X-ray sets, used with slower film receptors, were not manufactured with this in mind. A high-quality electronic timer capable of reproducible exposures at the 0.01 s level are now required. Focal spot size is also important, as the larger this is, the greater the penumbra effect on images. The effective focal spot size of new equipment should not be greater than 1 mm, and ideally be smaller.

A state-of-the art intraoral X-ray set will have:

- 60–70 kV
- constant potential generation
- rectangular collimation
- 20–30 cm X-ray source-to-skin distance
- electronic timer capable of very short exposures
- effective focal spot of 0.5–1 mm.

Irrespective of how modern the X-ray equipment, the final image is dependent upon excellent technique. To optimize technique, an intraoral radiographic facility requires the use of film holders with a beam-aiming device, in particular when rectangular collimation is used (Fig. 3-14).

Panoramic radiography

Many of the features highlighted for dental (intraoral) X-ray sets also apply to panoramic machines. Consequently, filtration and constant potential generation are just as important for panoramic X-ray systems. In terms of collimation, modern panoramic X-ray units (Fig. 3-15) should offer a feature of selectable field size limitation, whereby only selected areas are exposed. The common options include 'dentition only,' pediatric mode, right or left side only, and midline excluded, but some machines offer greater versatility to image only a group of teeth in one jaw (Fig. 3-16). Field size limitation is of great value in limiting dose, particularly when an area is subject to repeated radiologic review. Lecomber and co-workers[18] examined the 12 field size options of the Orthophos panoramic unit and showed that the 'dentition only' mode reduced effective dose by half, largely by a substantial reduction in radiation exposure to the salivary glands.

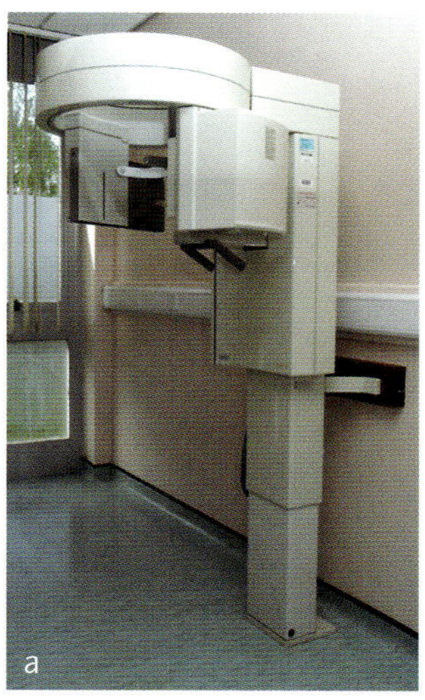

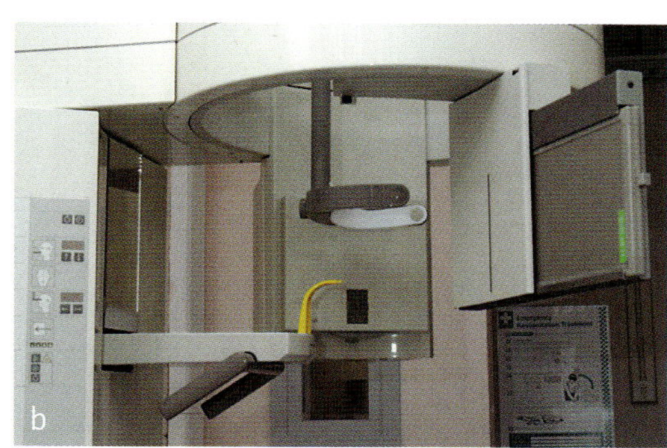

Fig. 3-15 A modern panoramic X-ray set (a) with close-up view of the principal components (b). (From Horner et al. [2007][15] with permission.)

Selection of exposure factors in panoramic radiography is usually a choice of voltage and, in some cases, current (milliamperage). In some machines, this choice is concealed behind pictograms (eg 'large man, normal man, little man' pictograms). In general radiography, however, automatic exposure control has become a commonplace means of taking the choice of exposure away from the operator. This involves a photodiode, or other detector, positioned behind the image receptor to measure the transmitted dose rate. When a preset maximum dose rate is reached, the exposure is terminated. While this is straightforward for simple radiography, it has been slow to be adopted into panoramic radiography, partly because of cost and partly because of the more complex exposure process of a scanning beam. In this case, the automatic exposure control does not terminate the exposure if the maximum is exceeded; rather, it adjusts the exposure for the next increment of the image. This feature has been incorporated into only a few panoramic radiography systems but has been demonstrated to give improvements in image quality.[19]

Studies have shown that the quality of panoramic radiographs is frequently poor, in part because of failures in patient positioning. To some extent, this reflects the use of older machines with poor patient aids to positioning. Modern panoramic machines feature positioning lights that are essential for accurate localization of the teeth in the center of the focal plane. 'Autofocus' technology is now pro-

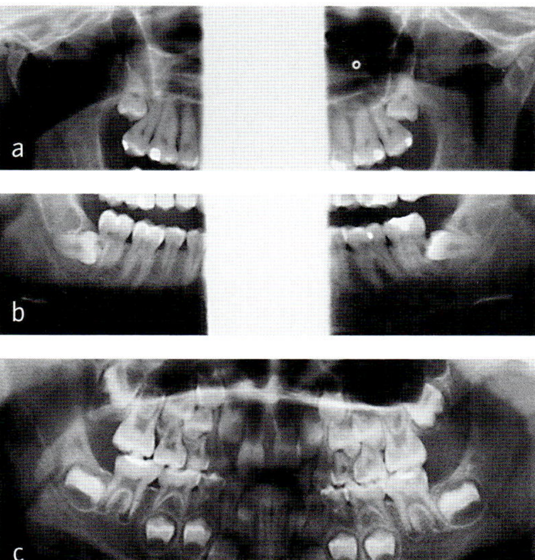

Fig. 3-16 Some examples of images obtained using selective field size limitation: (a) posterior maxilla; (b) posterior mandible; (c) pediatric mode. (From Horner et al. [2007][15] with permission.)

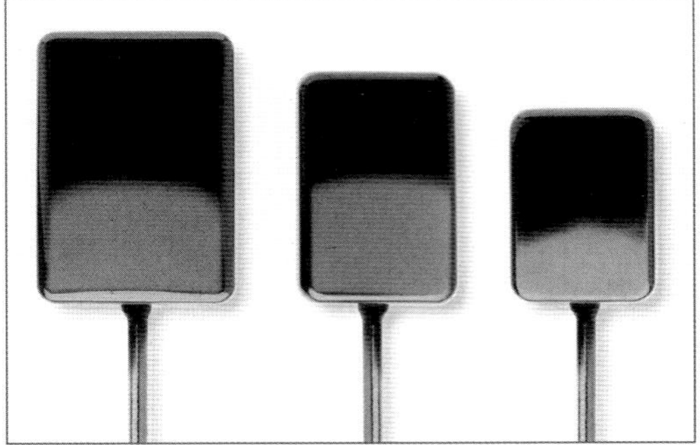

Fig. 3-17 Direct digital intraoral sensors. Three different size sensors from the same manufacturer. (From Horner et al. [2007][15] with permission. Courtesy of Schick Technologies, Long Island City, NY, USA.)

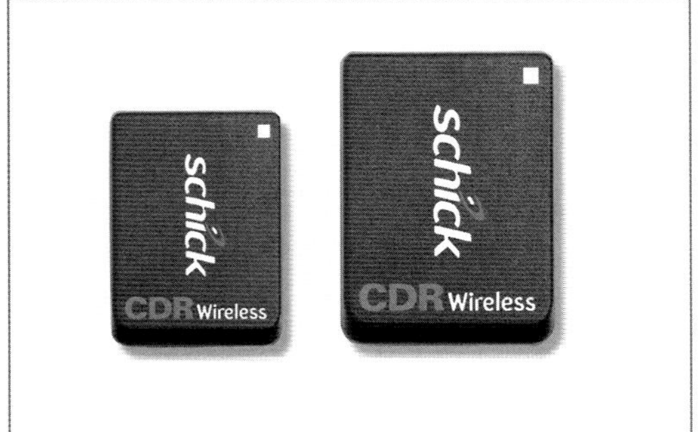

Fig. 3-18 Wireless direct digital sensors (From Horner et al. [2007][15] with permission. Courtesy of Schick Technologies, Long Island City, NY, USA.)

vided by one manufacturer of panoramic equipment. Once the patient has bitten into the special bite block, a laser beam passes to the block, allowing the distance to be calculated. Once this is done, the X-ray source/image receptor C-arm adjusts so that this distance, and that of the focal plane, is correctly positioned.

Digital imaging

As mentioned above, digital radiology came late to dentistry, but is increasingly the standard means of imaging in dental practice, both for intraoral and panoramic radiography. As systems become more refined and, increasingly, as younger dental clinicians have trained using digital radiography in dental school, this steady tide away from film and cassettes is likely to continue. Intraoral radiography is of two main system types: the solid-state (CCD and complementary metal oxide semiconductors) receptors and phosphor plate technology.[15] Both are applicable to intraoral and panoramic radiography but differ in their relative advantages and disadvantages.

For intraoral radiography, solid-state sensors have a range of external sizes (Fig. 3-17), but all are more bulky than a dental film packet or a phosphor plate. This presents challenges in positioning and there is evidence of a higher reject rate in clinical use. Paradoxically, the larger size of solid-state sensors does not reflect the image receptor area, which is usually significantly smaller than the external size. This emphasizes the importance of using careful technique, augmented with the appropriate sensor holder/beam-aiming device. A recent development has been systems that are not attached by cable to the computer. One such system is truly 'cable free' (Fig. 3-18), with the sensor itself having an internal power supply and the digital data being transmitted by radiofrequency waves. This is a significant advantage, as hanging cables present a hazard and can be prone to damage. The solid-state sensors are, however, always at risk of damage or, for cable-free sensors, accidental loss. Solid-state systems are usually presented as offering significant dose reductions relative to film, although the superiority is often exaggerated by using D-speed film for comparison. Generally, solid-state intraoral radiography can be used with a reduction of exposure factors, approximately 50% relative to F-speed film, although there is substantial variation between manufacturers.[20] Early solid-state systems suffered from a particularly narrow exposure latitude with saturation of the CCD if overexposed, producing areas of 'black-out'. This problem still appears to exist for some systems on the market. Farman and Farman[20] have presented a superb overview of digital intraoral X-ray systems, mainly solid state, comparing image-quality and exposure parameters.

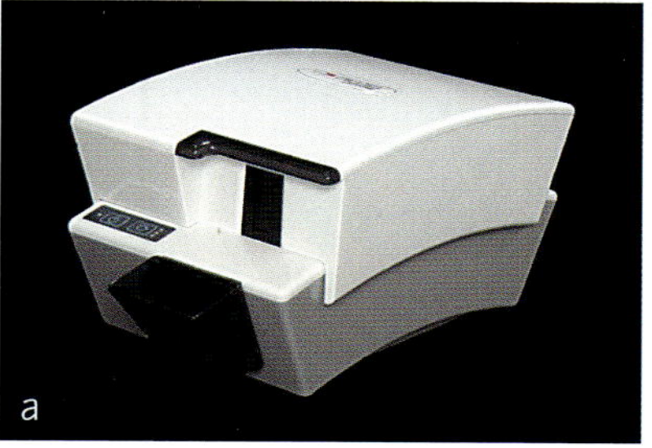

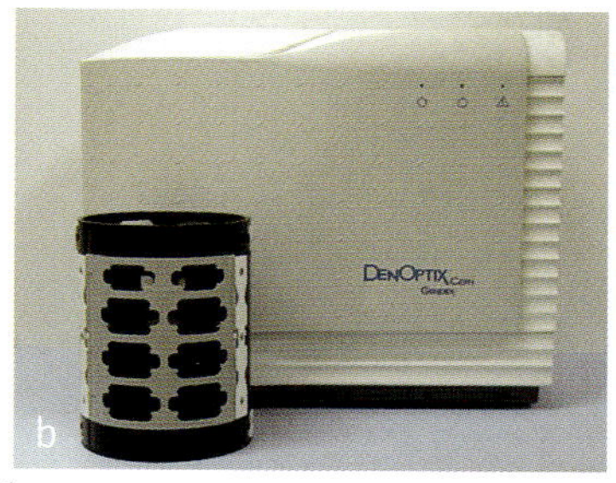

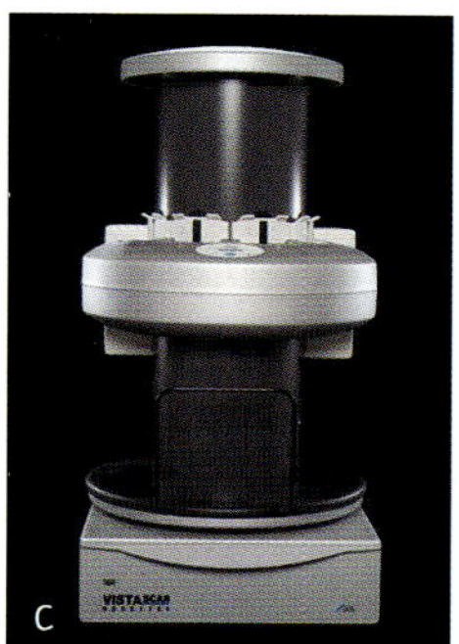

Fig. 3-19 Examples of three phosphor plate digital intraoral systems: (a) Digora Optime; (b) Gendex DenOptix; (c) Dürr VistaScan. (From Horner et al. [2007][15] with permission.)

In contrast, for phosphor plate systems (Fig. 3-19), there appears to be some distinct advantages. Practical radiographic technique is simpler because the plates resemble conventional intraoral film in size and thickness (Fig. 3-20). This means that existing film holder/beam-aiming devices can be used with little or no modification. Imaging plates, while not cheap, can be replaced at a fraction of the cost of a new solid-state sensor. There are more size options for phosphor plates, permitting occlusal views to be taken on some systems. There are, however, some drawbacks. Unlike solid-state technology, where images appear instantaneously on the computer monitor with no intermediate handling/processing stage, phosphor plates must be loaded into the scanner and processed, taking a minute or so of waiting and handling. The plates must be erased of all previous images prior to reuse, and while one system does this automatically, for others the plates must be placed on an illuminated viewing box for a period to ensure a 'clean' start. Plates can be damaged by rough handling, producing artefacts. In terms of radiation-dose implications, phosphor plates are remarkable for having very wide exposure latitude.[21] Dose reduction relative to intraoral film is possible, although care should be taken to avoid image noise, which will appear if very short exposures are used. The concern, however, is that the careless user may set excessively high exposures; the wide latitude means that acceptable image quality is maintained at substantially higher doses than necessary.

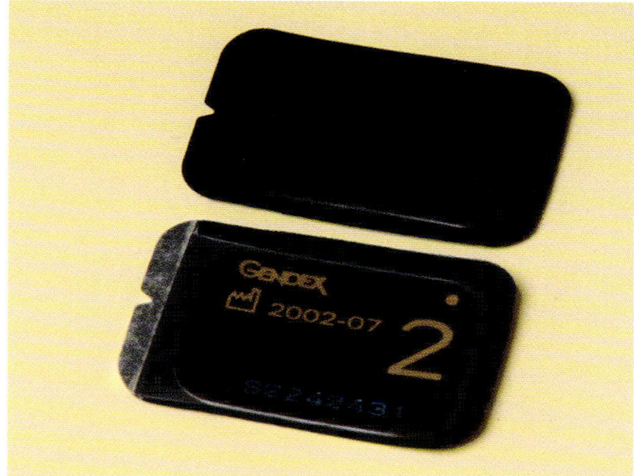

Fig. 3-20 Phosphor plates in a barrier envelope. The envelope protects the plate from light during radiography. (From Horner et al. [2007][15] with permission.)

Solid-state receptors are widely used for panoramic and cephalometric imaging. Large CCDs, matching the size of a panoramic radiograph, are not feasible to produce, but as the panoramic X-ray beam is slit-shaped, a correspondingly tall, thin CCD is used that moves in coordination with the scanning beam. This is a very simple and effective process, with no cassettes to be handled and an instant image. Phosphor plate technology is also straightforward to use, but handling of large imaging plates is more demanding for the user. It is important to understand that, regardless of the system used, extraoral digital imaging does not carry any guarantee of dose reduction, as the comparable analogue image receptor gains from using

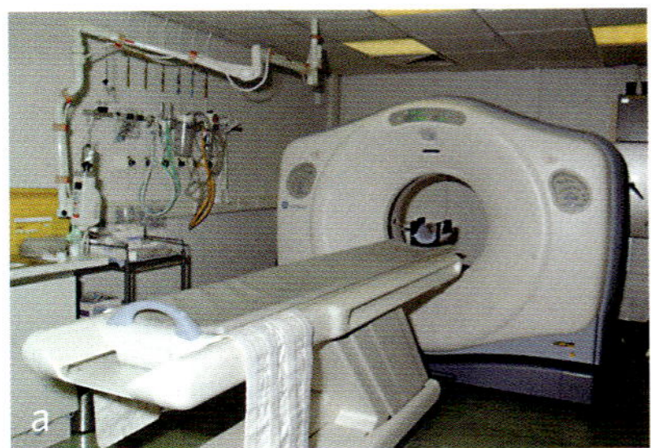

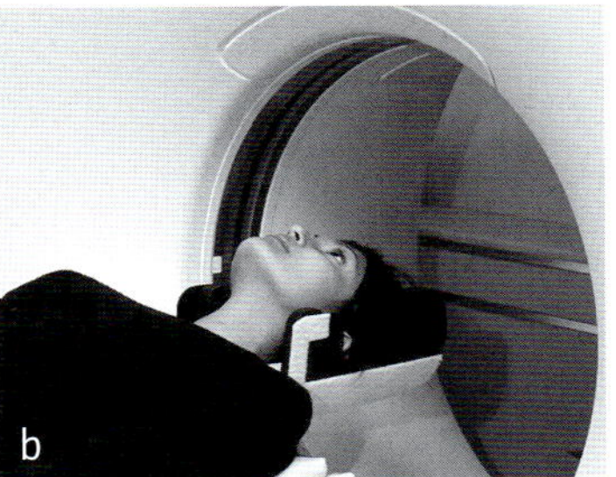

Fig. 3-21 (a) A computerized tomographic scanner. (b) The patient is positioned here for a maxillary scan. (From Horner et al. [2007][15] with permission.)

intensifying screens. Indeed, compared with the recommended film/screen speed rating for panoramic radiography, digital imaging may mean higher exposure factors must be used. It is, however, sometimes possible to reduce the radiation exposure factors with digital panoramic radiography at the expense of some increase in image noise.[22]

Further details on the technology underlying digital imaging are given by Horner and co-workers.[15]

Cross-sectional and volumetric imaging

For 100 years and more, dental imaging has been two dimensional, with subject depth reduced to subtle or imperceptible variations in image density. Thus, the 'skiagraph' (shadow picture) produced by the radiographic pioneers has remained the same. The ideal image, however, is one that accurately represents the true three-dimensional nature of the subject. In medical radiology, this ideal was finally achieved by the development of CT in the early 1970s. The basic principle of CT is that thin, cross-sectional images, usually in or close to the axial plane of the body, can be produced by complex mathematical analysis of X-rays transmitted through the body from multiple directions. In the original CT scanner, this was a lengthy process of taking 160 parallel readings over a 180 degree rotation at 1 degree intervals, followed by several hours of computer time in analyzing the data. In the subsequent 30 years, CT scanning has passed through four 'generations' of development, leading to the current 'state-of-the-art' spiral scanners, in which a continuous spiral rotation of the X-ray source and detectors is possible, synchronized with a uniform movement of the patient through the scanner aperture. Using such systems, scan times are extremely short, leading to fewer motion artefacts.

Although CT (Fig. 3-21) has been used by researchers for a variety of dental applications, principally in oral surgery, the main use of CT in everyday dentistry is in implant imaging.[23] When a dental implant is planned, dental clinicians must consider both the quality and quantity of bone at the proposed implant site. Most conventional dental images (periapical and panoramic radiographs) provide excellent information only in the plane of the dental arch, with no indication of buccolingual bone characteristics. Ingenious use of lateral cephalometric and occlusal radiographs can provide some of this missing information, but still in two-dimensions. CT scans of the jaws can be reconstructed from their native axial format into cross-sections that are perpendicular to the line of the dental arches (Fig. 3-22). An additional advantage of these images is that they can be displayed in 'life-size' form, whereas conventional radiographs are always magnified. Measurement of alveolar height, width and external contour are straightforward. As far as bone quality is concerned, it is also simple for the dental clinician to examine the images for the internal trabecular bone architecture at the implant site and the cortical bone thickness. In addition, anatomical relationships with important structures, such as the inferior dental canal, the maxillary sinus and the submandibular fossa, can be understood. CT is not, however, without

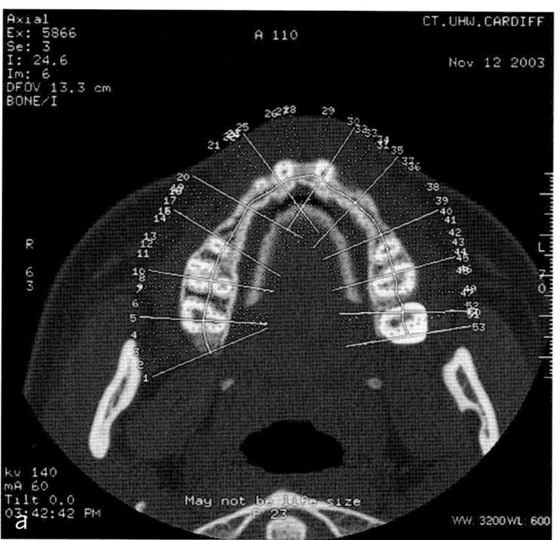

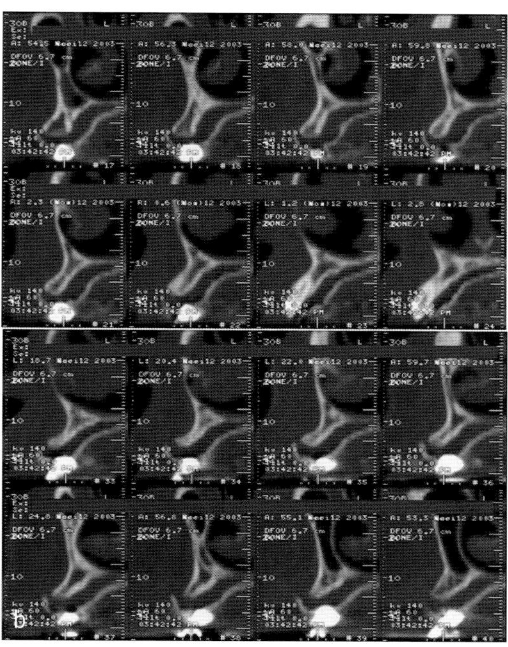

Fig. 3-22 Computerized tomography images of the maxilla. (a) A single axial slice, where image multiple points have been selected along the line of the alveolar ridge; (b) cross-sectional images produced by reconstructing the axial image dataset. (From Horner et al. [2007][15] with permission.)

drawbacks. It is essential for the dental clinician to be able to relate the CT images to the clinical situation. While this may be no problem for implants of a single tooth, where extensive spans of edentulous jaw are being treated with multiple implants, localizing the image to the mouth requires that the CT is performed with a stent containing radiopaque markers in the mouth. Motion artefacts are quite common and, depending on the direction of movement, can distort the true jaw shape. Metallic restorations may produce prominent artefacts. Finally, the radiation dose with CT is substantially higher than for dental radiography,[24] being equivalent to weeks or months of background radiation for the former compared with days for the latter; for implants of a single tooth, the risk-benefit ratio of CT becomes to justify.

CT-derived cross-sectional images are quite sufficient for most implant planning purposes. There are, however, a number of manufacturers who produce software that can take 'raw' CT data and transform these into a more extensive range of images, employing, for example, color to improve interpretation. This allows the dental clinician to perform 'virtual' implant placement and to select the optimal implant size and surgical approach.

In view of the cost and size of CT equipment, and the demanding quality assurance and maintenance requirements, there are only a few dental clinicians worldwide working in primary care who own a medical CT scanner. In some respects, this is a valuable restriction, as it prevents inappropriate use of this potentially high-dose technique. Regardless of this, it is counter-intuitive to suppose that dental clinicians, unlike their medical colleagues, would not value easier access to three-dimensional imaging in a wider range of clinical situations than implant treatment. The answer to this need will be addressed in the next section.

Cone beam computerized tomography

The most significant development in dental imaging since the introduction of panoramic radiography in the 1950s has been cone beam CT (CBCT).[25] This

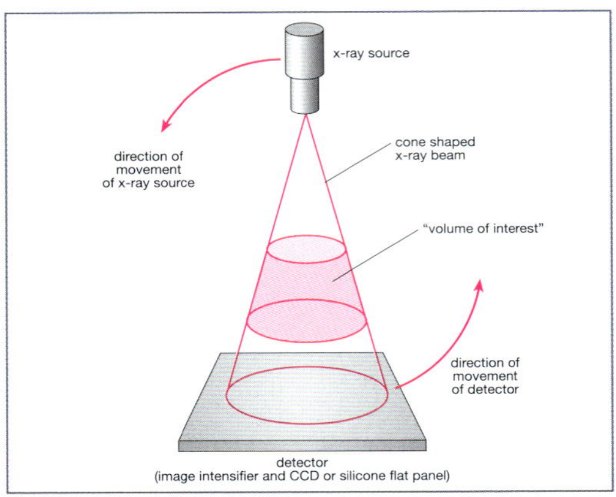

Fig. 3-23 The principle of cone beam computerized tomography. The X-ray source produces a cone-shaped X-ray beam that acquires a volume of the region of interest in a single rotation. (From Horner et al. [2007][17] with permission.)

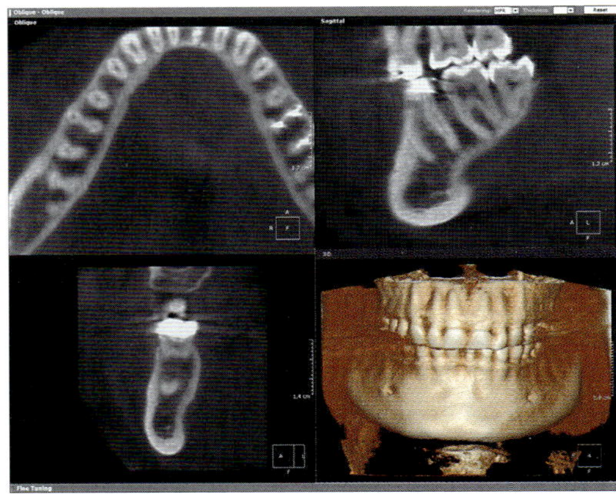

Fig. 3-24 TImage display with cone beam computerized tomography. From the top left, axial, sagittal, surface-rendered and coronal images are shown.

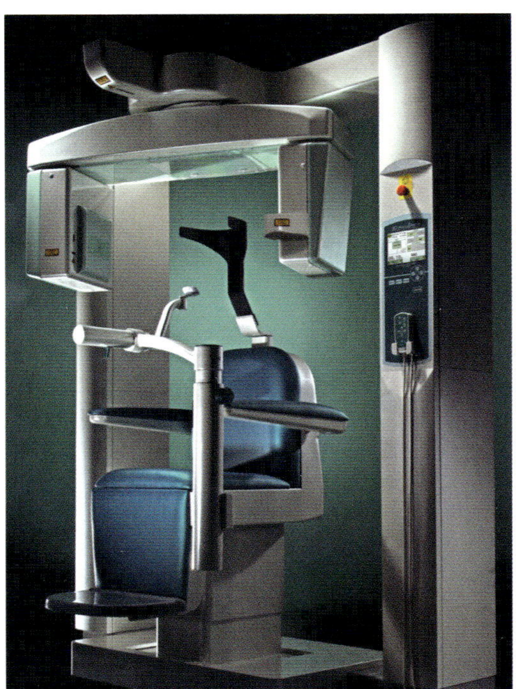

Fig. 3-25 A 'state-of-the-art' cone beam computerized tomography machine.

technique, also known as digital volumetric tomography, differs from conventional CT in both the X-ray beam and the detector. An X-ray source capable of producing a three-dimensional cone-shaped X-ray beam and a two-dimensional image detector rotate synchronously around the patient's head through 360 degrees (Fig. 3-23). At repeated intervals during the rotation, projection images are captured by either a flat-panel amorphous silicon detector or image intensifier/CCD combination. These image data are subject to sophisticated software programs, including back-filtered projection, to derive a three-dimensional image dataset that is cylinder-shaped (in one case spherical). This is then available for two-dimensional display in coronal, axial and sagittal planes and an option of a 'three-dimensional' surface-rendered image (Fig. 3-24). Scanning times are typically in the 10–40 s range. A key feature of CBCT, in contrast with CT, is that the volume elements (voxels) of patient data are isotropic (x, y and z axes are of the same length). This results in improved resolution, in the submillimeter range, with one current system being capable of 0.125 mm^3 voxels. In contrast, while conventional CT scanners have voxel x–y dimensions in the submillimeter range, the z-axis is usually 1–2 mm. A modern CBCT unit is shown in Fig. 3-25.

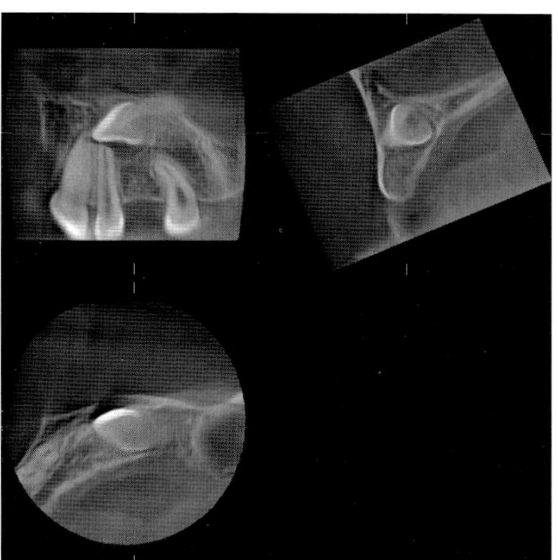

Fig. 3-26 Assessment of an impacted maxillary canine with resorption of the lateral incisor using cone beam computerized tomography. (Image courtesy of Professor Christina Lindh, Malmö University, Sweden.)

The field-of-view (volume) dimensions in CBCT depend upon the manufacturer's specifications but range from large volumes that can cover the entire head or maxillofacial region down to small-volume systems suitable for imaging one or two teeth. A few CBCT units have only a single volume size, but most offer some choice for the dental clinician to match to the clinical situation and these are to be preferred to avoid unnecessary X-ray exposure. Similarly, there is sometimes the facility to choose an image resolution. Higher resolution, all other factors remaining constant, usually means higher radiation exposures, so careful judgement is required to optimize radiation doses.

Unlike conventional CT, there is very limited latitude for imaging tissues of different attenuation. Soft-tissue differentiation is poor, but hard-tissue contrast is excellent. For dental applications, this is no problem, but CT remains superior for soft-tissue surgical applications. Because the dataset is three dimensional, resolution is consistent in all three planes and higher in the non-axial planes than that achievable in conventional CT using reconstruction techniques. An added advantage is that radiation doses with CBCT appear to be considerably lower than for conventional CT, although further research is needed to obtain data for the ever-increasing number of machines on the market and to clarify the best practice for optimization of doses.

At the time of writing, high-quality research on the clinical applications of CBCT is sparse, with most of the literature dominated by case reports and non-systematic reviews. The number of publications, however, is growing exponentially each month, and an evidence-based understanding of the role of CBCT in dentistry will emerge. At present, it is clear that the main applications of CBCT in current practice are in:

- orthodontics
- implant dentistry
- oral surgery
- endodontics.

The three-dimensional nature of CBCT means that it meets the desire of orthodontists to assess the developing dentition position accurately.[26] Research has demonstrated a high level of dimensional accuracy on CBCT images using dry skulls as a reference standard.

When dealing with potential root resorption associated with impacted teeth (Fig. 3-26), CBCT appears to offer sensitive diagnosis, although evidence is currently based largely on case series rather than diagnostic accuracy studies. 'Panoramic' and 'cephalometric' images can be reconstructed from volumetric datasets. Despite these apparent advantages, there is also significant concern about the radiation dose consequences of using CBCT in any 'routine' way for orthodontic assessment,[27] in particular in children, as has become widespread in the USA.

There is ample evidence that comprehensive conventional radiography is not always required in orthodontic assessment, so the need for three-dimensional data is far from obvious for most patients. Until research is carried out assessing the impact on management of CBCT in orthodontics,

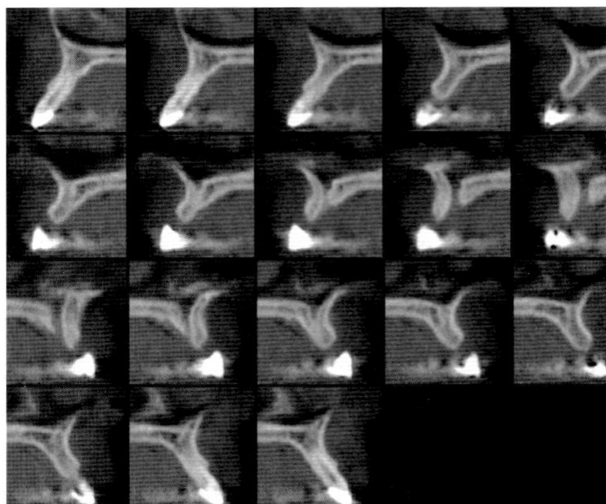

Fig. 3-27 Cross-sectional images from cone beam computerized tomography for implant planning in the maxilla. (From Horner et al. [2007][15] with permission.)

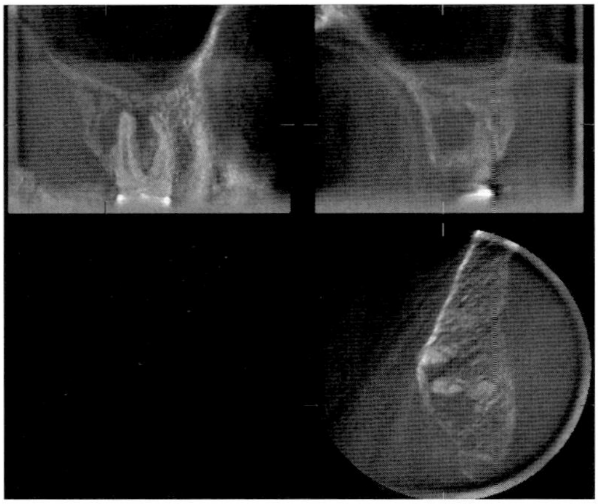

Fig. 3-28 Endodontic assessment of a maxillary molar tooth using cone beam computerized tomography. (Image courtesy of Professor Christina Lindh, Malmö University, Sweden.)

routine use cannot be justified and a cautious approach must be used.

For implants, the decision to use CBCT in planning (Fig. 3-27) is far easier to justify. Guidelines indicating the usefulness of conventional CT for some implant planning cases are already in existence.[28] CBCT offers improvements in both radiation dose and image quality, which means that it should be preferred. In the wider oral surgical field, this easy choice is often repeated. For assessment of the relationships between mandibular third molars and the inferior alveolar canal, for example, CBCT is clearly superior to the use of conventional CT, but it is also superior to using parallax radiography. It is, however, important to remember that CBCT currently shows soft tissues poorly; if a lesion or abnormal area appears to involve soft tissues and this is likely to be important in management, then conventional CT, or magnetic resonance imaging (MRI) would be preferred so that duplication of examinations is avoided.

An application of CBCT that has attracted a lot of interest is endodontics.[29] The good resolution of CBCT means that imaging of root canals is possible, which may be useful in complex canal systems, although the evidence is still limited (Fig. 3-28). Research suggests improved diagnosis of periapical pathosis, although study quality is limited at present. Evidence from case reports also suggests a significant value for identifying root perforations, which are elusive on periapical radiography.

Where CBCT is used for endodontics, it is important to use small-volume systems rather than the large-volume scanners, otherwise irrelevant areas will be exposed and radiation doses will be unacceptable, particularly as the high-resolution mode is invariably required.

There is no doubt that CBCT is an area of rapid development. There are currently around 20 scanners on the market. Prices will probably fall with time, as competition becomes more vigorous. There remains an urgent need for research focused on the impact of CBCT on patient management and for clear guidelines for dental clinicians to ensure appropriate use. Such research needs to be focused on children because of their greater radiation sensitivity and the heavy use of imaging in younger age groups in dentistry.

Non-ionizing radiation techniques

Magnetic resonance imaging

MRI involves placing a patient into an intense magnetic field and applying pulses of radiofrequency electromagnetic radiation. The applied radiofrequency radiation causes hydrogen nuclei (protons) to react by moving out of alignment with the magnetic field; once the external radiofrequency pulse ends, the hydrogen nuclei return to position, emitting their own radiofrequency pulse. As different tissues contain different quantities of hydrogen nuclei and in different molecular forms, the emitted radiofrequency reflects the body's internal structure, providing structural data that can be used to produce an image.

MRI was first used in medical imaging in the late 1970s and since then it has come to dominate much of radiologic practice, displacing the preeminence of CT because of its greater soft tissue contrast, its multiplanar imaging abilities and its nil radiation dose.

It can be used almost everywhere in the body but has particular value in neuroradiology, cancer imaging and diseases of muscles and joints. Redpath[30] has produced a useful review of MRI developments.

The use of MRI in dentistry is, in contrast, very limited. MRI equipment is extremely expensive and complex to maintain. As such, its major 'dental' uses are in maxillofacial medicine and surgery, with major applications in temporomandibular joint assessment, salivary gland imaging and in management of oral cancer.

Outwith these applications, the most interest in dental use has been in the field of implantology treatment planning.[31] The T1-weighted images show cortical bone and teeth as 'black' structures (Fig. 3-29). While the images seem to have comparable quality to CT, limitations on access to MR scanners, and claustrophobia and other contraindications to its use, mean that it remains a technique limited to a few specialized centers, with staff dedicated to its use.

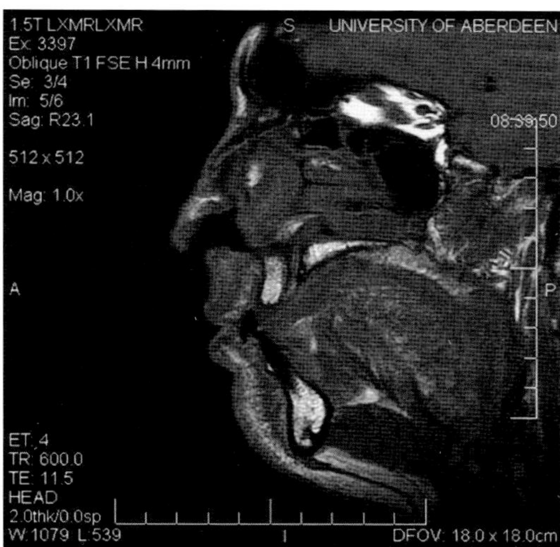

Fig. 3-29 Cross-sectional image produced by magnetic resonance imaging for mandibular implant planning. Note that cortical bone is black (no signal) and the medullary bone is bright (high signal). (From Horner et al. [2007][15] with permission.)

Ultrasound

Medical imaging with ultrasound is a well-established modality. It uses high-frequency sound (in the megahertz frequency range) that is applied to the body using a transducer containing a piezoelectric material. The sound is transmitted or reflected from different tissue types in different ways, giving characterization of the body part. Reflected sound is detected using the same transducer, giving 'real-time' imaging. Doppler flowmetry allows identification of blood vessels. In the maxillofacial region, ultrasound is a valuable tool for assessing the salivary glands and the neck.

Dentistry, however, involves an inappropriate environment for ultrasound because the sound waves are reflected well by hard tissues, including bone and teeth. Despite this, there has been some dental research in using ultrasound, notably for periapical diagnosis[32] and caries detection.[33] With the former, it appears that ultrasound can distinguish between granulomas and cysts effectively, although sound transmission seems to require a perforation of the buccal cortical plate of bone. As far as caries diagnosis is concerned, there is some in vitro evidence of diagnostic efficacy, but only limited clinical trials have been carries out. The findings of Matalon and co-workers,[33] using a commercially available 'ultrasonic caries detector,' suggest higher sensitivity than radiography, but a lower specificity.

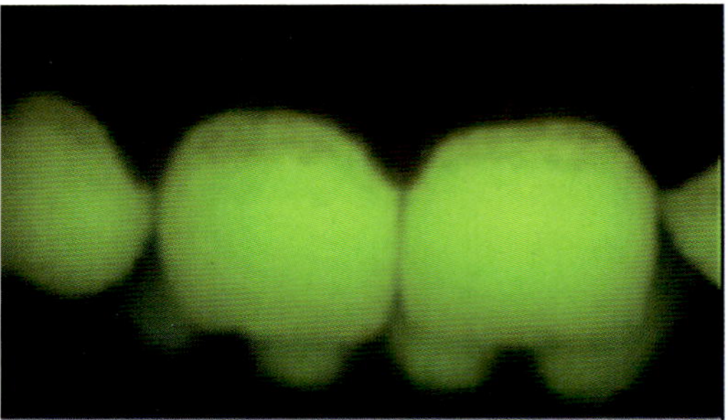

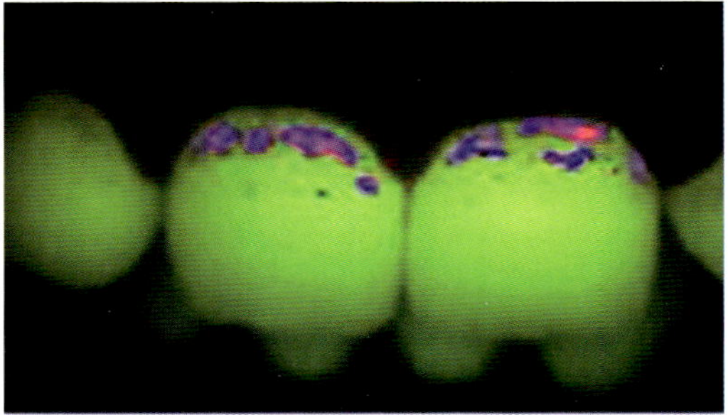

Fig. 3-30 Quantitative light-induced fluorescence (QLF) for detection of caries: (a) QLF image of anterior teeth; (b) QLF after image processing, clearly demarcating areas of enamel demineralization. (Images provided by Professor Roger Ellwood and Dr Iain Pretty, Colgate Palmolive Dental Health Unit, UK.)

Quantitative light-induced fluorescence

Visible light has been used as a means of caries detection in occlusal and smooth surfaces of teeth in the form of quantitative light-induced fluorescence (QLF).[34,35] When exposed to 370 nm blue light from a xenon source, enamel emits light in the green and red part of the spectrum. Demineralized enamel shows a reduction in this fluorescence. This image can be captured and subjected to image processing and analysis (Fig. 3-30). Reported sensitivities and specificities for QLF are comparable with other diagnostic systems, and intra- and inter-examiner variability appears to be excellent.[35]

Other systems

For other novel detection systems used for caries diagnosis that produce data but no image, such as electronic and laser fluorescence, the reader is referred to the excellent review by Pretty.[35]

Image analysis and computer-aided diagnosis

Unlike analogue imaging, digital imaging provides data in mathematical format; essentially, any image is a mass of numerical information. Each picture element (pixel) has a specific gray scale value corresponding to its X-ray attenuation characteristics. In such a form, images can be changed to optimize particular features: image processing. A very simple form of this is shifting the gray scale to alter apparent brightness or contrast. For example, while the image may contain a range of structures of widely differing X-ray attenuation, it is easy to limit the full gray scale, from white to black, over just a narrow part of this range, improving contrast for a particular type of structure at the expense of 'burning out' others that are not of interest. Image-processing facilities are always available on dental digital systems.

As van der Stelt[36] has pointed out, the division between image processing and image analysis is difficult to define, but the latter can be described as 'certain calculations extracting specific data from the image.' A very simple example invariably included in dental imaging software is length measurement, where the cursor marks are placed at two points and the number of pixels between these is automatically calculated. This is usually expressed in millimeters, but assumptions are made when relating pixels to true distance measurements, not least that the image is undistorted. For accurate results, the system must first be calibrated against an object of known length. Other commonly available image-analysis tools include angle and area measurements.

Digital subtraction radiography is a slightly more complex process. Digital images are taken of the same area at two different times. The images are then subtracted, pixel by pixel. If the gray scale values of every pixel are identical on the two

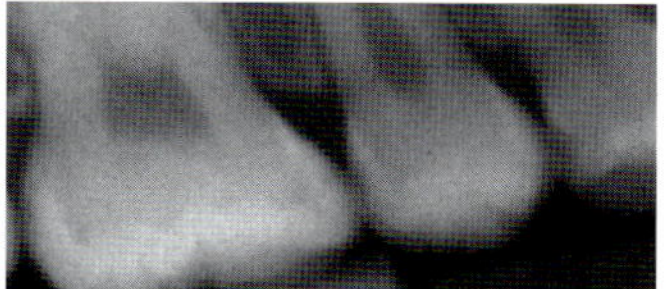
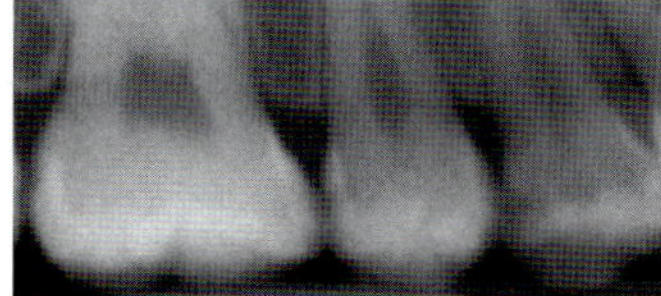
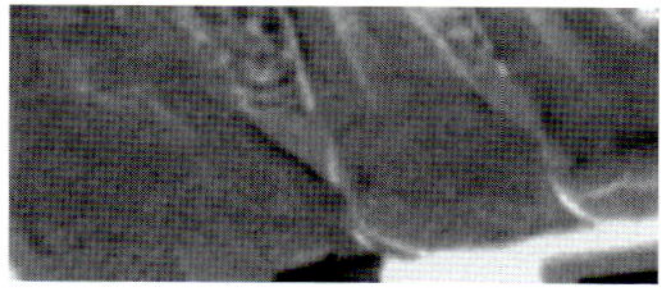

Fig. 3-31 Digital subtraction radiography as an aid to assessment of caries progression. (a) Part of baseline bitewing image; (b) part of bitewing image after 12 months; (c) subtraction image, showing areas of change in a dark shade of gray. Note the progression of the approximal caries and the occlusal caries lesion in the first premolar. (Images provided by Professor Roger Ellwood and Dr Iain Pretty, Colgate Palmolive Dental Health Unit, UK.)

images, the resulting image should be blank. If, however, there have been some changes, these will stand out on the subtracted image (Fig. 3-31). By using this method, it is possible to identify changes that would be undetectable to the observer. Digital subtraction radiography has been used for many clinical purposes in dentistry, including monitoring periodontal bone levels, caries progression/regression, periapical healing and tooth resorptions. It has remained, however, largely a research tool, principally because of the demands of ensuring that the imaging technique is precisely reproduced. More recently, software has been developed that permits non-identical images to be 'morphed' into each other, overcoming this barrier.

While digital subtraction radiography permits the dentist to identify features invisible to the eye, some more-sophisticated methods have been developed that have specific diagnostic applications. An example of this is computer-aided diagnosis of dental caries, a subject described in more depth by Wenzel.[37] Gakenheimer[38] has described a system that analyzes gray scale variation in an operator-defined region of the tooth and correlates this with a database of dental images of known caries status to produce a probability of caries being present. This system has been incorporated into one commercially available digital intraoral X-ray system. It is disappointing to note, however, that an independent study of diagnostic accuracy[39] found that the computer-aided diagnosis software performed less well than observers. Despite this, research continues in this area, with more promising results appearing with sophisticated image analysis techniques.[40]

More success has been achieved in using image-analysis methods for assessment of bone structure. Trabecular analysis systems have been devised for potential use in assessment of osseointegration around dental implants.[36] Recently, software that automatically detects and measures mandibular cortical width on panoramic radiographs has been described (Fig. 3-32), which, in conjunction with clinical information, has a high diagnostic validity for the detection of osteoporosis in women.[41] Apart from these developments, however, and despite anticipation of advances in computer-aided diagnosis over the last 20 years, progress has been disappointing.

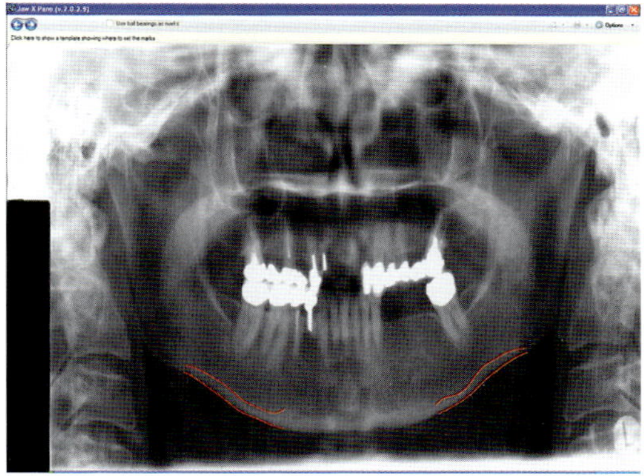

Fig. 3-32 Automated osteoporosis risk assessment using image analysis of panoramic radiographs. The software identifies and measures inferior cortical width and combines it with clinical data to derive a risk level. Jaw-X softbone image reproduced courtesy of Crebone AB, Sunbyberg, Sweden.

Vision 2020

From the preceding discussion in this chapter, it is clear that after 100 years of incremental change dental imaging is now undergoing a period of rapid transition. The advent of digital radiography and volumetric imaging offers enormous potential for image manipulation and analyses that were impossible with two-dimensional analogue image data. As such, it seems very likely that in the next decade or so we will move closer to a situation where images will cease to be passive reservoirs of information and move closer to becoming 'intelligent imaging systems.'

X-ray equipment and techniques

The world of dental imaging has been revolutionized by the introduction of CBCT. The attractiveness to dental clinicians of three-dimensional imaging seems likely to be a driver for more widespread use and greater versatility in clinical applications. As such, what is the future for conventional intraoral and panoramic X-ray equipment and techniques? Looking towards 2020, it seems possible that CBCT will have begun to displace these techniques.

The bulk of the diagnostic work carried out by non-specialist dental clinicians consists of caries and periapical diagnosis and the demonstration of periodontal bone levels. Small-volume CBCT already permits the dental clinician to produce volumetric data of a few teeth, giving three-dimensional 'periapical' and 'bitewing' images. The limited research available at the time of writing indicates improved detection of periapical pathosis. Studies also show greater sensitivity in detecting caries. There is currently limited research published on periodontal bone imaging, but it is hard to deny that three-dimensional imaging is superior to two-dimensional radiographs in demonstrating bone levels and complex infrabony defects.

The barriers to opening the floodgates to CBCT use today are threefold: cost, radiation dose and the paucity of knowledge about impact upon patient management. As far as cost is concerned, it is inevitable that CBCT will fall in cost as more manufacturers produce equipment. Systems of relatively low costs, essentially panoramic X-ray equipment incorporating a small-volume CBCT facility, are already on the market. Radiation dose is, however, a problem when large-volume CBCT equipment is used. Such equipment is only of value for orthodontists and surgeons and it is unacceptable to use large-volume imaging to examine a few teeth at the higher resolutions demanded by dental imaging. Consequently, it is likely that, in the future, a clear distinction will develop between large ('craniofacial') and small ('dental') CBCT, and separate equipment models will be manufactured for the two applications. Limiting volume size will also help to solve the potential problem of the competency of dental clinicians to evaluate the large-volume images that frequently show regions of the skull base, orbits and sinuses: areas that require specialist reporting by a radiologist. Further optimization of X-ray exposures are likely to be achieved through improvements in the efficiency of flat-panel detectors.

The remaining question relates to the impact of CBCT upon patient management. There is, at present, no published research that investigates whether three-dimensional information leads to changes in patient management compared with conventional techniques. At a time when cost and radiation dose are still concerns for CBCT use, such knowledge is essential to help in development of selection criteria. If, however, cost and radiation concerns are allayed by greater manufacturer competition and advances in technology, it is likely that the obstacles to replacing conventional radiographic techniques with CBCT will have disappeared.

Image-guided treatments

With the advent of dimensionally accurate, three-dimensional imaging in dentistry, there is a prospect of innovative applications. One especially interesting field of development is in image-guided treatment. Image-guided surgery is the use of a real-time correlation of the operative field to a preoperative imaging dataset that reflects the precise location of a selected surgical instrument in relation to the surrounding anatomic structures. Image guidance is not new to surgery. Any intervention in which the surgeon uses indirect visualization (endoscopy, fiber optics, ultrasound) to guide the operative procedure can be defined as image guided. These techniques are, however, real-time and the images do not detract from the primary importance of the operator's skill. Stereotactic surgery uses previously obtained images (CT or MRI) that can be related to the clinical situation at a later time, a method that has been widely used in neurosurgery and sinus surgery. To achieve this, there has to be a comprehensive three-dimensional dataset, a device that can be fixed to defined points on the patient and a probe or tool that is used to perform the surgical procedure. The CT or MRI is performed with the patient wearing a headset containing fiducial landmarks. At the time of surgery, this headset allows registration of the images to the patient. The operating instrument is also registered with the apparatus and its position can be related directly to the image data by the appearance and movement of crosshairs on the monitor.

What of image guidance in dentistry? The only substantial progress has been made in the field of implant surgery.[42] The simplest example is the use of so-called CAD/CAM surgical guides (computer-aided design/computer-aided manufacturing) produced by a 'three-dimensional printing' method called stereolithography. Preoperative CT data are processed to produce three-dimensional images with which the surgeon can carry out 'virtual surgery,' selecting the best sites for the implants and choosing their sizes. These data are then used to manufacture a surgical template containing metal sleeves that match the site and drill dimensions. True, real-time, image guidance has been developed more recently. With this technique, the patient wears a template during CT scanning and during surgery. This template, along with the surgical handpiece, contains infrared transmitters that permit cameras located in the operating room to follow movement and give feedback to the surgeon.[43]

Image-guided treatment today is in its infancy for non-implant dentistry. By 2020, however, it is possible that dental handpieces may be linked to three-dimensional images, each feeding information back to the other, facilitating accurate and minimal tooth preparation. The technology exists to make this dream a reality; all that it will take is the concerted efforts of teams of dental researchers, engineers and imaging scientists.

The intelligent imaging system

The 'state-of-the-art' in computer-aided diagnosis has been discussed above. It is clear that, at present, progress is limited to a few examples and the impact on most dental clinicians is minimal. With the ever-improving speed and processing capacity of computers, however, this situation may change. The most prevalent dental diseases – caries, periodontal disease and periapical inflammatory disease – produce structural alterations, principally by removal or addition of mineral. General-purpose segmentation algorithms can be applied to images to identify areas with different gray scale values or atypical structure. These methods can highlight areas for the dental clinician that warrant closer investigation. More complex image analytical techniques, such as active shape and active appearance modeling, may also have a role to play. This requires 'training' of software to recognize structures and their boundaries. Once this is achieved, the software can analyze subsequent images for the expected appearances and identify deviations from these, allowing subsequent measurements of density or distance that can automatically identify abnormality. Using such methods, it can be anticipated that by 2020 there will be an increasing availability of software programs aimed at specific diagnostic tasks. The interesting question is whether these will simply be 'advisory,' pointing the dental clinician to conduct further tests, or definitive, removing the role of the dental clinician as diagnostician.

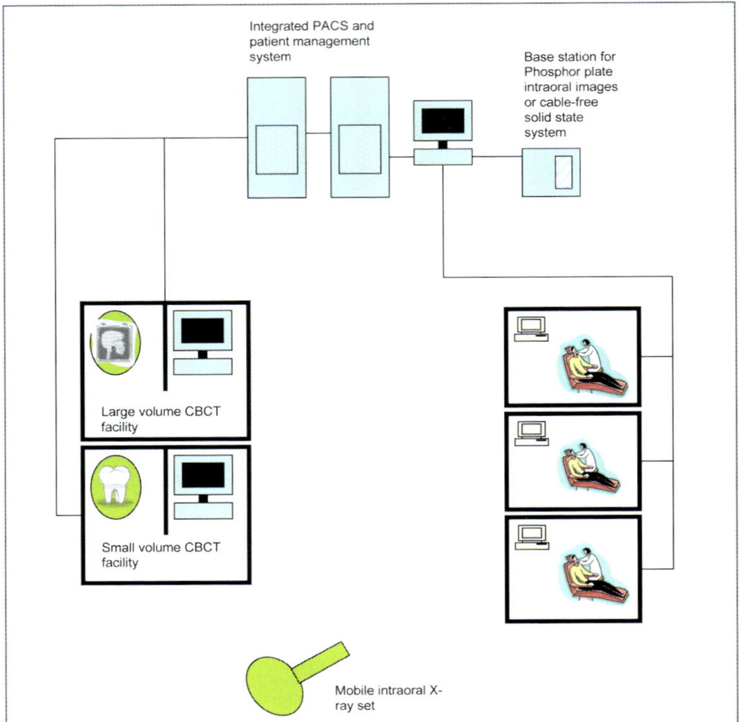

Fig. 3-33 The 2020 image-guided dental practice. This scenario anticipates developments in CBCT technology that overcome current radiation dose concerns and research evidence for cost-effectiveness over conventional imaging. A large- and a small-volume CBCT facility are shown; this presupposes a natural development towards 'craniofacial' and 'dental' CBCT machines. Each surgery has a networked computer for integrated patient records and images, along with facilities for image-guided interventions. The occasional need for intraoral radiography is satisfied with a mobile dental X-ray set and a phosphor plate or cable-free solid-state intraoral image receptor.

The image-guided dental practice in 2020

How then will the imaging element of a dental practice in 2020 differ from that today? We can only guess at the rate of progress in equipment and software that will occur in the next decade. In one respect, this will be dictated as much by the global economy as by demand from clinicians. We can, however, imagine a likely trend in imaging that may, at least in part, be achieved by 2020.

The look of a 2020 image-guided dental practice is summarized in Fig. 3-33. With suitable development in CBCT to limit doses, it is quite possible that intraoral radiography will become redundant, or at least rarely used. With the availability of small-volume CBCT systems, bitewing and periapical radiography may be rarely indicated because of the superior diagnostic accuracy of three-dimensional images. In endodontics, diagnostic working-length images will no longer be needed because of improvements in electronic apex location. It may be that a large small-surgery practice would maintain one mobile dental X-ray set for situations where CBCT was impractical, such as in young children or during surgery, in which case a cable-free solid-state or phosphor plate intraoral system for capturing images would be shared between the dental clinicians. Each surgery would be equipped with a high-resolution monitor and keyboards networked to a small picture archiving and communication system, which would be used to archive images and interface with the electronic patient record system. Software for computer-aided diagnosis would be integrated with the archiving and communication system, while facilities for image-guided dentistry may also be installed.

Predicting the future is a dangerous task. We are blind to the unexpected discovery that might take us down an entirely different path. Financial costs to dental clinicians may mean that such 'high-tech' facilities are available only to a few. Nonetheless, there is no doubt that imaging in dental practices in the next 10 or 20 years will play an increasingly important part of high-quality dental care.

References

1. Röntgen WC. On a new kind of rays. Nature 1896;53: 274–276.
2. Hirschmann PN. The next century. From the archives of dental radiology. Dentomaxillofac Radiol 1996;25:1–4.
3. Langland OE, Langlais RP. Early pioneers of oral and maxillofacial radiology. Oral Surg Oral Med Oral Pathol Oral Radiol Endod 1995;80:496–411.
4. Harrison F. The new photography and its application to dental practice. J Br Dent Assoc 1896;17:343–344.
5. Morton WJ. The X-ray is not necessarily dangerous. Dent Items Interest 1897;19:314.
6. Farman TT, Farman AG. Evaluation of a new F speed dental X-ray film. The effect of processing solutions and a comparison with D and E speed films. Dentomaxillofac Radiol 2000;29:41–45.
7. Rushton VE. Panoramic radiography: history and future development. In: Rushton VE, Rout PGJ (eds). Quintessentials of Dental Practice 20: Panoramic Radiology. London: Quintessence, 2006:1–15.
8. Tammisalo E, Hallikainen D, Kanerva H, Tammisalo T. Comprehensive oral X-ray diagnosis: Scanora multimodal radiography. A preliminary description. Dentomaxillofac Radiol 1992;21:9–15.
9. Langland OE, Langlais RP, McDavid WD, DelBalso AM. Panoramic Radiology. Philadelphia, PA: Lea & Febiger, 1989.
10. James JJ, Davies AG, Cowen AR, O'Connor PJ. Developments in digital radiology: an equipment update. Eur Radiol 2001;11:2616–2626.
11. Hounsfield GN. Computerized transverse axial scanning (tomography). 1 Description of system. Br J Radiol 1972; 46:1016–1022.
12. Mouyen F, Benz C, Sonnabend E, Lodter JP. Presentation and physical evaluation of RadioVisioGraphy. Oral Surg Oral Med Oral Pathol 1989;68:238–242.
13. Horner K, Shearer AC, Walker A, Wilson NHF. RadioVisioGraphy: an initial evaluation. Br Dent J 1990;168: 244–248.
14. Brettle DS, Workman A, Ellwood RP, Launders JH, Horner K, Davies RM. The imaging performance of a storage phosphor system for dental radiography. Br J Radiol 1996;69: 256–261.
15. Horner K, Drage N, Brettle DS. Quintessentials of Dental Practice 28: 21st Century Imaging. London: Quintessence, 2008.
16. Helmrot E, Carlsson GA, Eckerdal O, Sandborg M. Influence of scattered radiation and tube potential on radiographic contrast: comparison of two different dental X-ray films. Dentomaxillofac Radiol 1991;20:135–146.
17. Horner K. Review article: radiation protection in dental radiology. Br J Radiol 1994;67:1041–1049.
18. Lecomber AG, Downes SL, Mokhtari M, Faulkner KG. Optimisation of patient doses in programmable dental panoramic radiography. Dentomaxillofac Radiol 2000;29:107–112.
19. Eraso FE, Ludlow JB, Platin E, Tyndall D, Phillips C. Clinical and in vitro film quality comparison of manual and automatic exposure control in panoramic radiography. Oral Surg Oral Med Oral Pathol Oral Radiol Endod 1999;97: 518–523.
20. Farman AG, Farman TT. A comparison of 18 different x-ray detectors currently used in dentistry. Oral Surg Oral Med Oral Pathol Oral Radiol Endod 2005;99:485–489.
21. Berkhout WE, Beuger DA, Sanderink GC, van der Stelt PF. The dynamic range of digital radiographic systems: dose reduction or risk of overexposure? Dentomaxillofac Radiol 2004;33:1–5.
22. Gijbels F, Jacobs R, Bogaerts R, Debaveye D, Verlinden S, Sanderink G. Dosimetry of digital panoramic imaging. Part I: patient exposure. Dentomaxillofac Radiol 2005; 34:145–149.
23. Almog DM, Benson BW, Wolfgang L, Frederiksen NL, Brooks SL. Computerized tomography-based imaging and surgical guidance in oral implantology. J Oral Implantol 2006;32:14–18.
24. European Commission Directorate-General for Energy and Transport. Radiation Protection 136. European Guidelines on Radiation Protection for Dental Radiology. Luxembourg: Office for Official Publications of the European Communities, 2004.
25. Scarfe WC, Farman AG. What is cone-beam CT and how does it work? Dent Clin North Am 2008;52:707–730.
26. Müssig E, Wörtche R, Lux CJ. Indications for digital volume tomography in orthodontics. J Orofac Orthop 2005;66: 241–249.
27. Silva MAG, Wolf U, Heinicke F, Bumann A, Visser H, Hirsch E. Cone-beam computed tomography for routine orthodontic treatment planning: a radiation dose evaluation. Am J Orthod Dentofacial Orthop 2008;133:640.e1–5.
28. Harris D, Buser D, Dula K, Gröndahl K, Harris D, Jacobs R et al. EAO Guidelines for the use of Diagnostic Imaging in Implant Dentistry. Clin Oral Implants Res 2002;13: 566–570.
29. Patel S, Dawood A, Ford TP, Whaites E. The potential applications of cone beam computed tomography in the management of endodontic problems. Int Endod J 2007;40: 818–830.

30. Redpath RW. MRI developments in perspective. Br J Radiol 1997;70:S70–S80.
31. Gray CF, Redpath TW, Smith FW, Staff RT. Advanced imaging: magnetic resonance imaging in implant dentistry. Clin Oral Implants Res 2003;14:18–27.
32. Cotti E, Campisi G, Ambu R, Dettori C. Ultrasound real time imaging in differential diagnosis of periapical lesions. Int Endod J 2003;36:556–563.
33. Matalon S, Feuerstein O, Calderon S, Mittleman A, Kaffe I. Detection of cavitated carious lesions in approximal tooth surfaces by ultrasonic caries detector. Oral Surg Oral Med Oral Pathol Oral Radiol Endod 2007;109–113.
34. Bjelkhagen H, Sundström F, Angmar-Månsson B, Ryden H. Early detection of enamel caries by the luminescence excited by visible laser light. Swed Dent J 1982;6:1–7.
35. Pretty IA. Caries detection and diagnosis: novel technologies. J Dent 2006;34:727–739.
36. van der Stelt, PF. Better imaging: the advantages of digital radiography. J Am Dent Assoc 2008;139(Suppl):7S–13S.
37. Wenzel A. Bitewing and digital bitewing radiography for detection of caries lesions. J Dent Res 2004;83(Spec Iss C):C72–C75.
38. Gakenheimer DC. The efficacy of a computerized caries detector in intraoral digital radiography. J Am Dent Assoc 2002;133:883–890.
39. Wenzel A, Hintze H, Kold LM, Kold S. Accuracy of computer-automated caries detection in digital radiographs compared with human observers. Eur J Oral Sci 2002;110:1–5.
40. Li S, Fevens T, Krzyzak A, Li S. An automatic variational level set segmentation framework for computer aided dental X-rays analysis in clinical environments. Comput Med Imaging Graph 2006;30:65–74.
41. Devlin H, Allen P, Graham J, Jacobs R, Nicopoulou-Karayianni K, Lindh C et al. The role of the dental surgeon in detecting osteoporosis: the OSTEODENT study. Br Dent J 2008;204:E16.
42. Jabero M, Sarment DP. Advanced surgical guidance technology: a review. Implant Dent 2006;15:135–195.
43. Casap N, Wexler A, Persky N, Schneider A, Lustmann J. Navigation surgery for dental implants: assessment of accuracy of the image guided implantology system. J Oral Maxillofac Surg 2004;62:116–119.

CHAPTER 4

Restorative dentistry

Roland Frankenberger

Definition and background

Restorative dentistry, in most countries in the world, is the art and science of the restoration of decayed and otherwise damaged teeth using direct and indirect restorative materials. Cements, dental amalgam (amalgam) and resin-based composite materials are used for direct restorations, which still constitute the majority of restorations around the world.[1-4] Resin composites, ceramics and cast gold are used for the indirect approach, representing a more time-consuming and expensive treatment option.[1,5-8]

The effectiveness of restorative dentistry is largely measured in terms of the survival times and annual failure rates of restorations.[1] Increasingly, however, the success of restorations is measured also in terms of patient satisfaction and effects on remaining tooth tissues, with the minimum intervention approach having been extensively investigated since the early 1980s.[1,9-13]

Although most of the available filling materials are able to act successfully as durable restorative systems, bonded materials, in particular, still suffer technique sensitivity.[2,14-21] The difference between conventional treatment concepts, such as those applied in the use of amalgam, and modern adhesive concepts using resin-based materials is substantial. Conventional concepts are largely mechanistic (Fig. 4-1) whereas the concepts for the operator-sensitive bonded restorative materials are largely based on the biomechanics of tooth–restoration interfaces. As widely reported and accepted, however, success in restorative dentistry is not determined solely by which material is used and the procedures adopted; the other key variables are the patient and the operator.

Education is of fundamental importance to the quality of restorations; however, dental clinicians receive different levels of continuing education for the many, varied developments in materials, techniques and treatment concepts.[4,22] Furthermore, in many dental schools, students now complete fewer restorations than previously, limiting experience prior to graduation. In addition to these difficulties, teachers are not consistent within and between countries in what they teach and what they expect of their students.

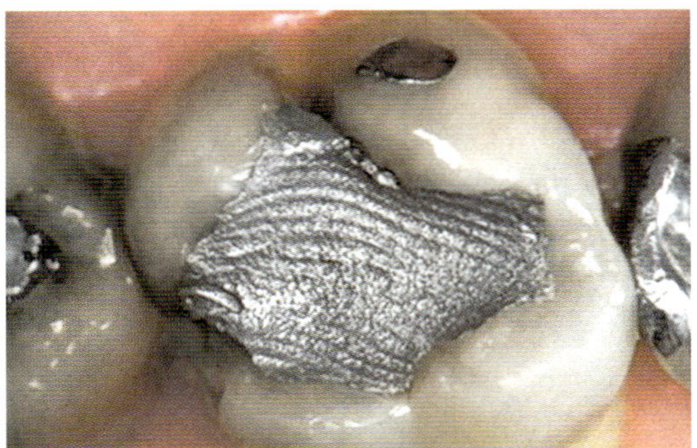

Fig. 4-1 Amalgam restoration after 10 years, presumably placed using suboptimal instrumentation – a finger tip!

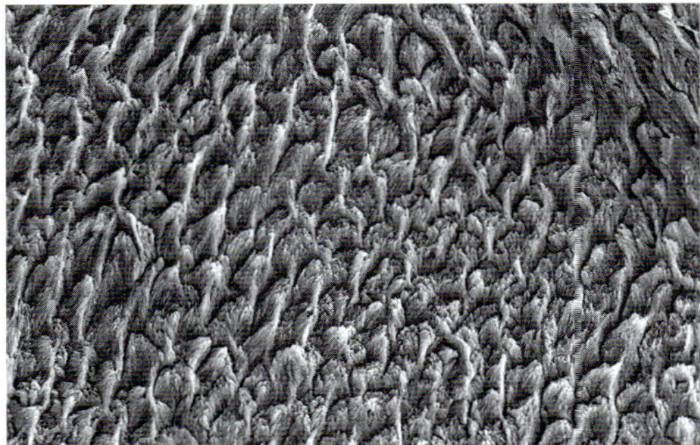

Fig. 4-2 Enamel surface after 15 s etching with 35% phosphoric acid.

Historical milestones

1818: Amalgam is found suitable for restoring teeth

Regnart, Bell and Taveau are reported to be the dental clinicians who pioneered the worldwide use of dental amalgam. Restorations with amalgam were quickly established to be a cost-effective and durable means of restoring decayed and damaged teeth. This view continues to be widely held today, in particular given the qualities and performance of non-gamma-2 amalgam alloys.

1948–1955: Hagger and Buonocore make the first steps toward adhesive dentistry

Hagger in 1948,[23] following over 100 years of conventional restorative dentistry, pioneered adhesive concepts based on chemical interactions between restorative materials and tooth tissues. Buonocore, who has received considerably more credit for his work than Hagger, introduced enamel etching and bonding.[24,25] Stemming from a comparison between phosphoric acid and phosphomolybdateoxalic acid for etching, Buonocore found phosphoric acid to be the solution of choice for the durable bonding of resins to enamel.[24,25] Notwithstanding a reduction in the concentration of phosphoric acid to 35% from 85%, as used by Buonocore, this approach to enamel etching is applied worldwide to this day (Fig. 4-2). Buonocore's concurrent work on bonding to dentin did not enjoy similar success, with breakthroughs in this field not occurring until some 30 years later.

1972: Wilson and Kent introduce glass-ionomer cements

The first successful approach to deve oping a fluoride-releasing material, to supersede silicate cements, was reported in 1972, when glass-ionomer cements were introduced to the scientific community.[26] Although materials of great interest (Fig. 4-3), glass-ionomer cements suffer from relatively poor flexural strength and from flexural fatigue behavior, limiting their application in clinical practice.[27] However, fluoride release gives glass-ionomer cements great appeal for use in older patients, children and irradiated patients.[17,27–30]

1987: Mörmann and Brandestini introduce computer-assisted design/computer-assisted manufacture

The introduction of computer-assisted design/computer-assisted manufacture (CAD/CAM) was a revolution in restorative dentistry,[31,32] but wide-

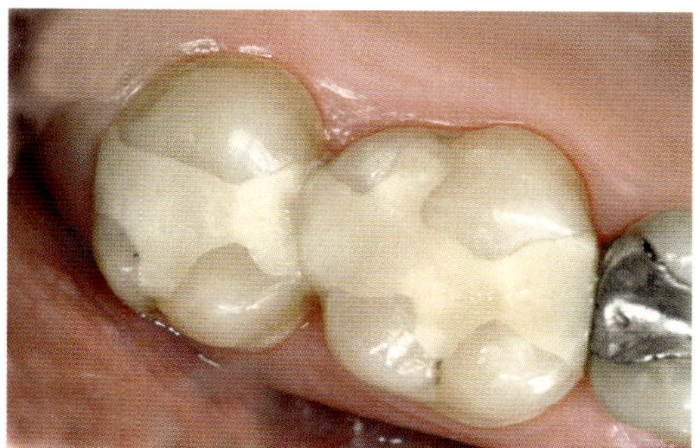

Fig. 4-3 Three-year-old glass-ionomer cement restorations in upper molars.

spread acceptance of the principal system (Cerec, Sirona) took more than a decade. Today, chairside-prepared CAD/CAM ceramic inlays perform exceptionally well, even when luting gaps of < 100 μm are present at the time of placement.[33] CAD/CAM is a tool predicted to find increasing application in clinical practice. The opportunity to provide an indirect restoration in one visit, avoiding the need for provisional restorations and laboratory costs, let alone return visits, offers many advantages to both the patient and the clinician.

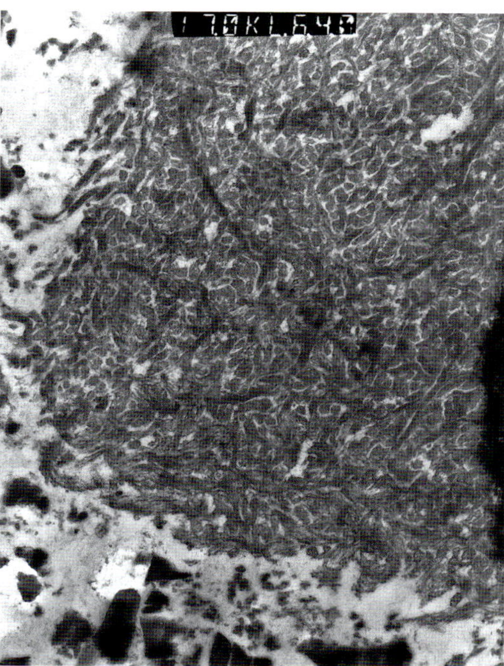

Fig. 4-4 The hybrid layer: the basis of bonding between resin and dentin.

1990/1991: Fusayama and Nakabayashi describe the hybrid layer

Traditionally, it was unthinkable to acid etch dentin, given fears of killing the dental pulp; all exposed dentin, in particular all operatively exposed dentin, was covered (protected) with liners and bases. The change in thinking to acid-etched dentin being the substrate of choice for the resin bonding of restorations was dramatic.[34] The key to this development was the realization of the importance of the interfacial (hybrid) layer between exposed collagen of the dentin substrate and the resin included in the dental adhesive system (Fig. 4-4).[35] Adhesion mediated by the hybrid layer underpins the ever-expanding application of tooth-colored resin-bonded materials, including the restoration of posterior teeth with composites.[9,12,16,36]

1992: Kanca describes the 'wet bonding' technique

When dentin is etched, successful bonding is typically dependent on the meticulous application of the wet bonding technique.[37] It remains difficult, however, to persuade dental clinicians to bond to a wet surface. The use of rubber dam and the creation of dry conditions continues to be widely considered to be a prerequisite for bonding to enamel, making it all the more difficult to explain the wet bonding technique: bonding to a moist rather than dry dentinal surface. This approach is critical to clinical success in terms of limiting post-operative hypersensitivity caused by dentin being dried in a similar manner to enamel following etching (Fig. 4-5).[2,14,15,21,37,38] While the use of phosphoric acid and resin remains the most effective

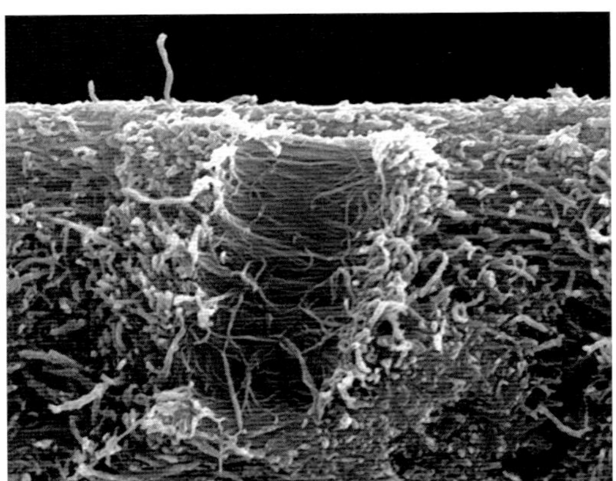

Fig. 4-5 Demineralized dentin surface. Without wet bonding, the limiting collagen network would be subjected to collapse. Scanning electron microscope, 1:7000.

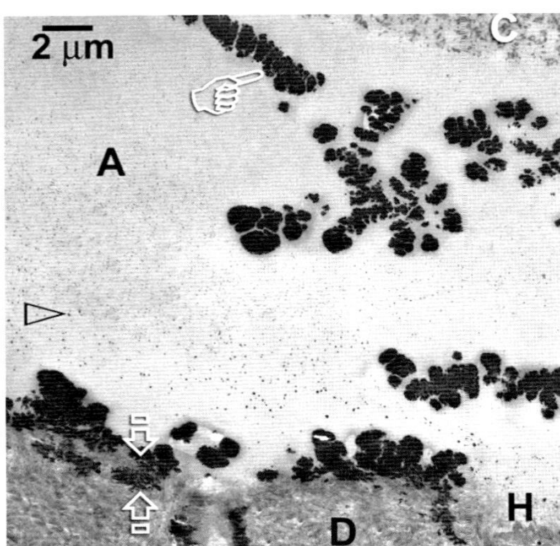

Fig. 4-6 Massive water treeing within an all-in-one adhesive interface.[46] A, adhesive; D, underlying dentin; H, hybrid layer; C, resin composite. Transmission electron microscopy, 1:3000.

means of bonding enamel, in particular enamel margins, it remains a challenge to identify the materials best suited to achieve reliable dentin bonding.[39] In the quest to achieve this goal, the recognition of the importance of wet bonding is a special milestone in the history of adhesive dentistry.

2003: Tay and Pashley discover 'water trees'

The confidence in hybrid layers, in particular to counteract shrinkage stresses in resin composites, was increasingly questioned when manufacturers decided to rationalize and otherwise simplify adhesive systems and procedures.

Such developments led to the so-called all-in-one adhesive systems, promising reliable bonding to enamel and dentin in one step only. As a consequence, bond strengths to enamel and dentin, restoration margin qualities and clinical outcomes were disappointing.[2,9,14,15,39–53] One of the reasons for these detrimental consequences is the considerable permeability of one-step adhesives. This permeability allows water sorption into the adhesive interface. This sorption may be seen by transmission electron microscopy as 'water treeing' highlighted by silver nitrate staining (Fig. 4-6).[2,46–54]

2007: Tay and Pashley introduce ethanol wet bonding

Tay, Pashley and colleagues introduced ethanol wet bonding as a way to avoid the water treeing dilemma. Ethanol wet bonding is effectively critical point drying in the clinical situation to create durable bonding to dentin.[51] It is a proven concept; however, it requires meticulous technique and, contrary to market demands, is relatively time consuming.

2007 Peumans and Van Meerbeek demonstrate the clinical effectiveness of 'mild' two-step self-etch adhesives

By means of a clinical trial, Peumans, Van Meerbeek and colleagues demonstrated the clinical effectiveness of the 'mild' pH, self-etch approach, employing a two-step hydrophobic bonding agent that did not

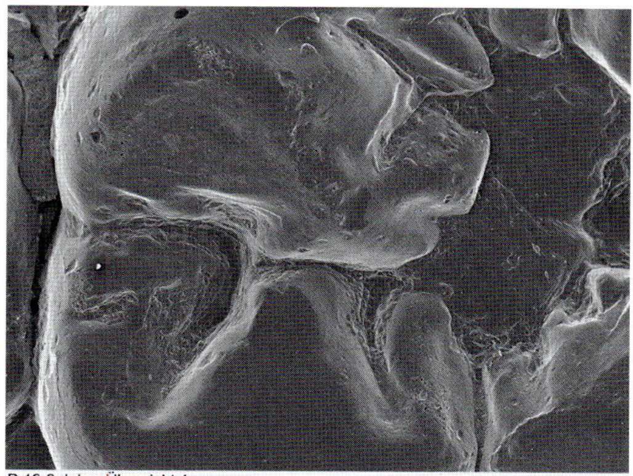

Fig. 4-7 Scanning electron micrograph following of a replica of a two-year-old glass-ionomer cement restoration placed by atraumatic restorative treatment (ART).

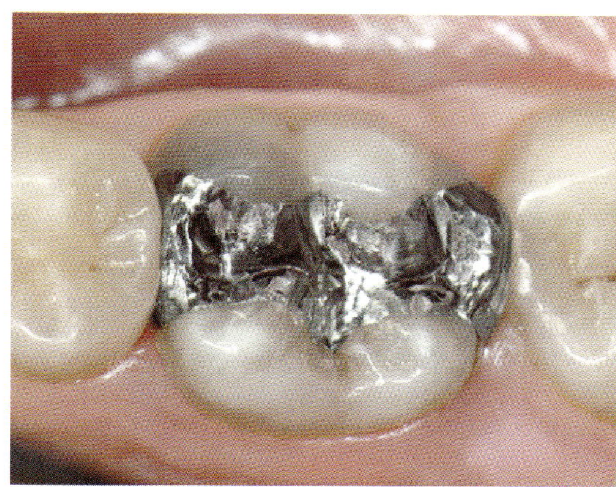

Fig. 4-8 A restoration of dental amalgam.

require initial phosphoric acid etching of enamel margins.[38] This approach provides a good compromise between effective bonding and ease and speed of use.

Treatment concepts

Direct restorations

Cements and atraumatic restorative treatment

In developing countries, dental care, including the management of caries, may need to be undertaken in locations with no electrical or water supply. Under such circumstances, a restorative technique involving only hand instrumentation and the direct placement of a material such as a viscous glass-ionomer cement is of considerable interest. The atraumatic restorative treatment (ART) concept has been shown to be an effective form of such treatment.[55-57]

There is, however, a huge difference in success rates between occlusal and occlusoproximal restorations using this approach, with occlusal restorations being much more successful (Fig. 4-7).

Dental amalgam

Despite the publicity surrounding resin composites and their esthetic qualities, dental amalgam should not be underrated as a restorative material (Fig. 4-8).[1,3,58,59] The problem with amalgam, however, is its diminishing acceptability to patients. Apart from the silver-gray metallic appearance, many patients have concerns regarding mercury release from amalgam. Latest studies pertaining to this issue support the view that such concerns are unfounded.[60]

Nevertheless, a number of countries, in particular the Scandinavian countries, have banned the use of amalgam, typically as a consequence of discontinuing the use of elemental mercury in manufacturing and other processes. Such arrangements may well become increasingly widespread, limiting the availability of amalgam for use in clinical practice.

Teaching the use of amalgam, which has been discontinued in some dental schools and limited in others to amalgam replacement procedures, introduces students to classical principles of cavity preparation. The value of such teaching will be

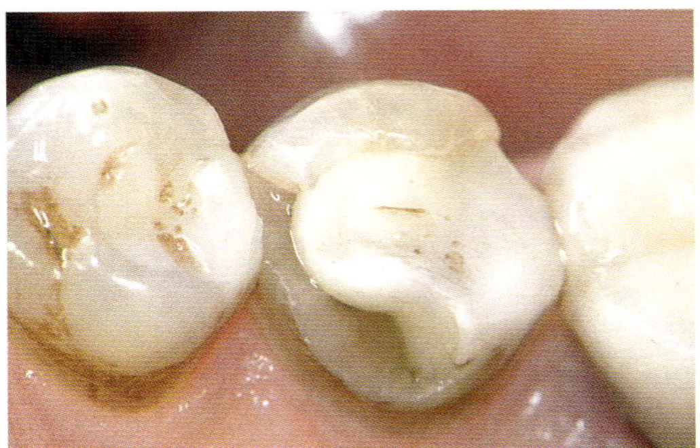

Fig. 4-9 Catastrophic restoration failure in a tooth restored with a direct resin composite.

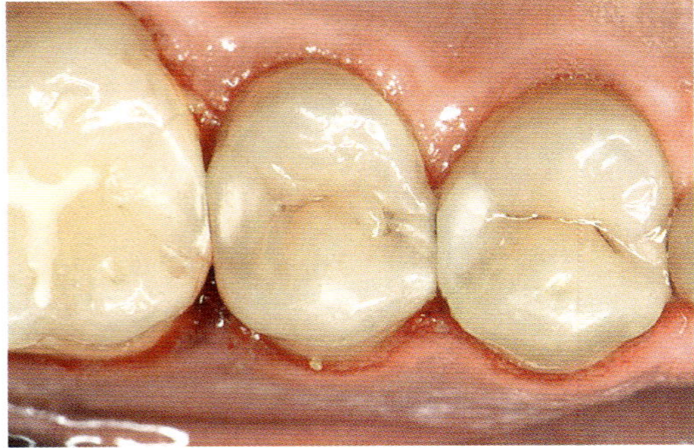

Fig. 4-10 Three minimally invasive, proximal slot resin composite restorations (distally in the premolars, mesially in the molar) 12 years after placement

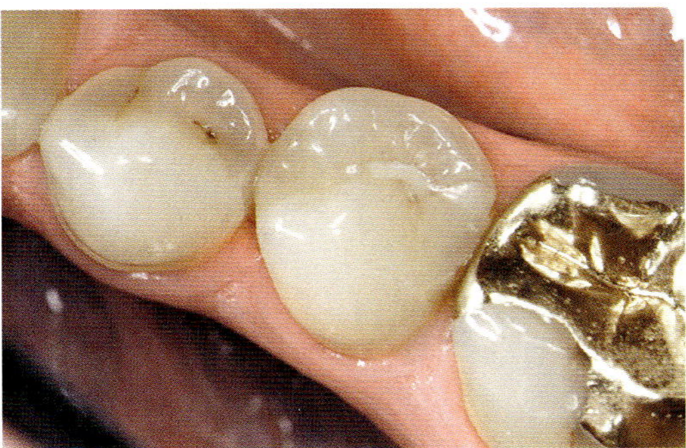

Fig. 4-11 A minimally invasive mesio-occlusal-distal resin composite restoration in a second premolar 10 years after placement.

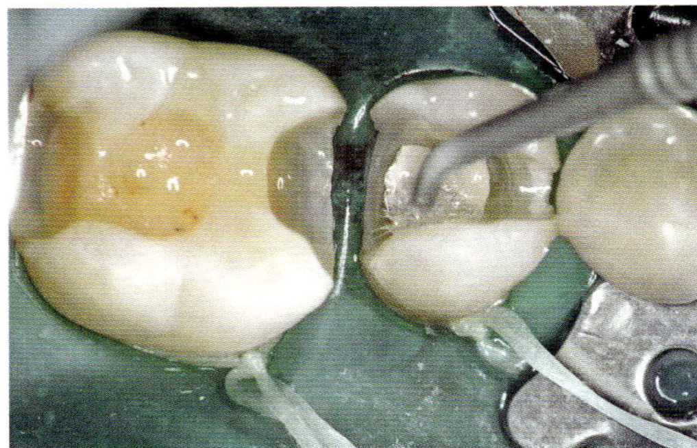

Fig. 4-12 Medium to large caries lesion in the first molar and an extensive preparation in the endodontically treated premolar.

increasingly questioned with the expanding use of tooth-colored restorative materials in combination with minimal interventive techniques.

Resin composites

Directly applied resin composites are capable of being bonded to enamel and dentin with excellent esthetic outcomes. The opportunity to meet esthetic expectations of patients together with the opportunity to save remaining tooth tissues are major advantages. Other aspects of resin composites are less favorable, especially polymerization shrinkage, which may result in stresses in the restored tooth unit, if not marginal gap formation and crack formation, in particular at the base of weakened cusps.

Notwithstanding these inherent limitations, resin composites when used correctly may perform as well as amalgam in clinical service.[1,9,10,12,16,17,45,61,62] The challenge in using resin composites lies in overcoming technique sensitivity, related primarily to bonding techniques.[14,15,20,21] In this regard, the operator has an immense influence on the clinical outcome of bonded restorations, with bonded resin composites being as challenging, if not more challenging, than bonded ceramics.

While clinical results with correctly applied resin composites are very good, both initially and over the long term,[12,16,17,59,63] catastrophic failures can occur when fundamental prerequisites are neglected (Fig. 4-9).[12,62]

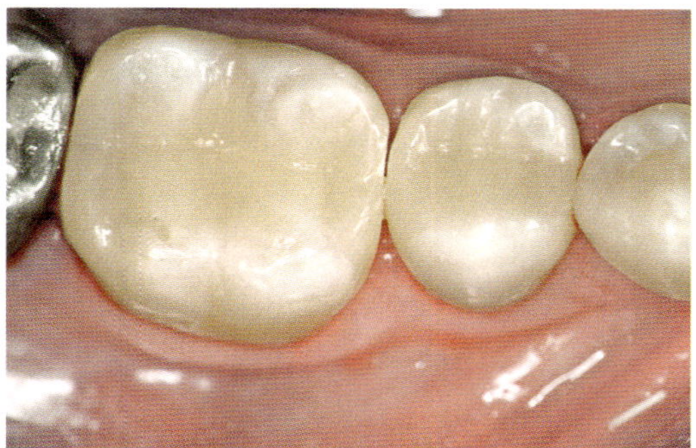

Fig. 4-13 Resin composite restorations in 1997.

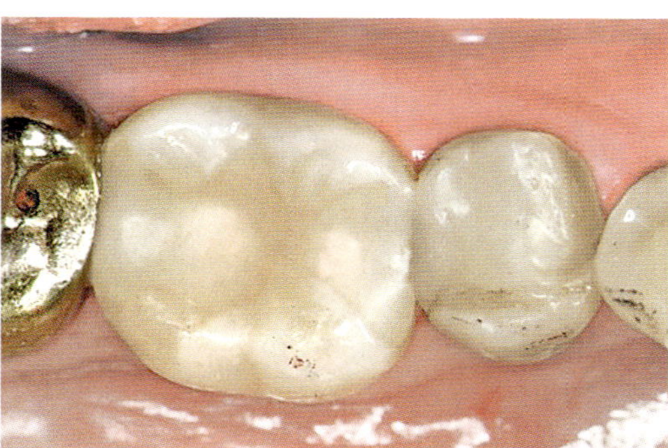

Fig. 4-14 The resin composite restorations in Fig. 4-13 after seven years (2004).

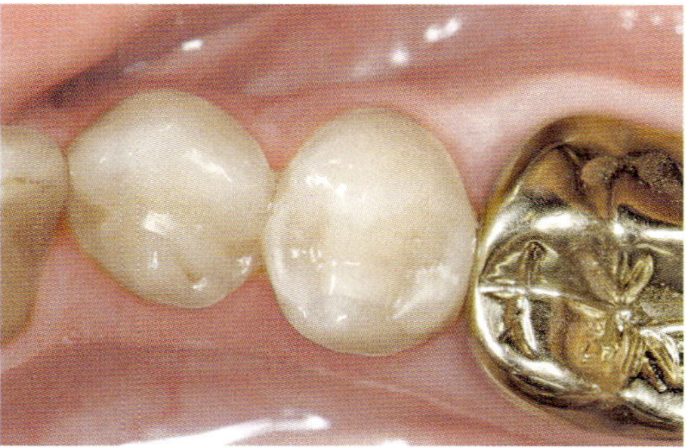

Fig. 4-15 Resin composite inlay in a second premolar after 10 years of clinical service.

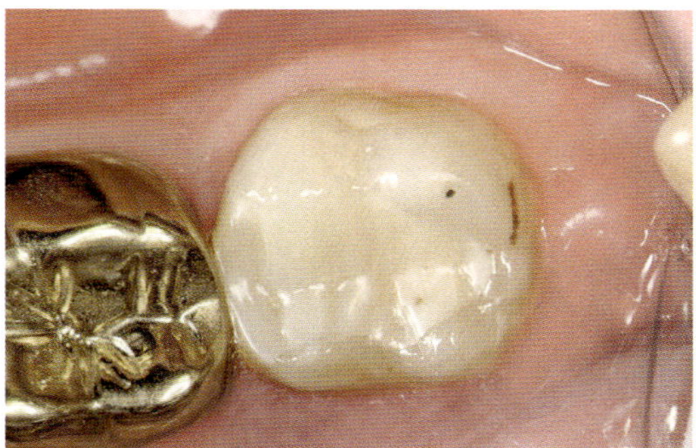

Fig. 4-16 Resin composite inlay in the second molar after 10 years of clinical service.

In a situation such as that illustrated in Fig. 4-9, an alternative approach should have been considered.

Despite the limited data available from prospective randomized, controlled clinical trials, small, minimally invasive resin composite restorations play an important part in the modern clinical practice of restorative dentistry (Figs 4-10 to 4-14).

It has been well established over many years that the minimal interventive approach (Figs 4-10 and 4-11) is very successful.[2,9,16,17] With larger restorations, it is sometimes difficult to achieve durable results, given the challenge of managing polymerization shrinkage in extensive preparations (Fig. 4-12) and the possibility of wear in situations in which the restorations are subjected to heavy occlusal loading. Under such circumstances, an indirect approach may be indicated, if not at the time of restoring the tooth then subsequently when the direct restoration begins to demonstrate signs of wear or other deterioration. In this way, the direct restoration is transitional, possibly becoming the core to support the indirect restoration (Figs 4-13 and 4-14).

Indirect restorations

Resin composite inlays

Resin composite inlays (Figs 4-15 and 4-16) have been reported to be a successful alternative to

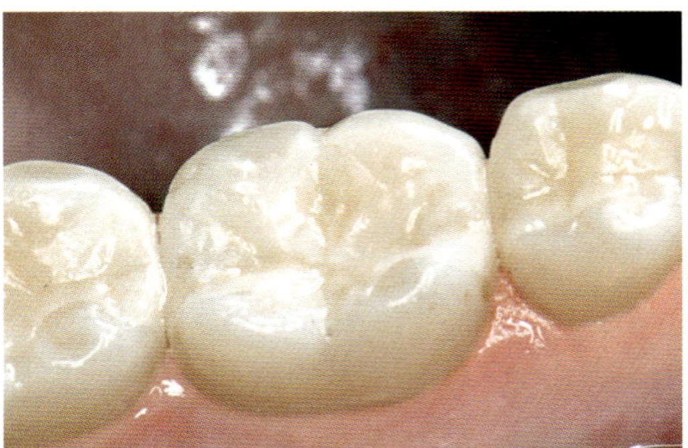

Fig. 4-17 Glass ceramic inlays after 12 years of clinical service.

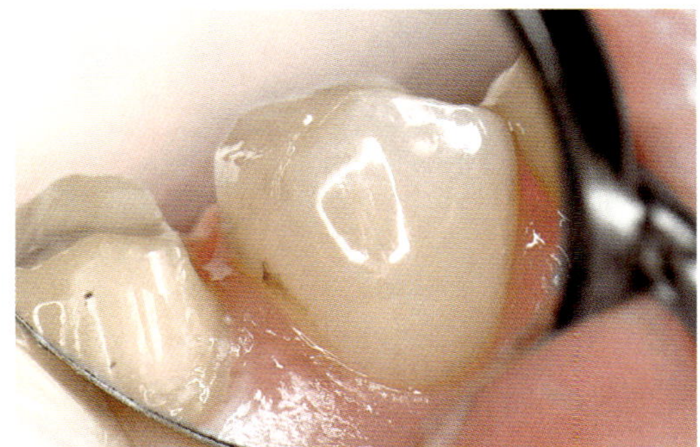

Fig. 4-18 Small marginal enamel fractures following the placement and occlusal loading of a provisional restoration.

ceramic inlays.[8,16] This is, in part, because the cost difference between resin composite and ceramic inlays is relatively small and because both ceramic and resin composite inlays have their own specific limitations. When resin composite, rather than ceramic, is to be used to restore a tooth that requires extensive preparation, there may be fewer difficulties at the time of placement as the resin composite is more forgiving and easier to adjust and refinish than ceramic.

Ceramic inlays and onlays

There are many more long-term clinical trials published in respect of ceramic inlays than for indirect resin composite restorations.[1,5–7,16,33,36,64–70] One of the reasons for this may be that patients who meet the inclusion criteria and enter clinical trials of ceramic inlays are less likely to default than if indirect resin composites were to be tested.[7]

From the data available, it is apparent that ceramic inlays (Fig. 4-17) and onlays may be one of the most successful forms of indirect, tooth-colored restoration, with annual failure rates of 1–2%.[1,7,16,66,68] Failures with ceramic inlays and onlays are mainly related to fracture of the restoration or endodontic problems.[1,7,16,66,68] A major issue with ceramic inlays and onlays remains the possibility of enamel in antagonist teeth suffering atypical wear, in particular if the occlusal contacts of the restoration had to be adjusted at the time of placement.[71]

Laboratory-made ceramic inlays

Ceramic inlays produced by an experienced technician can have the marginal accuracy of cast gold restorations. From the clinical standpoint, such accuracy enhances the excellent tissue response to ceramic restorations and, subject to the configuration of the margin, greatly improves the prognosis of the restored tooth unit.

A persistent difficulty when providing laboratory-made ceramic inlays is the limitation of provisional restorations. Such restorations may suffer leakage and provide limited, if any, mechanical protection to the remaining tooth tissues (Frankenberger et al., unpublished results). Problems of leakage may be readily overcome by sealing the dentin with an adhesive prior to the placement of the provisional restoration (immediate dentin sealing[72]) or placing a layer of flowable resin composite (the resin-coating technique[73]). With regard to the lack of mechanical protection for the remaining tooth tissues, notably weakened cusps and enamel margins (Fig. 4-18), the only way to overcome this poorly recognized and underestimated problem is to provide onlays rather than inlays, but this is much more destructive of tooth tissue.

Chairside ceramic inlays

CAD/CAM ceramic inlays systems, such as Cerec (Sirona), have been controversial since their introduction more than 20 years ago. The 'better the fit, the better the clinical outcome' theory had to be set aside to allow the clinical application of the CAD/CAM approach to develop. During the early stages of the CAD/CAM revolution, clinical outcomes were always reported to be favorable, despite relatively poor marginal fit. The failure rate of early CAD/CAM inlays could be as low as 1% after 18 years of clinical service. Subsequent work has confirmed that the quality of the marginal fit of CAD/CAM inlays may be less critical than the leakage and cuspal damage that occurs during the provisional restoration phase of the provision of laboratory-made inlays: a factor in favor of chairside inlay systems.

Cast gold inlays

Although increasing overshadowed and rejected in favor of esthetic alternatives, it must not be forgotten that cast gold inlays and onlays may be the restorations with the most favorable survival prognosis.[1,5,16] An annual failure rate of approximately 0.5% with gold inlays, possibly after many years of clinical service, is a near perfect clinical outcome.[1,5,16] This also holds for partial cast gold crowns used in the restoration of endodontically treated teeth.

Vision 2020

This book was written in 2008 with a view to predicting the nature of dentistry 12 years later, in 2020. If the book had been written in 1996, it might have predicted for 2008 more than has come to pass, largely because a number of key issues remain to be addressed. These issues are the barriers to significant developments in restorative dentistry between now and 2020. If solutions are not found, the art and science of restorative dentistry may not progress a great deal, if at all. In contrast, overcoming the barriers may open up many new exciting opportunities.

Technique sensitivity of adhesive systems

Compared with conventional techniques using amalgam or traditional cements, adhesive techniques are far more technique sensitive.[9,14,16,35,37,43,58] When the same adhesive-dependent material suffers 2.6% or 24.6% four-year failure rates when used by two different operators, technique sensitivity is clearly a major issue. Indeed, technique sensitivity is considered to be compromising the worldwide acceptance and greater success of modern approaches to the restoration of teeth and, as such, is viewed as the principal barrier to major new developments in restorative dentistry.

The etch-and-rinse technique is often put forward as a major reason for the technique sensitivity of adhesive procedures. After etching dentin with phosphoric acid, the use of an appropriate wet bonding technique is important, especially when two-step etch-and-rinse techniques are employed, which can leave dentin dry, possibly dessicated.[14,15,18] It is a fallacy that the introduction of self-etch adhesives helped to solve the problem of technique sensitivity.[20,43,52] This may be more a marketing tool to promote the sales of self-etch products than a clinical reality. Moreover, it is well established that the use of self-etching adhesives may compromise restoration-enamel bonding, in particular the marginal bonding and sealing of restorations,[46] encouraging clinicians to attempt selective etching of enamel. This is impossible to achieve clinically as unintentional etching of dentin will occur during rinsing. It is also widely accepted that self-etch adhesives do not work well on dentin previously etched by the application of phosphoric acid.

The situation with all-in-one adhesives is similar to that for self-etching adhesives. All-in-one adhesives suggest quick and reliable bonding, but, at best, bonding with such systems requires more than one application and, as a consequence, placement time is considerably prolonged.[43,46,74]

Given the above, one of the greatest challenges facing manufacturers of dental adhesives remains the reduction of the technique sensitivity of adhesive materials; achieving this will improve clinical outcomes globally.

Antibacterial adhesives and resin composites

Antibacterial properties have for several decades been described as a very important attribute of restorative materials.[58,62] Amalgam has been considered to have some antibacterial effects and glass-ionomer cements have been reported to be somewhat antibacterial,[28,75] but resin composites lack such qualities.

Attempts have been made to give resin composites antibacterial properties; however, the first attempt to market such a composite led to clinical results such as those seen in Fig. 4-7.[12,62] Despite such outcomes, it should remain a goal for researchers and manufacturers to develop resin composites and associated adhesive systems with good antibacterial properties. Clearfil Protect Bond (Kuraray, Tokyo, Japan) is certainly a step in the right direction; however, given that this system has a tendency to suffer shade drift following photopolymerization, its application may be limited to an effective means of cavity disinfection.[76]

Results of investigations in collaboration with a company providing antibacterial nano-silver and microsilver particles, which can be incorporated into resin composites, have been promising, both in terms of reduced bacterial adhesion and the survival of bacteria on composite surfaces and bone cements.[77,78]

Self-adhesive low-shrink composites

RelyX Unicem (3MESPE), developed by Hecht, was the first self-adhesive luting composite to remain in the dental market for more than five years. Several studies have reported promising dentin-bonding performance, and RelyX Unicem has become one of the most widely used materials for the luting of all types of crown.[79,80] It is also well known, however, that enamel bonding with this material is relatively poor, possibly insufficient to guarantee long-term cuspal stabilization when used to lute ceramic inlays in large cavities on the mesio-occlusal-distal surface of a tooth.[79,80]

Notwithstanding some limitations in the best materials currently available, an important first step has been taken towards self-adhesive resin composites. More developments can be expected in this field in the next decade. This will also be true for self-adhesive resin composites for use as restorative materials. Such materials should find special application in the further development of minimal interventive operative dentistry.

The first low-shrink resin composite (Filtek Silorane; 3MESPE) took more than a decade to develop, and in the development process there were difficulties in ensuring that the material had a reliable bonding mechanism. Nevertheless, it seems to be only a matter of time until it is possible to have low-shrink resin composite systems, together with convenient and reliable adhesives.

Innovative adhesion concepts

With modern materials and approaches to the adhesive bonding of direct and indirect materials, it is possible to achieve good clinical outcomes. But there are two main areas of difficulty:

- technique sensitivity
- biodegradation of the hybrid layer over time.

It is possible to envisage ways to reduce technique sensitivity and, in turn, improve the long-term stability of the hybrid layer. For example, electric devices may be used to improve resin penetration[54,81] or agents such as chlorhexidine may be incorporated in adhesive systems to suppress the action of matrix metalloproteinases released from etched dentin over time.[72-84]

It is, therefore, possible to address limitations in systems identified during 15 years of hybrid layer research and to improve stepwise the clinical performance of bonded restorations. Plans by manufacturers to develop materials, are, however, driven by market demands and the need to be profitable.

These plans and the clinical priorities identified by research in dental schools may not always match up. For example, when findings regarding marginal quality obtained with different adhesives over the 15 years of evolution of adhesive systems are examined, performance, in general, may appear to have decreased instead of steadily improving (Fig. 4-19). The thrust of development has been focused on the simplification and speed of use of adhesives rather than on enhancing clinical outcomes.

An alternative approach may be to invent completely new ways of developing an adhesive bond between tooth tissues and resin composites and ceramics.[85] Initial steps have been taken to incorporate adhesive proteins into restorative materials, with the prospect of new concept materials and techniques being available by 2020.

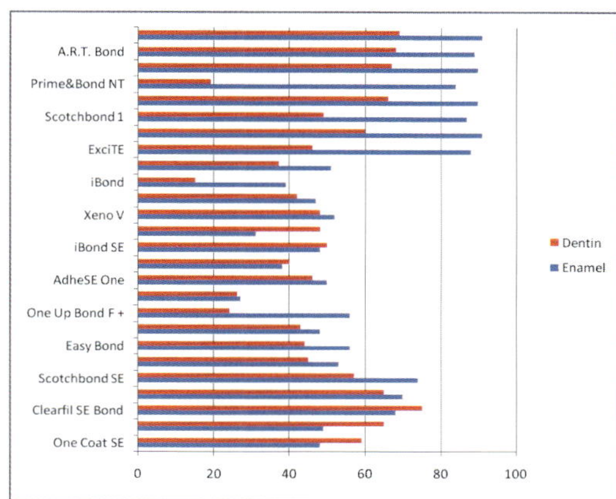

Fig. 4-19 Summary of findings for margin quality of different adhesives having been tested over 15 years in the materials science laboratories at the University of Erlangen. Results after thermomechanical loading (100,000 cycles, 50 N/2500 thermocycles). Methodology according to Frankenberger and Tay.[46] (Courtesy of R Frankenberger and U Lohbauer.)

Restoration repair kits

Given the limitations of all existing restorative materials and types of restoration, dental practitioners are trapped in a cycle of repeat dentistry. More often than not, practitioners find themselves replacing restorations rather than treating primary caries. Unfortunately, this situation is aggravated by dental clinicians receiving more remuneration for replacing rather than maintaining restorations, let alone preventing secondary disease.[6,43,44,48] In other words, it is more lucrative to undertake procedures that further compromise teeth than to practice modern approaches aimed at preserving as many teeth and as much tooth tissue as possible. The replacement of restorations, possibly to improve appearance only, means either sacrificing sound tissue and losing whatever benefits there may have been from an initial minimal interventive approach[86] or spending more time and undertaking more detailed procedures than were required to place the restoration initially. Under such circumstances, it is essential that there is further investigation and development of effective repair procedures.[6,30,45,48,87] In addition, procedures for the maintenance and refurbishment of restorations, in particular tooth-colored restorations, will become increasingly important over the next 10 or so years. Indeed, certain manufacturers have already started to introduce restoration repair kits. By 2020, such kits will be commonplace in general dental practice.

Concluding remarks

Restorative dentistry, which has advanced greatly in the last 30 or so years, may look forward to many new opportunities and successes, subject to certain barriers to progress being overcome. Of these barriers, technique sensitivity is the most challenging and important.

References

1. Hickel R, Manhart J. Longevity of restorations in posterior teeth and reasons for failure. J Adhes Dent 2001;3:45-64.
2. Peumans M, Kanumilli P, De Munck J, Van Landuyt K, Lambrechts P, Van Meerbeek B. Clinical effectiveness of contemporary adhesives: a systematic review of current clinical trials. Dent Mater 2005;21:864-881.

3. Wilson NH, Burke FJ, Mjör IA. Reasons for placement and replacement of restorations of direct restorative materials by a selected group of practitioners in the United Kingdom. Quintessence Int 1997;28:245–248.
4. Wilson NH, Mjör IA. The teaching of Class I and Class II direct composite restorations in European dental schools. J Dent 2000;28:15–21.
5. Federlin M, Wagner J, Manner T, Hiller KA, Schmalz G. Three-year clinical performance of cast gold vs ceramic partial crowns. Clin Oral Invest 2007;11:345–352.
6. Frankenberger R, Petschelt A, Kramer N. Leucite-reinforced glass ceramic inlays and onlays after six years: clinical behavior. Oper Dent 2000;25:459–465.
7. Kramer N, Frankenberger R. Clinical performance of bonded leucite-reinforced glass ceramic inlays and onlays after eight years. Dent Mater 2005;21:262–271.
8. Leirskar J, Nordbo H, Thoresen NR, Henaug T, von der Fehr FR. A four to six years follow-up of indirect resin composite inlays/onlays. Acta Odontol Scand 2003;61:247–251.
9. De Munck J, Van Landuyt K, Peumans M, Poitevin A, Lambrechts P, Braem M et al. A critical review of the durability of adhesion to tooth tissue: methods and results. J Dent Res 2005;84:118–132.
10. Deligeorgi V, Mjör IA, Wilson NH. An overview of reasons for the placement and replacement of restorations. Prim Dent Care 2001;8:5–11.
11. Frankenberger R, Kramer N, Pelka M, Petschelt A. Internal adaptation and overhang formation of direct Class II resin composite restorations. Clin Oral Invest 1999;3:208–215.
12. Kramer N, Garcia-Godoy F, Frankenberger R. Evaluation of resin composite materials. Part II: in vivo investigations. Am J Dent 2005;18:75–81.
13. Kramer N, Garcia-Godoy F, Reinelt C, Frankenberger R. Clinical performance of posterior compomer restorations over 4 years. Am J Dent 2006;19:61–66.
14. Ferrari M, Tay FR. Technique sensitivity in bonding to vital, acid-etched dentin. Oper Dent 2003;28:3–8.
15. Frankenberger R, Kramer N, Petschelt A. Technique sensitivity of dentin bonding: effect of application mistakes on bond strength and marginal adaptation. Oper Dent 2000; 25:324–330.
16. Manhart J, Chen H, Hamm G, Hickel R. Buonocore Memorial Lecture. Review of the clinical survival of direct and indirect restorations in posterior teeth of the permanent dentition. Oper Dent 2004;29:481-508.
17. Manhart J, Garcia-Godoy F, Hickel R. Direct posterior restorations: clinical results and new developments. Dent Clin North Am 2002;46:303–339.
18. Perdigao J, Frankenberger R. Effect of solvent and rewetting time on dentin adhesion. Quintessence Int 2001;32:385–390.
19. Schoch M, Kramer N, Frankenberger R, Petschelt A. Direct posterior composite restorations with a new adhesive system: one-year results. J Adhes Dent 1999;1:167–173.
20. Van Landuyt KL, Mine A, De Munck J, Countinho E, Peumans M, Jaecques S et al. Technique sensitivity of water-free one-step adhesives. Dent Mater 2008;24:1258–1267.
21. Van Meerbeek B, Van Landuyt K, De Munck J, Hashimoto M, Peumans M, Lambrechts P et al. Technique-sensitivity of contemporary adhesives. Dent Mater J 2005;24:1–13.
22. Gordan VV, Mjör IA, Blum IR, Wilson N. Teaching students the repair of resin-based composite restorations: a survey of North American dental schools. J Am Dent Assoc 2003; 134:317–323.
23. Hagger O. New catalyst for polymerization of ethylene at room temperature. Helv Chim Acta 1948; 31:1624–1630.
24. Buonocore MG. A simple method of increasing the adhesion of acrylic filling materials to enamel surfaces. J Dent Res 1955;34:849–853.
25. Buonocore MG, Matsui A, Gwinnett AJ. Penetration of resin dental materials into enamel surfaces with reference to bonding. Arch Oral Biol 1968;13:61–70.
26. Wilson AD, Kent BE. A new translucent cement for dentistry. The glass ionomer cement. Br Dent J 1972;132: 133–135.
27. Lohbauer U, Frankenberger R, Clare A, Petschelt A, Greil P. Toughening of dental glass ionomer cements with reactive glass fibres. Biomaterials 2004;25:5217–5225.
28. Al-Naimi OT, Itota T, Hobson RS, McCabe JF. Fluoride release for restorative materials and its effect on biofilm formation in natural saliva. J Mater Sci Mater Med 2008; 19:1243–1248.
29. Lee HS, Berg JH, Garcia-Godoy F, Jang KT. Long-term evaluation of the remineralization of interproximal caries-like lesions adjacent to glass-ionomer restorations: a micro-CT study. Am J Dent 2008;21:129–132.
30. Mjör IA, Gordan VV. Failure, repair, refurbishing and longevity of restorations. Oper Dent 2002;27:528–534.
31. Mörmann WH, Brandestini M. [Cerec-System: computerized inlays, onlays and shell veneers.] Zahnarztl Mitt 1987;77:2400–2405.
32. Mörmann WH, Brandestini M, Lutz F. [The Cerec system: computer-assisted preparation of direct ceramic inlays in 1 setting.] Quintessenz 1987;38:457–470.
33. Reiss B. Clinical results of Cerec inlays in a dental practice over a period of 18 years. Int J Comput Dent 2006;9: 11–22.
34. Fusayama T, Nakamura M, Kurosaki N, Iwaku M. Non-pressure adhesion of a new adhesive restorative resin. J Dent Res 1979;58:1364–1370.
35. Nakabayashi N, Ashizawa M, Nakamura M. Identification of a resin-dentin hybrid layer in vital human dentin created *in vivo*: durable bonding to vital dentin. Quintessence Int 1992;23:135-141.
36. Breschi L, Mazzoni A, Ruggeri A, Cadenaro M, Di Lenarda R, De Stefano Dorigo E. Dental adhesion review: aging and stability of the bonded interface. Dent Mater 2008;24: 90-101.

37. Kanca J, III. Resin bonding to wet substrate. 1. Bonding to dentin. Quintessence Int 1992; 23:39–41.
38. Peumans M, De Munck J, Van Landuyt K, Lambrechts P, Van Meerbeek B. Five-year clinical effectiveness of a two-step self-etching adhesive. J Adhes Dent 2007; 9:7–10.
39. Frankenberger R, Kramer N, Petschelt A. Fatigue behaviour of different dentin adhesives. Clin Oral Invest 1999; 3:11–17.
40. Carvalho RM, Chersoni S, Frankenberger R, Pashley DH, Prati C, Tay FR. A challenge to the conventional wisdom that simultaneous etching and resin infiltration always occurs in self-etch adhesives. Biomaterials 2005;26:1035–1042.
41. Frankenberger R, Kramer N, Ebert J, Lohbauer U, Kappel S, ten Weges S et al. Fatigue behavior of the resin-resin bond of partially replaced resin-based composite restorations. Am J Dent 2003; 16:17–22.
42. Frankenberger R, Pashley DH, Reich SM, Lohbauer U, Petschelt A, Tay FR. Characterisation of resin–dentine interfaces by compressive cyclic loading. Biomaterials 2005; 26:2043–2052.
43. Frankenberger R, Perdigao J, Rosa BT, Lopes M. 'No-bottle' vs 'multi-bottle' dentin adhesives: a microtensile bond strength and morphological study. Dent Mater 2001; 17:373–380.
44. Frankenberger R, Strobel WO, Kramer N, Lohbauer U, Winterscheidt J, Winterscheidt B et al. Evaluation of the fatigue behavior of the resin-dentin bond with the use of different methods. J Biomed Mater Res B Appl Biomater 2003; 67:712–721.
45. Frankenberger R, Strobel WO, Lohbauer U, Kramer N, Petschelt A. The effect of six years of water storage on resin composite bonding to human dentin. J Biomed Mater Res B Appl Biomater 2004; 69:25–32.
46. Frankenberger R, Tay FR. Self-etch vs etch-and-rinse adhesives: effect of thermo-mechanical fatigue loading on marginal quality of bonded resin composite restorations. Dent Mater 2005; 21:397–412.
47. Nikolaenko SA, Lohbauer U, Roggendorf M, Petschelt A, Dasch W, Frankenberger R. Influence of c-factor and layering technique on microtensile bond strength to dentin. Dent Mater 2004; 20:579–585.
48. Tay FR, Frankenberger R, Krejci I, Bouillaguet S, Pashley DH, Carvalho RM et al. Single-bottle adhesives behave as permeable membranes after polymerization. I. In vivo evidence. J Dent 2004; 32:611–621.
49. Tay FR, Lai CN, Chersoni S, Pashley DH, Mak YF, Suppa P et al. Osmotic blistering in enamel bonded with one-step self-etch adhesives. J Dent Res 2004; 83:290–295.
50. Tay FR, Pashley DH. Water treeing: a potential mechanism for degradation of dentin adhesives. Am J Dent 2003; 16: 6–12.
51. Tay FR, Pashley DH, Kapur RR, Carrilho MR, Hur YB, Garrett LV et al. Bonding BisGMA to dentin: a proof of concept for hydrophobic dentin bonding. J Dent Res 2007; 86: 1034–1039.
52. Tay FR, Pashley DH, Suh B, Carvalho R, Miller M. Single-step, self-etch adhesives behave as permeable membranes after polymerization. Part I. Bond strength and morphologic evidence. Am J Dent 2004; 17:271–278.
53. Tay FR, Pashley DH, Suh BI, Carvalho RM, Itthagarun A. Single-step adhesives are permeable membranes. J Dent 2002; 30:371–382.
54. Breschi L, Mazzoni A, Pashley DH, Pasquantonio G, Ruggeri A, Suppa P et al. Electric-current-assisted application of self-etch adhesives to dentin. J Dent Res 2006; 85:1092–1096.
55. de Souza EM, Cefaly DF, Terada RS, Rodrigues CC, de Lima Navarro MF. Clinical evaluation of the ART technique using high density and resin-modified glass Ionomer cements. Oral Health Prev Dent 2003; 1:201–207.
56. Kalf-Scholte SM, van Amerongen WE, Smith AJ, van Haastrecht HJ. Atraumatic restorative treatment (ART): a three-year clinical study in Malawi – comparison of conventional amalgam and ART restorations. J Public Health Dent 2003; 63:99–103.
57. Wang L, Lopes LG, Bresciani E, Lauris JR, Mondelli RF, Navarro MF. Evaluation of Class I ART restorations in Brazilian schoolchildren: three-year results. Spec Care Dentist 2004; 24:28–33.
58. Mjör IA. Minimum requirements for new dental materials. J Oral Rehabil 2007; 34:907–912.
59. Mjör IA, Dahl JE, Moorhead JE. Age of restorations at replacement in permanent teeth in general dental practice. Acta Odontol Scand 2000; 58:97–101.
60. Yip HK, Li DK, Yau DC. Dental amalgam and human health. Int Dent J 2003; 53:464–468.
61. Blum IR, Mjör IA, Schriever A, Heidemann D, Wilson NH. Defective direct composite restorations: replace or repair? A survey of teaching in Scandinavian dental schools. Swed Dent J 2003; 27:99–104.
62. Braun AR, Frankenberger R, Kramer N. Clinical performance and margin analysis of Ariston pHc versus Solitaire I as posterior restorations after 1 year. Clin Oral Invest 2001; 5:139–147.
63. Frankenberger R, Kern M. Dentin adhesives create a positive bond to dental hard tissue. Int J Comput Dent 2003; 6:187–192.
64. Kramer N, Ebert J, Petschelt A, Frankenberger R. Ceramic inlays bonded with two adhesives after 4 years. Dent Mater 2006; 22:13–21.
65. Manhart J, Chen HY, Neuerer P, Scheibenbogen-Fuchsbrunner A, Hickel R. Three-year clinical evaluation of composite and ceramic inlays. Am J Dent 2001; 14:95–99.
66. Pallesen U, van Dijken JW. An 8-year evaluation of sintered ceramic and glass ceramic inlays processed by the Cerec CAD/CAM system. Eur J Oral Sci 2000; 108:239–246.
67. Thordrup M, Isidor F, Horsted-Bindslev P. A 3-year study of inlays milled from machinable ceramic blocks representing 2 different inlay systems. Quintessence Int 1999; 30: 829–836.

68. Thordrup M, Isidor F, Horsted-Bindslev P. A 5-year clinical study of indirect and direct resin composite and ceramic inlays. Quintessence Int 2001;32:199–205.
69. van Dijken JW. Resin-modified glass ionomer cement and self-cured resin composite luted ceramic inlays. A 5-year clinical evaluation. Dent Mater 2003;19:670–674.
70. van Dijken JW, Ormin A, Olofsson AL. Clinical performance of pressed ceramic inlays luted with resin-modified glass ionomer and autopolymerizing resin composite cements. J Prosthet Dent 1999;82:529–535.
71. Krämer N, Kunzelmann K-H, Taschner M, Mehl A, Garcia-Godoy F, Frankenberger R. Antagonist enamel wears more than ceramic inlays. J Dent Res 2006;85:1097-1100.
72. Magne P. Immediate dentin sealing (IDS): A fundamental procedure for indirect bonded restorations. J Esthet Restor Dent 2005;17:144-154.
73. Jayasooriya PR, Pereira PN, Nikaido T, Tagami J. Efficacy of a resin coating on bond strength of resin cements to dentin. J Esthet Restor Dent 2003;15-105-113.
74. Frankenberger R, Garcia-Godoy F, Lohbauer U, Petschelt A, Kramer N. Evaluation of resin composite materials. Part I: in vitro investigations. Am J Dent 2005;18:23–27.
75. Gama-Teixeira A, Simionato MR, Elian SN, Sobral MA, de Cerqueira Luz MA. *Streptococcus mutans*-induced secondary caries adjacent to glass ionomer cement, composite resin and amalgam restorations in vitro. Braz Oral Res 2007;21:368–374.
76. Gondim JO, Duque C, Hebling J, Giro EM. Influence of human dentine on the antibacterial activity of self-etching adhesive systems against cariogenic bacteria. J Dent 2008;36:241-248.
77. Alt V, Bechert T, Steinrücke P, Wagener M, Seidel P, Dingeldein E, Domann E, Schnettler R. An *in vitro* assessment of the antibacterial properties and cytotoxicity of nanoparticulate silver bone cement. Biomaterials 2004;25:4383-4391.
78. Bürgers R, Frankenberger R, Eidt A, Rosentritt M, Bechert T, Hahnel S, Schweikl H. Anti-adherence activity and bactericidal effect of microparticulate silver additives in composite resin material. Arch Oral Biol, submitted.
79. Frankenberger R, Lohbauer U, Schaible RB, Nikolaenko SA, Naumann M. Luting of ceramic inlays *in vitro*: marginal quality of self-etch and etch-and-rinse adhesives versus self-etch cements. Dent Mater 2008;24:185–191.
80. Hikita K, Van Meerbeek B, De Munck J, Ikeda T, Van Landuyt K, Maida T et al. Bonding effectiveness of adhesive luting agents to enamel and dentin. Dent Mater 2007; 23:71–80.
81. Pasquantonio G, Tay FR, Mazzoni A, Suppa P, Ruggeri A, Jr, Falconi M et al. Electric device improves bonds of simplified etch-and-rinse adhesives. Dent Mater 2007;23: 513–518.
82. Carrilho MR, Carvalho RM, de Goes MF, di Hipolito, V, Geraldeli S, Tay FR et al. Chlorhexidine preserves dentin bond in vitro. J Dent Res 2007;86:90–94.
83. Hebling J, Pashley DH, Tjaderhane L, Tay FR. Chlorhexidine arrests subclinical degradation of dentin hybrid layers *in vivo*. J Dent Res 2005;84:741–746.
84. Pashley DH, Tay FR, Yiu C, Hashimoto M, Breschi L, Carvalho RM et al. Collagen degradation by host-derived enzymes during aging. J Dent Res 2004; 83:216–221.
85. Dental adhesives of the future. J Adhes Dent 2002;4: 91-103.
86. Frankenberger R, Krämer N, Ebert J, Lohbauer U, Käppel S, ten Weges S, Petschelt A. Fatigue behavior of the resin-resin bond of partially replaced resin composite restorations. Am J Dent 2003;16:17-22.
87. Krejci I, Lieber CM, Lutz F. Time required to remove totally bonded tooth-colored posterior restorations and related tooth substance loss. Dent Mater 1995;11:34-40.

CHAPTER 5

Prosthodontics

William R. Laney

Definition

The aspect of healthcare concerned with the mouth and related structural components known as dentistry began as oral prosthetics.

A prosthesis is an artificial replacement for a missing body part. Therefore, a dental prosthesis replaces teeth and their supporting structures, while a maxillofacial prosthesis is a replacement for not only teeth but also missing parts of the jaw, face, head and neck.

Prosthodontics is the dental specialty pertaining to the diagnosis, treatment planning, rehabilitation and maintenance of the oral function, comfort, appearance and health of patients with clinical conditions associated with missing or deficient teeth and/or maxillofacial tissues and using biocompatible substitutes.[1] The broad spectrum of dental prostheses includes removable, both complete and partial prostheses, and fixed complete and partial restorations. Maxillofacial prostheses likewise can be fixed or removable, depending on their sources of support and the structures to be replaced.

Fixed prosthodontics includes prostheses retained by a dental cement, screws (in the case of certain types of endosseous implant) and friction. Removable partial dentures are supported by natural teeth, endosseous or transosteal implants, and the residual soft tissues and bone. Complete removable denture prostheses are supported by residual tissues, or may be fixed or removable when supported by endosseous implants.

Historical milestones

The evolution and development of what is now known as prosthetic dentistry occurred over more than three centuries. Early procedures for filling edentulous spaces, resulting from tooth loss or defect, can be traced to centuries BC.[2] Loose natural teeth were stabilized by silver or gold wire, and replacement units were extracted teeth from other mouths, carved ivory or wood replicas, which were wired to existing teeth. The metal of choice for early frameworks was gold wire or bands, which were used to retain tooth replacements or crown forms attached by wire, rivet and, later, solder.

Progress in prosthetic dentistry was limited until the eighteenth century publications of the Frenchman Pierre Fauchard, who documented improvements, in particular with respect to fixed prostheses.[3] By the middle 1700s, the works of Fauchard, Mouton and Boudet had described methods for fixed replacements using silk ligature, gold round wire or bands to secure mineral (porcelain), ivory, reshaped animal or transplanted human teeth. Many of these methods were used to secure crude facial and maxillofacial prostheses to obturate soft tissue and bony defects created by trauma or disease.

Attempts to improve the esthetic quality of tooth replacements led to the increased use of porcelains in the late eighteenth century and early nineteenth century. Chemant and Fonzi produced porcelain teeth with platinum pins. Later, Logan fused porcelain to platinum posts and Land fused porcelain crowns and inlays.

The technical need to move from the mouth to the laboratory bench was recognized by Fauchard. To expedite the production of removable complete dentures, early experimentation with articulators was reported by such pioneers as Balkwill, Gritman, Hayes, Snow and Stephan, whose hinge articulator with an arbitrarily fixed condylar path of 20 degrees was used extensively by dental laboratories until the mid twentieth century.

Subsequent articulator design evolved from the turn of the twentieth century and was influenced by various theories of occlusion. The Hagman Balancer and the Monson devices arose from those advocating the 'spherical' theory, while the 'adaptable' philosophy was espoused by such early workers as WE Walker, von Spee and Christensen. Subsequently, the 1926 concept of Rudolph Hanau, who proposed the 'quint' of factors affecting occlusion (condylar guidance, compensating curve, incisal guidance, cusp height and plane of occlusion), resulted in such adaptable articulators as the Gysi Adaptable, Hall-House, Wadsworth and Hanau instruments.

The search for a more practical denture base material resulted in the discovery of hard rubber, or vulcanite, by Goodyear in 1855. This material was later refined and produced commercially by SS White. The substance was workable, durable, reasonably accurate and cost-effective, but it lacked esthetic qualities. It was subsequently replaced by methyl methacrylate resin in 1937 and this has remained the material of choice because it is light in weight, relatively color stable and translucent, and easily processed, repaired or revised.

The era of modern prosthodontics began around 1950. It was heralded by significant advancements in diagnosis and treatment planning, rotary instrumentation for tooth preparation, operative techniques and procedures, patient pain management, infection control and improved restorative and laboratory materials. High-speed rotary instrumentation, initially using ball-bearing handpieces and later air-driven turbines, along with more effective evacuation equipment led to much improved and patient-friendly operational chair design and chairside assistance. 'Four-handed' dentistry was more efficient and enabled the clinician to produce more and better treatment for more patients. New and more accurate materials were developed for impressions, investments, ceramics, luting agents and metal castings. Waxes, plaster, modeling compound and zinc oxide pastes previously used for impressions were augmented by the reversible and irreversible hydrocolloids, mercaptan rubbers and silicones produced shortly after the Second World War.

Some of the new products were developed in response to evolving theories of impression making, pressure versus non-pressure; others were advocated for their improved accuracy in recording tooth preparations or maxillomandibular jaw relationships. Treatment and the dental image in the healthcare arena were enhanced by improvements in medication for sedation and pain relief, and antibiotics for infection prevention or control.

Since 1980 and into the early twenty-first century, biologically and physiologically generated prostheses have become more predictable and versatile by virtue of significant advances in scientific and technical knowledge. Preprosthetic surgi-

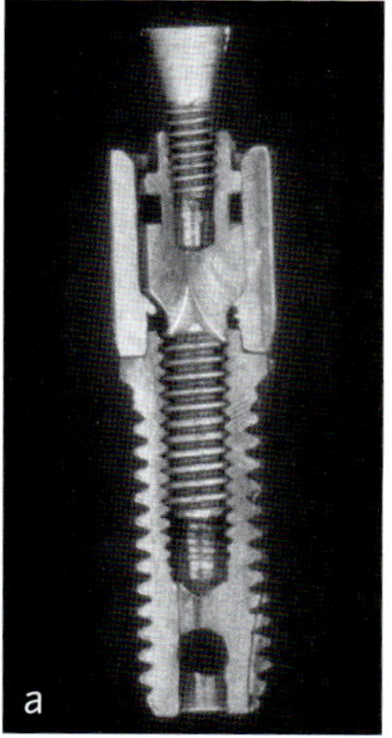

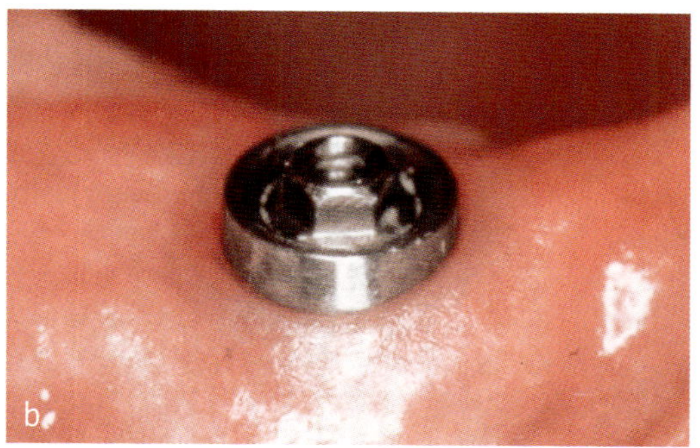

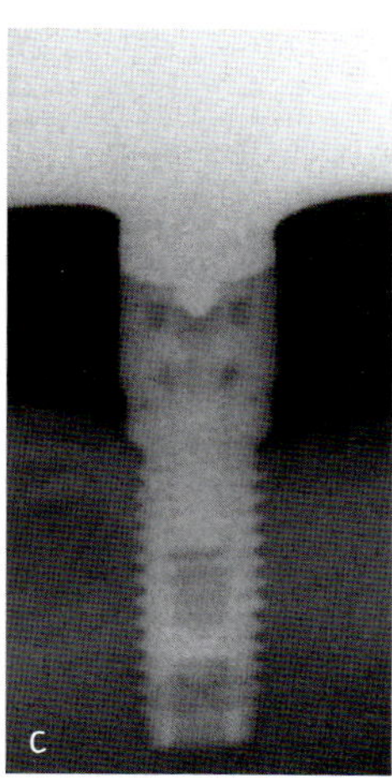

Fig. 5-1 (a) Basic titanium implant with sealed abutment and abutment screw. **(b)** Osseointegrated titanium endosseous implant with attached abutment. **(c)** Radiograph of integrated implant with bar attachment.

cal procedures have evolved to improve denture-bearing areas using bone and soft tissue grafts to enhance clinical outcomes. More dramatic and consistent outcomes have, however, been produced by the introduction and application of 'osseo-integration' in implant dentistry (Fig. 5-1).[4] In this period, the endosseous dental implant renaissance together with improved surgical procedures and computerized imaging have significantly increased restorative treatment options. Given a competitive market, new components and design choices appear regularly. Consequently, clinicians are provided with new opportunities for treating conditions previously committed to less-favorable outcomes with conventional restorations.

Treatment concepts

The demand for removable prosthodontic units remains strong among the world's edentulous and partially edentulous populations. Edentulism has been a key indicator of the oral health status of global populations and is regarded by many to be associated with reduced quality of life. Recent decades have witnessed a general decline in the incidence of edentulism as the result of better education, emphasis on preventive measures and improved materials and technologies. For example, edentulism prevalence at least halved between 1979 and 2002 among all ages, sexes and regions of Australia.[5] In a study of tooth loss among Finnish adults from 1978 to 1997, edentulism decreased from 14% to 6%, with the change being most marked in females. During the same period, the number of people with a complete natural dentition increased from 60% to 80%.[6]

A review of the dental literature in 2006 revealed that, in European countries, the frequency of adult wearers of removable dental prostheses varied from 13 to 29%, with 3 to 13% of edentulous patients using complete dentures in both jaws.[7] In individuals ≥ 65 year of age in the USA, over 40% were edentulous in 1993 and only 2% had all 28 permanent teeth. Generally, Caucasians had more teeth than Afro-Americans and edentulism was more common among those with less education and income, suggesting that cost has been the principal barrier to dental care for many Americans.[8] In a 1983 report on the provision of prosthodontic services by specialists and general practitioners, Douglas claimed that 19.5% the adult population of the USA between 55 and 64 years of age needed complete dentures.[9]

As longevity improves in increasingly large worldwide populations, the need for prosthodontic treatment continues to be high. For edentulous patients,

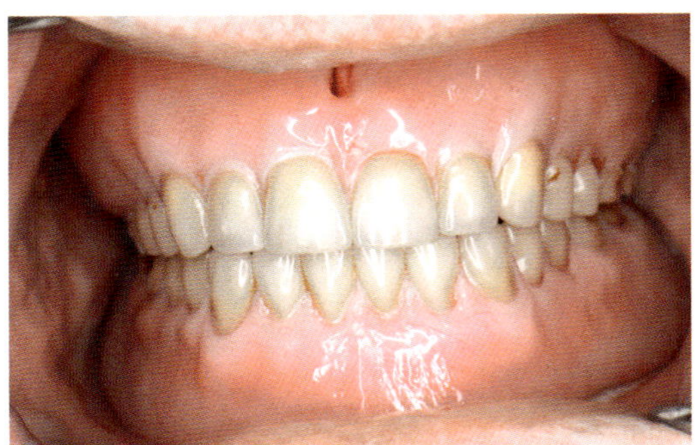

Fig. 5-2 Complete maxillary and mandibular conventional dentures.

the conventional removable complete denture is the treatment of choice given accessibility, convenience and cost. Constructed using acrylic resin, denture prostheses can be functional, esthetic, repairable and capable of restoring masticatory function and facial form at a moderate cost (Fig. 5-2). Because of the general downward trend in the prevalence of edentulism, schools of dentistry have placed less emphasis in the curricula on complete dentures, shifting the educational burden to other institutions, agencies, technical facilities or, more commonly, dental practitioner instructors lacking all the relevant knowledge, understanding and skills. Therefore, conventional removable complete denture restoration quality has tended to become the victim of change.

To alleviate the detrimental anatomic and physiologic changes associated with natural tooth loss, attempts to improve potential denture-bearing areas through preprosthetic surgical procedures have evolved over time (Fig. 5-3). While these measures, including bone and soft tissue grafting, have been helpful, recent advances have provided more predictable results in shorter time frames, thus reducing overall treatment time and patient discomfort and inconvenience.

Since the introduction of osseointegration in the 1980s, treatment options for tooth replacement have become more predictable and versatile.[4] Brånemark and colleagues in Sweden noted that healing bone was found to accept biologically and physiologically titanium screw-type endosseous implants placed in the jaw bone using an atraumatic surgical procedure.[4] Those patients who previously had experienced difficulties with prostheses supported by soft tissues and bone now

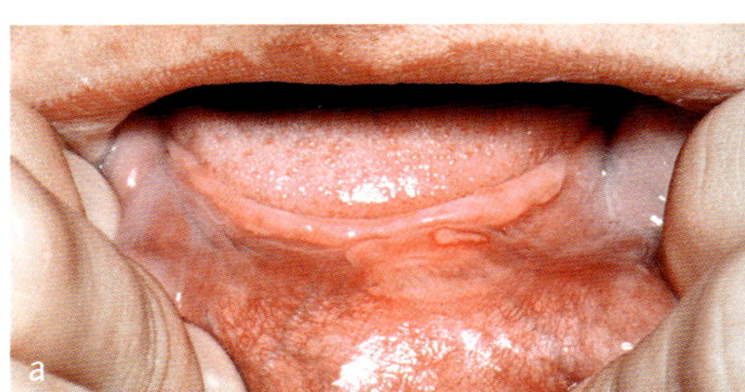

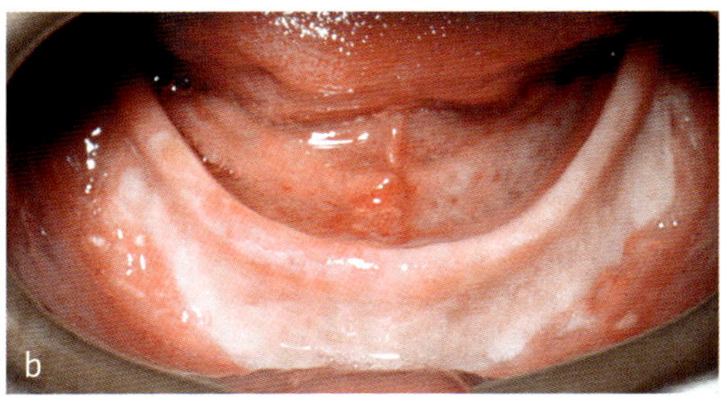

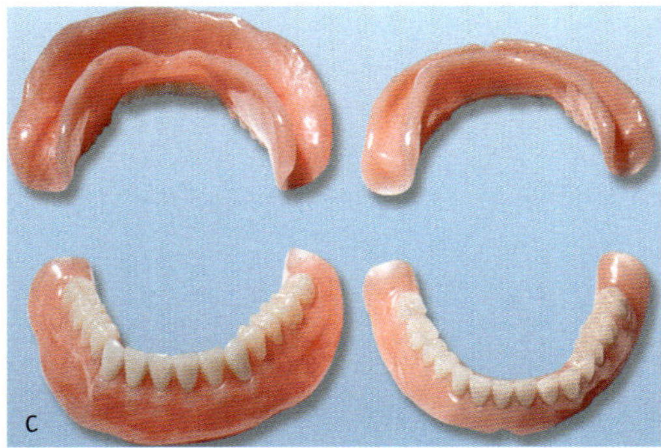

Fig. 5-3 (a) Preoperative intraoral condition of mandibular anterior sulcus obliteration. **(b)** Vestibuloplasty with split thickness skin graft. **(c)** Resultant prosthesis. Note improved extension buccally and lingually. Preoperative (right) and postoperative (left) prosthesis.

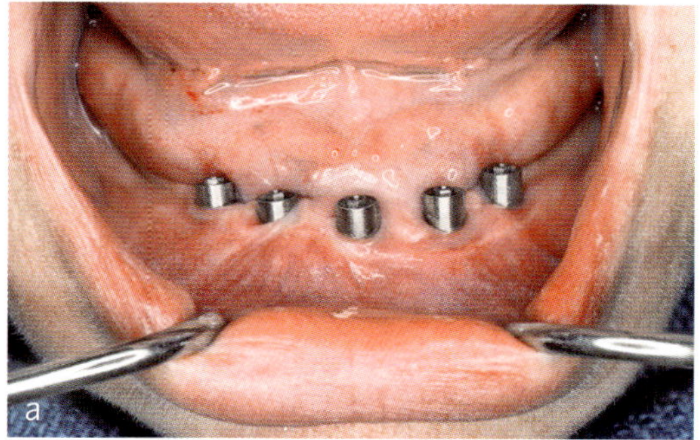

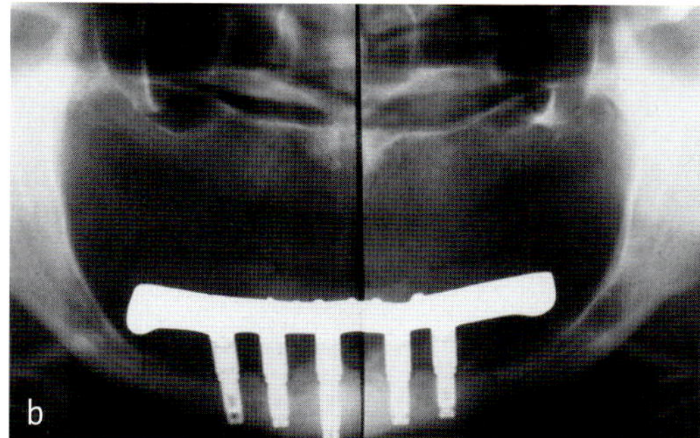

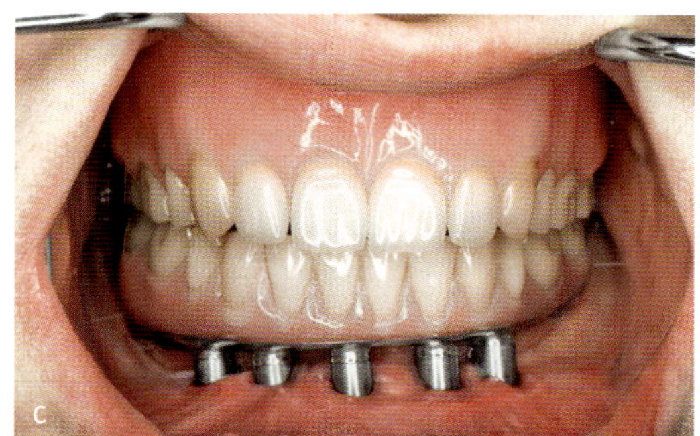

Fig. 5-4 (a) Edentulous mandible with five intraforaminal implants. **(b)** Radiograph of cast bar connected to implants and abutments. **(c)** Completed mandibular 'tissue-integrated prosthesis' opposing a conventional maxillary denture.

have the opportunity to benefit from enhanced stability and function through implant-supported prostheses, which can be fixed or removable (Fig. 5-4).

Osseointegration treatment options have been extensively facilitated by improved diagnostic imaging methods and computer-assisted surgical implant placement in edentulous patients. Implant position and location are critical in prosthesis design. Advances in imaging permit virtual surgical planning and the integration of navigational procedures in precise, preplanned surgical procedures.[10] In addition, advances in surgical procedure and technique have made implant placement possible in an expanded range of sites, using procedures such as residual ridge and maxillary sinus augmentation, incorporating autogenous bone and bone substitutes. These procedures provide additional opportunities for implant placement in regions of the jaw where bone loss has been substantial.[11] Distraction osteogenesis in the mandibular arch can also add vertical and horizontal bone volume for implant placement in selected patients.[12]

A useful treatment option for patients nearing the edentulous state continues to be the overdenture.[13] Before accepting an edentulous condition, patients may benefit psychologically through the retention of strategic teeth or retained roots. Indicated for mandibular arches, in particular, with large edentulous areas and minimal remaining tooth support, the overdenture can provide satisfactory retention and stability for what could otherwise be a difficult complete denture. Appropriately prepared remaining mandibular canines have usually been considered appropriate for overdenture support because of their position in the jaw, root length and size, potential for preservation of the remaining anterior alveolar ridge and tactile discrimination.

For patients with adequate financial resources or circumstances making them eligible for subsidized care, the placement of two endosseous implants in

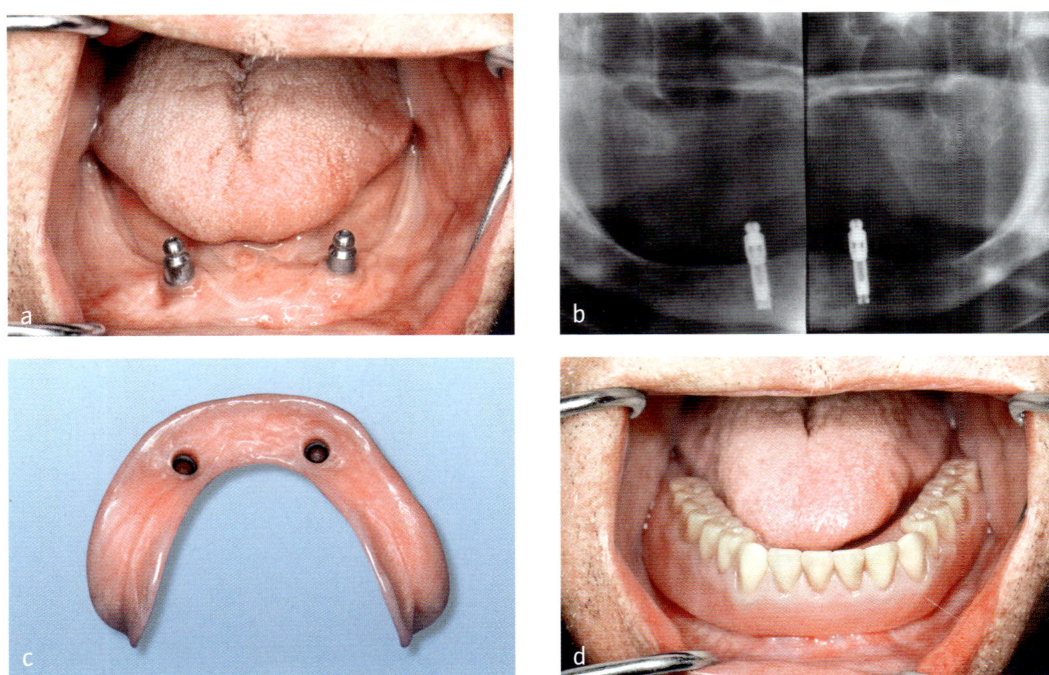

Fig. 5-5 (a) Endosseous implants in mandibular canine regions. **(b)** Radiograph confirming osseointegration. **(c)** Mandibular overdenture stabilized and retained by O-rings. **(d)** Overdenture in place.

the mandibular canine regions can also serve well as overdenture abutments. Special abutment attachments, such as elastic O-rings, can be utilized to provide retention and stability (Fig. 5-5). Magnets, Zest anchor and stud attachments are examples of other connecting mechanisms that can be used for retention.[14] Alternatively, two canine implant replacements may be splinted with a connecting bar to which bar clip attachments in the prosthesis base can be used to provide support and retention (Fig. 5-6). Various bar-sleeve systems such as the Dolder and Hader systems are common technical options.[15] Given concerns regarding the quality and resorption of bone in the maxilla following tooth loss, the provision of overdentures in the maxilla is an advantageous approach to treatment.[16]

Excessive loss of bone resulting from jaw atrophy, trauma or ablative surgery can effectively be managed by strategic endosseous implant placement and a removable overdenture.[17] Advances in laboratory technology have expanded to include procedures for jaw implants to provide support and retention for fixed and removable prostheses in edentulous patients. When connected by a bar, strategically placed endosseous implants in the maxilla can provide a fixed base for milled frameworks for removable prostheses. Electrical discharge machining (spark erosion) is the process of removing metal using a series of electrical sparks to erode material from a workpiece in a liquid medium under controlled conditions.[18-20] Thus, any shape can be reproduced using a single electrode to provide a precisely fitting frame for mechanical or frictional retention to a bar (Fig. 5-7). Replacement teeth can be arranged to functional and esthetic advantage, while enabling the patient to remove the prosthesis for care and maintenance.

A survey in the USA from 1971 to 1974 provided age-specific data regarding prosthodontic treatment needs. The findings indicated that the most common need for younger adults was removable and fixed partial dentures.[21] Treatment related to removable partial dentures was required by 73/1000 population. While some clinicians have demonstrated that the replacement of an absent molar tooth is not necessarily required for a patient's perception of adequate masticatory function, removable partial dentures remain the treatment of choice, in particular in clinical situations involving the loss of more than one but not all of the natural teeth. It is not uncommon to hear the question, 'Why replace missing teeth other than for esthetic appearance and speech?' While appearance may be the primary concern of patients, restoration of arch continuity is important in returning the dentition to an optimal functional state. Functional stimulation contributes to the

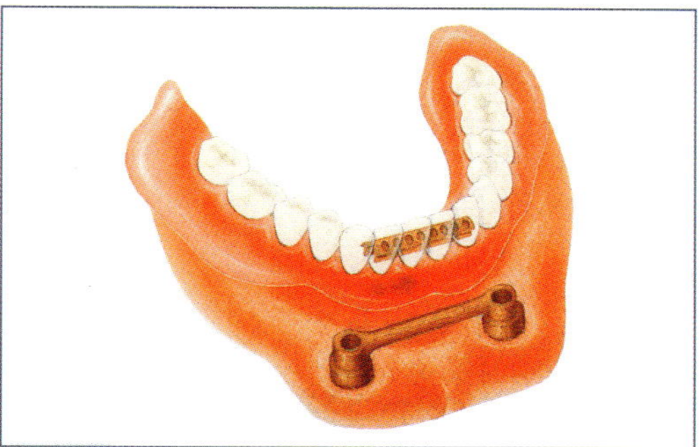

Fig. 5-6 Schematic of overdenture retained by clip on bar-connected implants. (Reproduced from Preiskel [1996][15] with permission.)

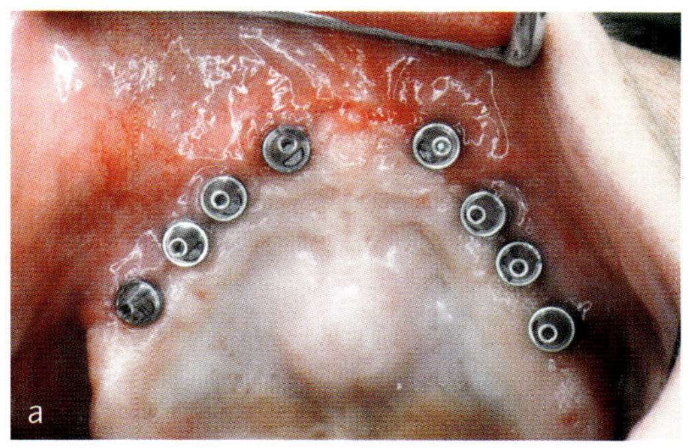

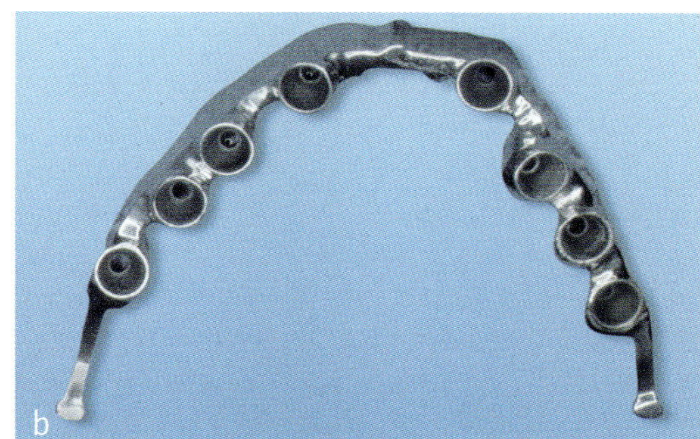

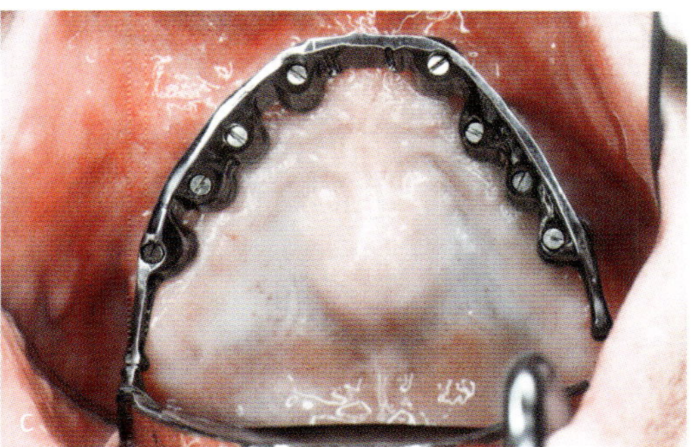

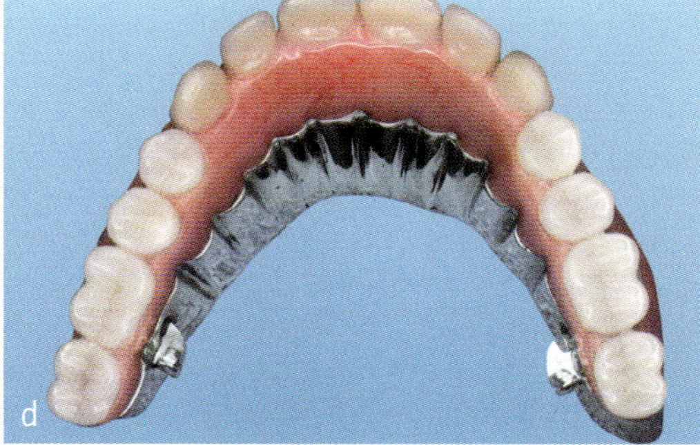

Fig. 5-7 (a) Abutments attached to endosseous implants. **(b)** Milled bar. **(c)** Screw-retained bar. **(d)** Completed bar-supported and retained overdenture with palatal clips for locking in place.

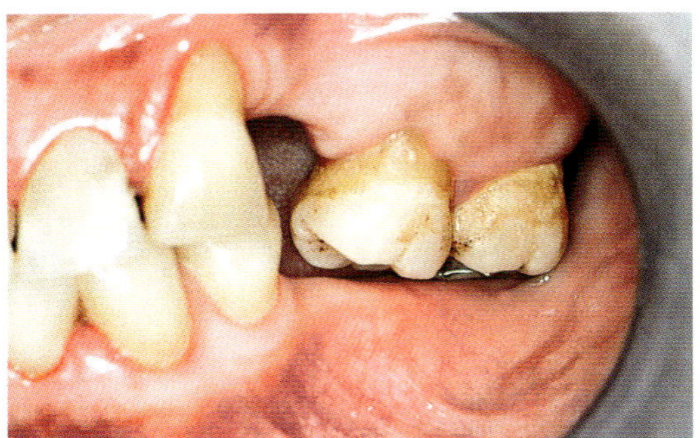

Fig. 5-8 Extrusion of maxillary molars into mandibular edentulous space. (Reproduced from Preti [2008][55] with permission.)

retention of residual bone, which is essential for removable partial denture support. Soft tissues in the edentulous area can also undergo change through the loss of attached mucosa, to leave a readily traumatized, sparsely keratinized mobile mucosa. Tooth replacement can also prevent passive eruption of the opposing dentition into edentulous spaces (Fig. 5-8).

Conventional removable partial dentures traditionally have a cast metal framework and are generally designed with multiple incisal, lingual or occlusal rest preparations in abutment teeth or restorations for support and indirect retention. Direct retention is usually provided by circumferential or bar clasps (Fig. 5-9). Vertical guide planes created on strategic tooth or restoration surfaces assist retention and influence movement control by directing the path of insertion and removal of the prosthesis (Fig. 5-10). Components of the partial denture are connected by cast lingual bars (mandible) and either anterior or posterior palatal bars in the maxillary arch. While not common, in clinical situations involving flaring of the remaining teeth, hinged labial major connectors with bar clasping attached to the framework can be used advantageously to utilize extensive infrabulge contours (Fig. 5-11). The hinged connector facilitates the placement and removal of the prosthesis by the patient. In edentulous areas, bases may be made of frame-retained acrylic resin or cast metal where space adaptation and added strength are design factors.

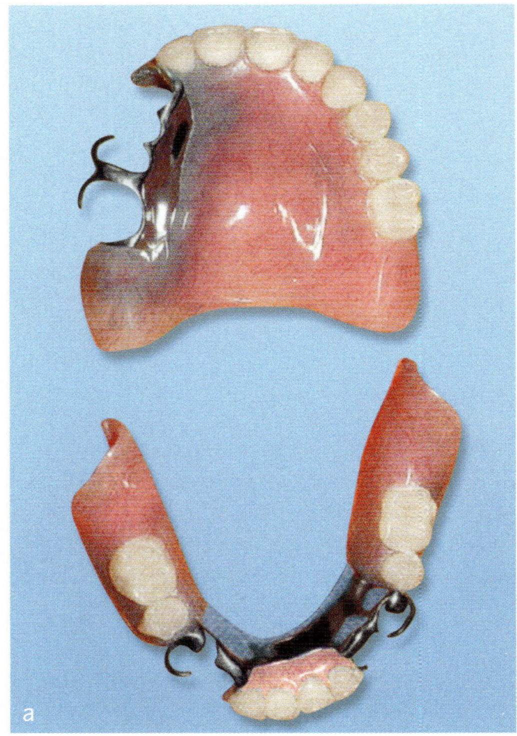

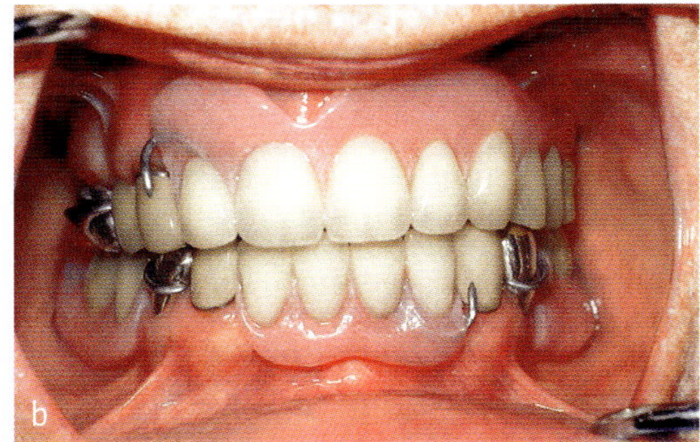

Fig. 5-9 (a) Conventional removable partial dentures with circumferential/bar clasp retention. **(b)** Prosthesis in place. (Reproduced from Carr et al. [2005][58] with permission from Elsevier.)

When abutment teeth require crown restorations, have insufficient crown length or clasp retention may be esthetically objectionable, internal precision attachments offer a treatment alternative

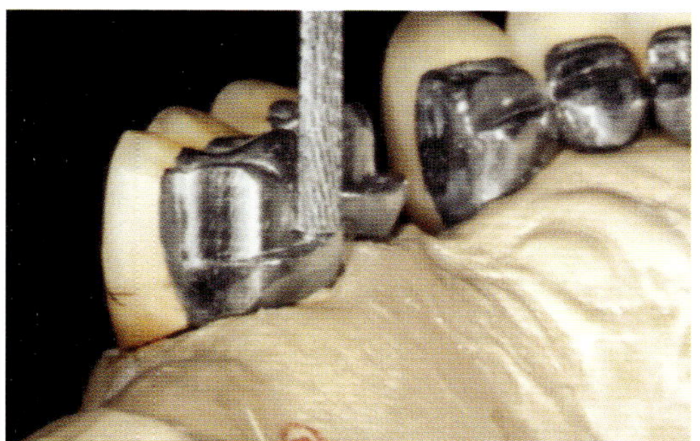

Fig. 5-10 Vertical guide planes milled into cast crown restoration. (Reprinted from Chaiyabutr and Brudvik [2008][57], ©2008, with permission from Elsevier.)

(Fig. 5-12). Since the path of prosthesis insertion is critical when using this approach, the female housing for the attachment must be incorporated in the crown restoration using surveyor guidance during construction. Torsional forces on the prosthesis are usually reduced by some capacity for vertical displacement, depending on the nature of any distal extensions. In the maxilla, full cast metal palatal coverage can serve as the major connector (Fig. 5-12a).

Removable partial dentures are designed to distribute occlusal and functional loads to the broadest base support possible. It is neither possible nor desirable to eliminate prosthesis movement with a removable restoration. The remaining teeth and edentulous ridge supporting structures can, however, be protected and preserved by appropriate design features that encourage the dissemination of inherent functional loads across the full extent of the available supporting bone.

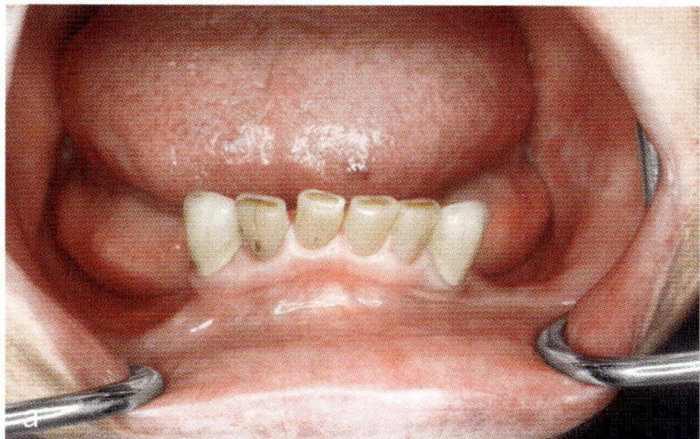

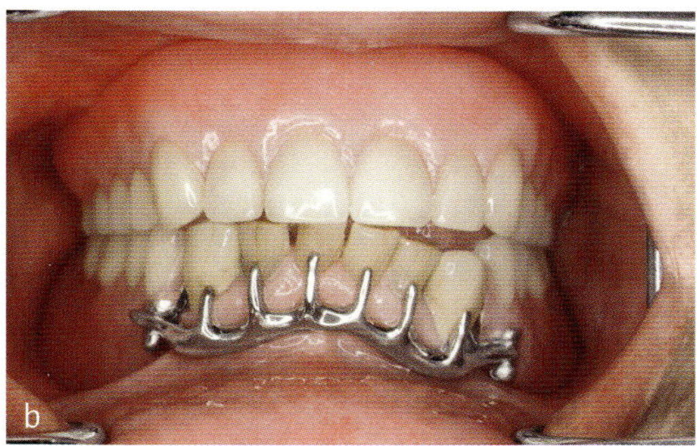

Fig. 5-11 (a) Flared mandibular incisors. **(b)** Hinged labial connecting bar with bar clasps hidden by lower lip.

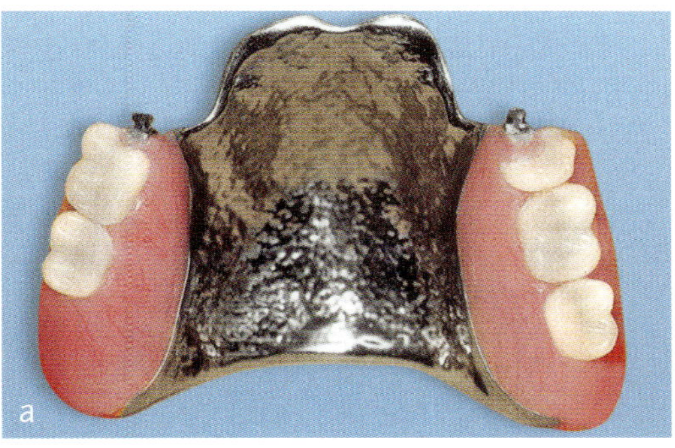

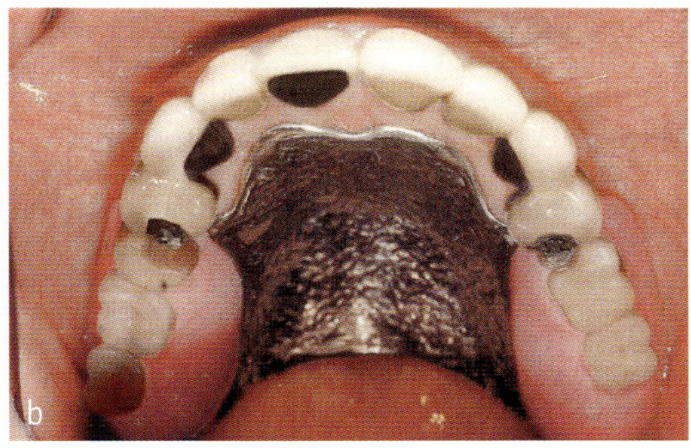

Fig 5-12 (a) Maxillary removable partial denture and intraoral retainers and full palatal coverage, including male components that seat in intracoronal rests. (b) Prosthesis seated. (Reproduced from Carr et al. [2005][58] with permission from Elsevier.)

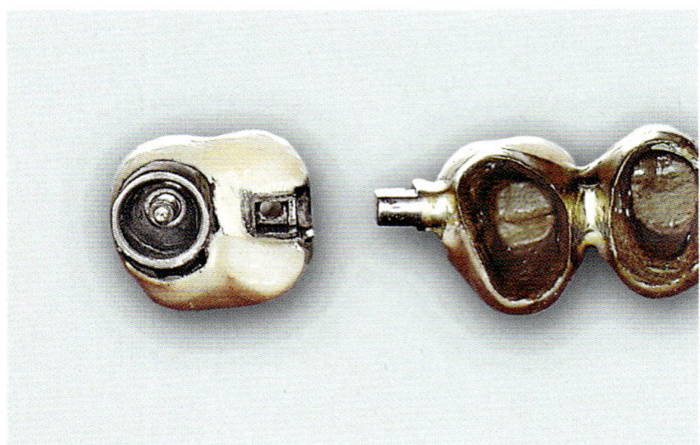

Fig 5-13 Tooth-implant-supported fixed partial prosthesis before placement. (Reproduced from Preti [2008][57] with permission.)

Following the success of implant support and retention in the treatment of the edentulous mandible, osseointegration was extrapolated for application to partially edentulous jaws.[22] Long-term evidence has demonstrated that equivalent or superior success can be expected with osseointegrated implants in partially edentulous patients, as achieved in edentulous mouths. Rapid technological advances and industrial competition have led to component design and the production of hardware that facilitates implant placement in nearly every region of the jaws. Patient demand for enhanced dental attractiveness, wherever possible improving on the previous natural appearance, has stimulated the research and development of advanced procedures and materials to provide the extraordinary outcomes currently observed.

With implant component design being so numerous and varied, removable partial prostheses have been largely replaced by fixed restorations supported by free-standing implants or the combined use of tooth and implant abutments. Whereas the periodontal ligament accommodates slight tooth movement in function, implants are essentially rigid in bone, within which functional load may be absorbed differentially (Fig. 5-13). Natural tooth intrusion can be a complicating factor in dual-supported restorations. This was reflected at the 2006 State of the Science on Implant Dentistry Consensus Conference (Section 3 Report),[23] which urged caution when considering tooth and implant support for the same restoration, given that long-term outcomes did not appear to be the same as when implant support alone was used.

The patient-driven emphasis on esthetic treatment outcomes has been accompanied by the expectation of reduced treatment time. The convenience factor has changed the procedural *modus operandi* and, because of improved implant surface treatments and new bone regenerative products, wound healing has been expedited. As a consequence, immediate functional loading techniques have evolved for selected clinical situations, with varying degrees of success. The Section 1 Report from the State of the Science on Implant Dentistry Consensus Conference[24] covered data from 19 clinical trials, with patient follow-up periods of one to ten years. The results suggested that overall performance was not significantly different between implants loaded early or immediately and those loaded after conventional healing periods. Concurrent advances in laboratory and materials science, clinical techniques and skills, and adjunctive multidisciplinary improvements, have refined expected outcomes in fixed prosthodontic treatment.[25] In 1998, the success and failure rates after 20 years of service for fixed partial dentures provided by general practitioners was reported from a review of 140 fixed prostheses, involving 557 retainers and 383 pontics.[26] When failed prostheses were considered, a cumulative success rate of 65% was found, with one third of the original restorations having been lost. While most of these restorations have since been replaced, considerable improvements in treatment outcomes could be expected using modern materials and techniques.

A lasting prerequisite for the planning of any treatment involving multiple units is accurate diagnostic casts mounted on an articulator appropriate for diagnostic waxing and the possible construction of provisional restorations. The preplanning for a desirable, mutually protected occlusal scheme will involve anterior tooth contact and the disengagement of posterior teeth during eccentric mandibular movements, together with posterior teeth contact to prevent excessive occlusal loading of the anterior teeth during function.

Although questionable periodontally involved teeth may receive added scrutiny in light of newer implant options, periodontal health is still essential for the maintenance of good oral health. Such procedures as endodontic therapy, crown lengthening, orthodontic realignment and root amputation, while previously considered desirable, are increasingly contraindicated in favor of implant options. Prior to 1980, the restoration of a short-span edentulous space with adjacent virgin teeth would have involved conservative, yet adequate, tooth preparation for prosthetic retainers. Currently, a treatment plan for the same clinical situation would in most cases involve the placement of one or two implants to provide free-standing support and retention for the replacement teeth, assuming the availability of adequate bone quality and quantity. Proven bone substitutes and/or guided regenerative therapy could be considered if the site were less than ideal for implant placement.

Maxillofacial prosthetics

The area of prosthodontics that has benefited most from advances in implant surgery and technologies has been maxillofacial prosthetics. Intraoral and facial defects resulting from surgery, trauma or congenital causes were previously managed prosthodontically by means of prostheses supported and retained predominantly by teeth (Fig. 5-14).[27] When the jaw was edentulous, the engagement of hard and soft tissue undercuts, the use of adhesives and adjunctive technical and surgical measures were employed to obtain retention and support, but often without significant success. The current approach to treatment will in all probability include implant placement for the support and retention of fixed and/or removable prostheses in one or both jaws. Should bone quality or quantity create treatment-planning obstacles, augmentation, regenerative and distraction surgical procedures could be undertaken prior to implant placement and the provision of prostheses.

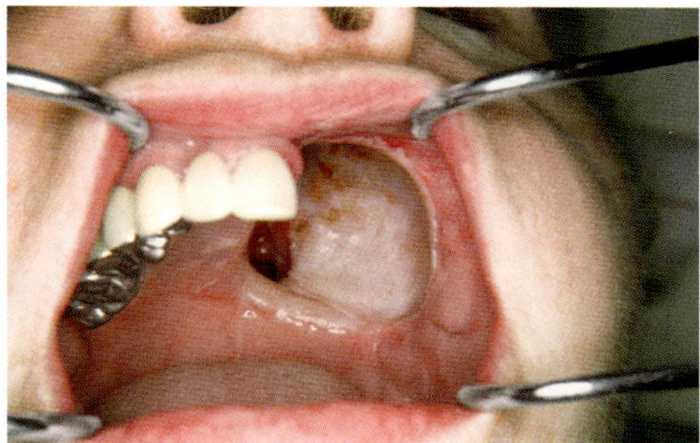

Fig 5-14 Remaining maxillary teeth splinted and contoured with cast crown restorations designed to provide guiding planes and surfaces in harmony with configuration of the acquired defect.

The management of congenital defects in children and adolescents has undergone considerable change. Following early jaw segment control, programmed lip and palate defect closure and velopharyngeal flap surgery to improve speech, the need for prosthetic obturators for patients with cleft lip and palate has declined. Therefore, relatively few adults with congenital defects present with unrepaired defects.[28] Those who do require prosthodontic restoration can be treated with advanced surgical procedures that will include grafting and endosseous implant placement (Fig. 5-15).

The use of titanium implants to retain extraoral maxillofacial prostheses has been facilitated by the design and production of flanged implants that are skin penetrating (Fig. 5-16).[4] These implants were originally developed to retain bone-conducting hearing aids retained by transepithelial penetrating implants placed in the mastoid process. Subsequently, this application of multiple implants joined by a connecting bar has provided a framework for the retention of auricular, nasal and orbital silicone prostheses. These prostheses have far superior fixation, marginal adaptation and patient convenience for placement, removal and site maintenance. Long-term data cite variable outcomes, in particular for orbital prostheses.[29] The majority of long-term outcomes for facial prostheses with implant retention have, however, been favorable.

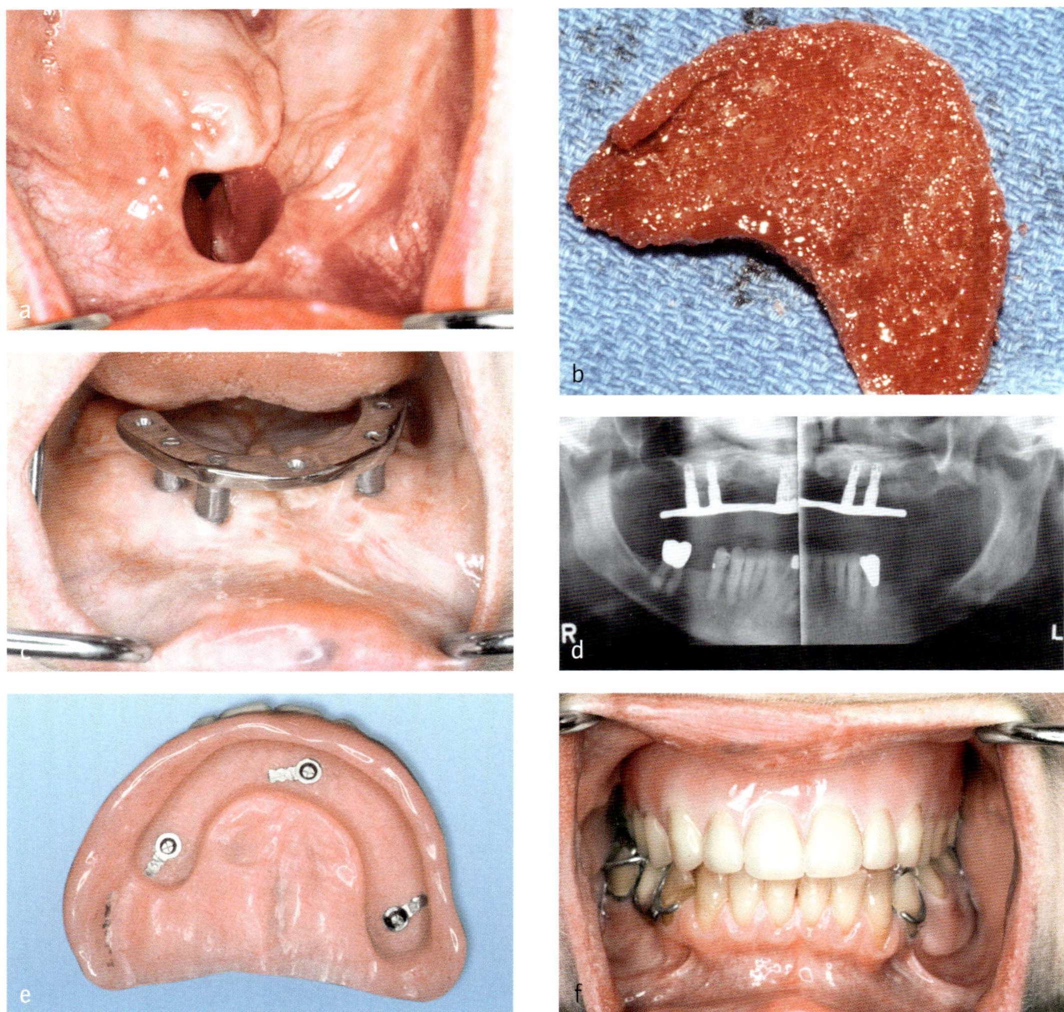

Fig. 5-15 **(a)** Congenital cleft lip and palate. **(b)** Bone graft to close palatal defect. **(c)** Implant placement with connecting bar containing female CEKA attachments. **(d)** Panoramic radiograph of maxillary implant support. **(e)** Prosthesis base with male CEKA attachments. **(f)** Completed maxillary overdenture and mandibular removable partial denture.

Ceramics

The emphasis on esthetics in response to patient demand has resulted in vast improvements in restorative materials, ranging from acrylic resin and resin composites to highly refined ceramics.[30] Improved metal-ceramic techniques and materials, more predictable procedures for producing complete ceramic crown restorations and machinable ceramics have increased the treatment options for esthetic enhancement and biological acceptance. Less-invasive tooth-preparation techniques can accommodate patient desires for improved esthetics without undertaking full-crown restorations. Porcelain laminate veneers for maxillary anterior teeth are a commonly used treatment option (Fig. 5-17).

When ceramics are the restorative option of choice, the selected material must provide specific esthetic and physical properties that positively influence the intended treatment goal and its potential for success.[31] Ceramics are the most consistently predictable esthetic dental material, suffering minimal degradation over time. Whereas metal-ceramic restorations (Fig. 5-18) continue to be the standard of excellence, because of their time-proven performance and versatility, all-ceramic materials are being developed to take full advantage of their benefits in terms of color match and marginal fit.

Ultimately, crown performance is determined by a complex set of interactions between crown material and geometry, the characteristics of crown support, structure, luting agent and clinical loading history. Different failure modes exist for mono- and

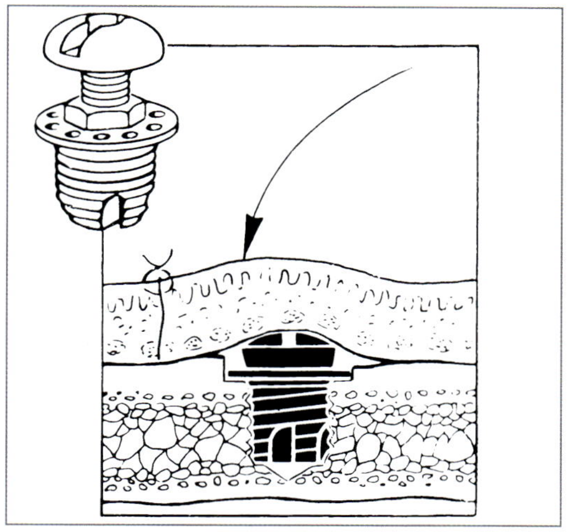

Fig. 5-16 Schematic of the short-flanged endosseous implant placement and cover screw at first stage of surgery. (Modified from Tjellstrom [1985][60] with permission.)

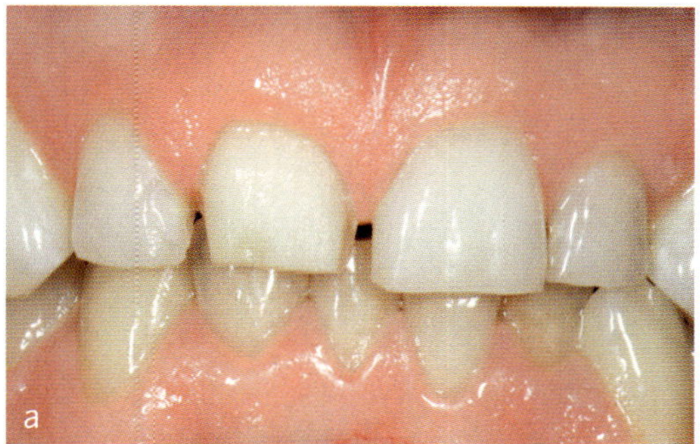

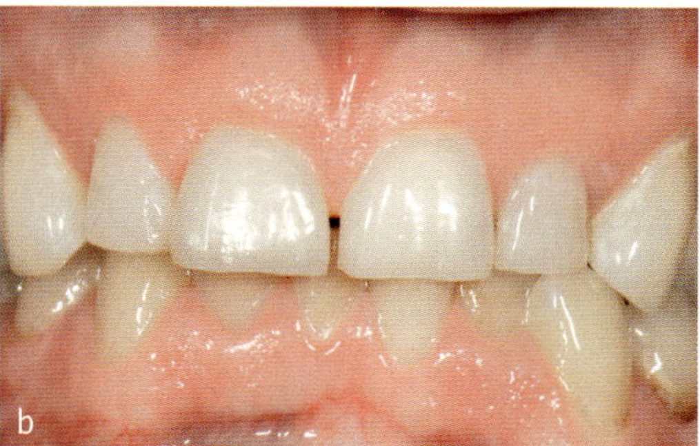

Fig. 5-17 (a) Ceramic veneer preparation in tooth enamel. **(b)** Completed ceramic veneer luted to acid-etched enamel. (Courtesy of KA Malament.)

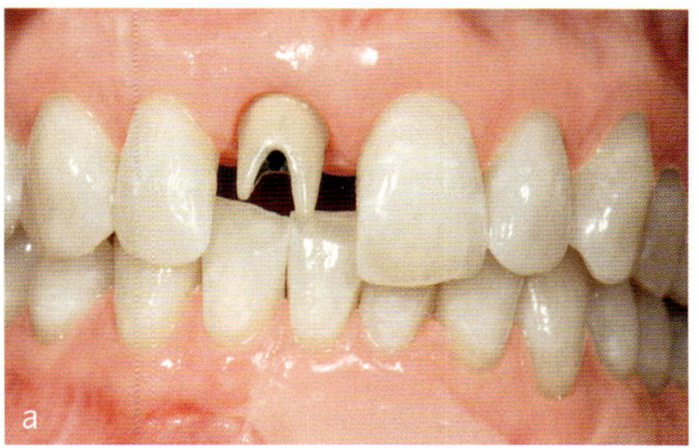

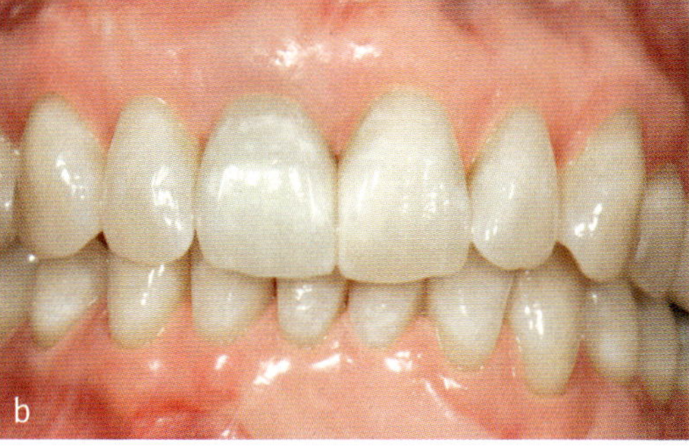

Fig. 5-18 (a) Metal-ceramic custom abutment for large screw access opening. Implant placed following central incisor extraction and bone graft to site. **(b)** Completed all-ceramic crown luted to metal-ceramic custom abutment. (Courtesy of KA Malament.)

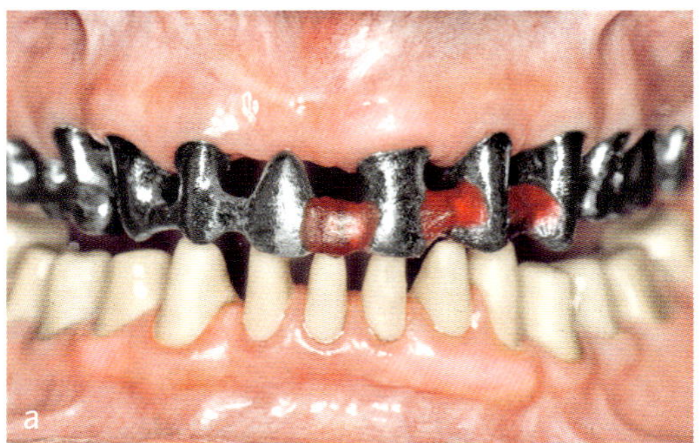
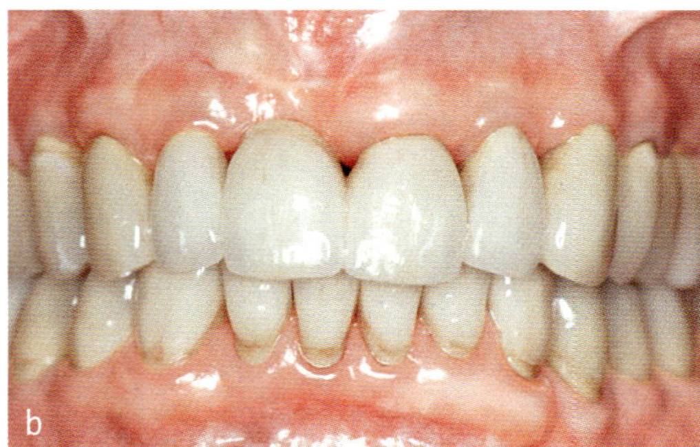

Fig. 5-19 (a) Clinical situation requiring complete maxillary and mandibular reconstruction. Maxillary framework for metal-ceramic restoration. Mandibular restorations alumina all-ceramic. **(b)** Completed reconstruction. Ceramic restorations as either metal or alumina cores have feldspathic ceramics overlaid on the cores. Completed restorations are bilayered ceramics. (Courtesy of KA Malament.)

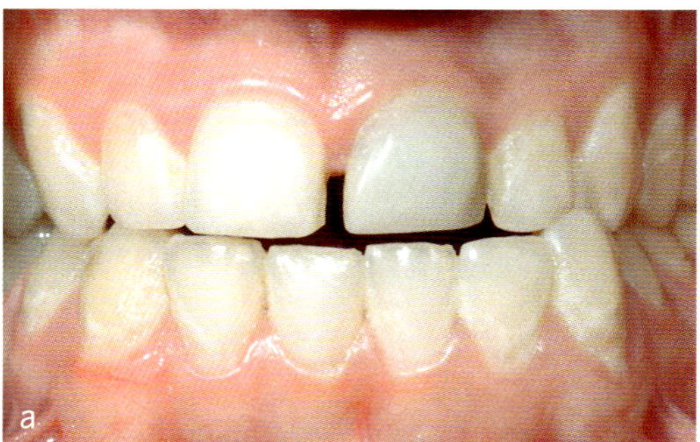
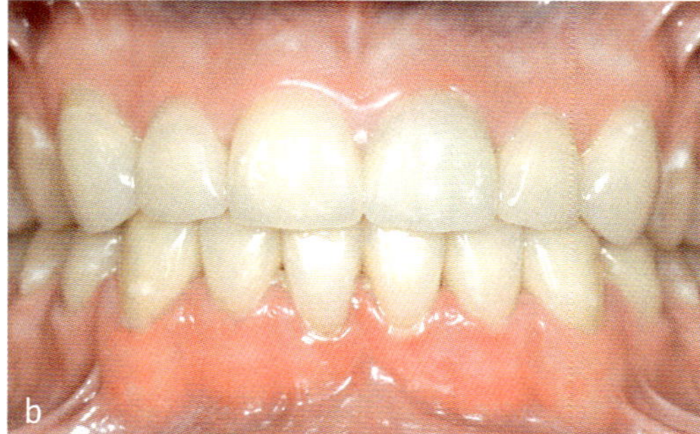

Fig. 5-20 (a) Patient requiring orthodontic therapy and complete tooth coverage restorations for treatment of extensive caries. **(b)** Completed maxillary and mandibular anterior are ceramic restorations. (Courtesy of KA Malament.)

bilayer all-ceramic crown-luting systems (Fig. 5-19). Factors involved include the resistance to crack (fracture) initiation and propagation, as influenced by physical properties; material thickness; crown/tooth geometry; cement modulus and lute thickness; damage induced by shaping, manufacture, surface treatments and clinical adjustments; and fatigue in a wet environment.

Gold restorations continue to demonstrate excellent long-term clinical performance because of, among other factors, their intimate margin adaptation. As with gold restorations, most ceramics exhibit a positive biologic response. They resist the adverse effects associated with colonization by microorganisms in the intraoral environment, since minimal pellicle and plaque adheres to highly glazed ceramic materials.[32] All-ceramic materials exhibit little, if any, of the physical degradation that might adversely affect tissue response (Fig. 5-20).

High-strength ceramic materials are often crystalline or biphasic, resulting in altered coloration and opacity. This requires veneering porcelain to mask the strong core material; however, each element of the resulting bilayer exhibits different properties and behaviors. Application of layering and veneering materials to achieve suitable shade match requires technical skill (Fig. 5-21). The bilayer of the high-strength all-ceramic crown restoration is similar to the structure of the natural tooth, in which enamel is attached to the vital dentin layer. This is significant for long-term function, since cracks generally initiate in the fit (high-tensile

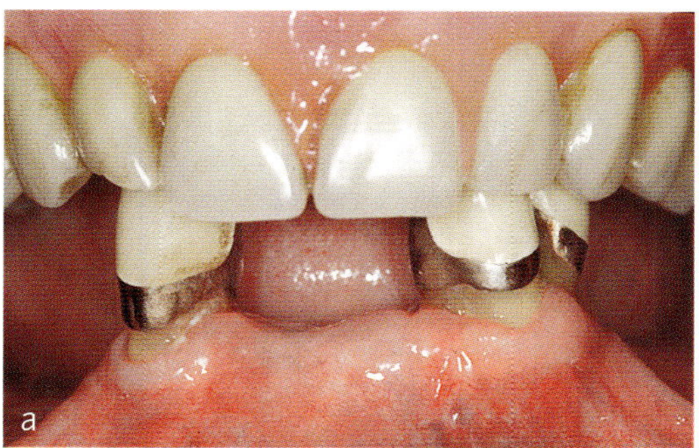

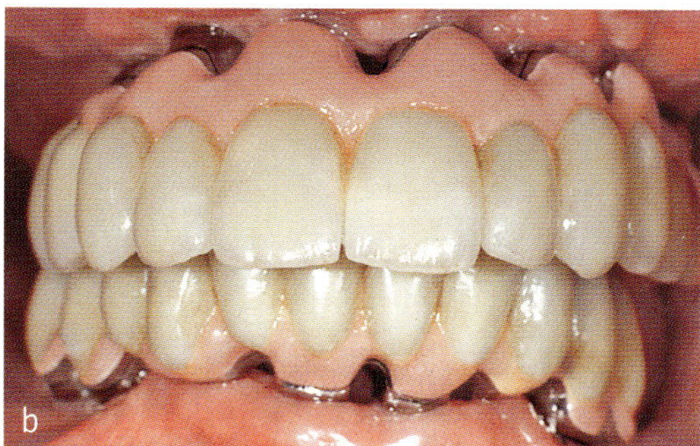

Fig. 5-21 (a) Edentulous maxilla with remaining mandibular teeth severely periodontally involved and requiring removal. **(b)** Completed maxillary and mandibular metal-ceramic implant-supported restorations. Gingival and tooth-colored feldspathic ceramics were used in the construction. (Courtesy of KA Malament.)

stress) surface of the crown, whether it is constructed in layers or as a ceramic monolith.[33] Once a crack initiates, it propagates typically unnoticed until catastrophic failure occurs.

While it is widely believed that the use of a ceramic material with enhanced physical properties will significantly increase the long-term survival of all-ceramic restorations, this is not always the case.[34] Investigators have used various methods to measure 'strength factors;'[35] yet without accounting for toughness and crack resistance, the tests may provide little insight into clinical performance.

Ultimately, any ceramic restoration is at its best prior to placement, after which the restoration must withstand wear, crack propagation, torsional forces, microbiological contamination, continued fatigue and accumulated damage.[36] All-ceramic bilayered restorations of feldspathic ceramic fused to alumina or zirconia, and produced by computer-aided design and manufacture, are becoming more popular.[37] Previously, three ceramic materials have been used extensively: IPS Empress,[36-40] In-Ceram[41] and Dicor.[42-44] These ceramic materials were developed with differing formulations and physical properties, along with research to monitor long-term survival of different types of restoration in large patient populations over extended periods of time. Survival data[45-50] have shown that restorations of these ceramic materials had least favorable performance when used to restore molar teeth.

Vision 2020

The repair and replacement of natural teeth will continue because of trauma, disease, congenital conditions and lack of patient motivation to maintain their dentition. The prevalence of tooth loss, in particular loss resulting in edentulism, will decline in the general population but will continue to exist in low-income and poorly educated and motivated sectors. Unless some spectacular breakthrough occurs in the development of materials and in laboratory or clinical procedures, the lost wax-casting technique will continue to provide the basis for framework construction for fixed and removable prostheses for the foreseeable future. Digital innovations can be foreseen to augment, or for certain applications replace existing equipment and instruments in the laboratory. Improvements in the strength, cost, versatility and esthetic properties of restorative materials will occur over time. Electronically enhanced articulator simulation of mandibular movements, to facilitate the development of specific occlusal schemes in the laboratory, remains a goal.

Further research and development will determine the extent of ongoing improvements in treatment outcomes. In recent years, improved data-collection methods have enabled dental treatment protocols to become more evidence-based. Patient satisfaction and their assessment of the functional and esthetic treatment outcomes have gained importance as factors in determining the success of treatments. Therefore, new, enhanced means of documenting treatment outcomes will be developed to meet patient expectations better and, in turn, will increase the evidence base of the clinical practice of prosthodontics.

A prediction of continued progress in prosthodontic diagnostic methods, treatment planning and clinical practice over the next decade can be made without hesitation. Advancements will be more significant and rapid in some areas than in others. For example, recent developments in electronics have resulted in digital applications for chairside clinical and diagnostic procedures, laboratory processes and product development.

Diagnosis and treatment planning have become more precise because of improved imaging technology and equipment. The charge-coupled device and the complementary metal-oxide semiconductor are the most commonly used image receptors in direct digital systems.[51] A primary advantage of these systems is the immediate display of the captured image. This permits the clinician to determine the acceptability of the image and allows the patient better understanding of their dental status in real-time. Both intra-and extraoral applications of the equipment are available; however, the cost of the equipment can be considerable compared with conventional film-based systems. In a 2005 survey of dental practitioners, some 25% of the respondents reported using some form of digital radiographic systems, while another 18% were planning to purchase digital equipment in the following year.[51] Improved equipment and increased use should ultimately reduce costs to both the clinician and the patient, while providing a more timely and effective service.

Virtual reality software will provide a chairside educational opportunity for patients to understand the conditions in their mouths, become educated as to causes and possible solutions to their problems, and compare potential changes in form and function based on possible interventions.[52] Communication among care providers can be expedited, which could ultimately enhance the integration of dentistry into a more holistic healthcare system. The potential of these diagnostic and treatment planning adjuncts cannot be overstated.

Electronic technology has led to the computer-aided design and manufacture of various abutment and crown restorations. This technology has seen increasing use for laboratory procedures. While this concept has frequently been used in prosthodontic practice, not many clinicians have yet accepted impression-recording techniques by means of digital devices.[53] The digital method seems to be simpler to use, with less material and paraphernalia required for its application. The cost of equipment purchase and its complexity have, however, discouraged some from adopting the technique, even though savings on time and material could pay for the equipment in approximately three years. The procedure involves a learning curve, and while the accuracy seems comparable to conventional methods and materials, intraoral camera use can be uncomfortable for some patients, and data on equipment maintenance are not yet available.

Continued improvements in dental ceramics can be expected. The recent significant advances driven by materials science, industry and skilled clinicians provide the impetus for further research and development in this aspect of prosthodontics. This trend can be expected because of the increased interest in predictability and versatility of fixed restorations supported by both teeth and endosseous implants. Patient demand for more lifelike esthetic restorations in an appearance-conscious trendy society is not likely to wane.

The progress in endosseous implant-supported prosthetic restorations over the past quarter of a century has been remarkable. This restorative technique will continue to expand while undergoing ongoing improvements. Titanium has been acknowledged to be a biocompatible material for implantation in bone, with favorable soft tissue response at sites where implants breach the oral mucosa. Implant strength sufficient to support appropriately designed prosthetic restorations has been demonstrated during long-term functional loading. Monitoring of the osseointegration status appears to be an achievable clinical goal, such that guidelines could be developed to provide guidance on implant size, type and surface coating for particular bone densities, prosthesis configuration and anticipated load.[52]

Furthermore, postprosthetic monitoring would enable the regular assessment of integration strength in response to specific prosthesis design and loading mode.

The desire of both patients and clinicians to reduce the time necessary for successful completion of treatment involving implants has prompted a trend in immediate restoration placement with immediate or early loading. To accomplish these goals, bone of optimal quality and quantity is needed. Approximate host site determination has been enhanced by affordable three-dimensional imaging, and implant placement procedures have been rationalized with added precision using computer-driven intra-active navigational methods and prefabricated surgical guides.[10] In selected situations, less-invasive surgical procedures involving flapless methods can be employed.

In response to the objective of expediting bone healing, an emphasis on implant surface preparation and characteristics has emerged. Immediate or early implant loading with certain prostheses has successfully been achieved with roughened implant surfaces, compared with longer periods required for the osseointegration of turned or machined surfaces. Current interest has focused on nanotechnology, which has been defined as 'research and technology development at the atomic, molecular, or macromolecular levels, in the length scale of approximately 1-100 nanometer range, to provide a fundamental understanding of phenomena and materials at the nanoscale and to create and use structures, devices and systems that have novel properties and functions because of their small and/or intermediate size'.[55] Recent studies involving nanotechnology have revealed the influence of nanoscale surface topography, or nanotextures, on cell behavior, suggesting that the osseointegration process could be managed by implant surface treatments employing this technology.[56] Prosthodontic researchers have hypothesized that titanium implants with varied topographic surfaces could affect gene expression not usually involved in bone wound healing.[55,56] Thus, titanium implants with specific surface preparation could directly affect the initiation and progress of the osseointegration process when inserted into bone.

Surface topography management in combination with the administration at the implant site of bioactive substances related to bone morphogenetic proteins to promote bone healing represent an active phase of investigation with promise for future implant generations. The importance of these investigations to the advancement of prosthodontics cannot be overstated.

The dental community generally has previously resisted embracing implant dentistry because of historical reports of implant failures. Since the early 1980s, however, impressive long-term clinical data have provided sufficient evidence to demonstrate scientifically the predictability of titanium endosseous implants. With improved knowledge and understanding of implants through new and expanded programs of education, more prosthodontists and dental practitioners in general will accept the proven implant concept and utilize implant-assisted prosthetic restorations. Patient demand for these services will increase, providing third-party financial support becomes available for a greater population of patients in need of prosthodontic care.

Preventive measures to limit tooth loss and minimally invasive procedures to improve the preservation of tooth structure and reduce tooth loss continue to be desirable goals in restorative dentistry. Beyond the implant era, tissue engineering could provide promise for the future. Until tissue and organ stem cell research has advanced to a more predictable phase, the growth and maturation of tooth buds in situ remains a distant goal for tooth replacement.

Acknowledgement

The text and illustrations pertaining to ceramics were provided by Dr Kenneth A. Malament, who is in specialty private practice in Boston, MA, USA, and is also a Clinical Professor, Department of Graduate Prosthodontics, Tufts University School of Dental Medicine, Boston, MA, USA.

References

1. Glossary of prosthodontic terms. J Prosthet Dent 2005; 94: 10–92.
2. Johnson WW. The history of prosthetic dentistry. J Prosthet Dent 1959;9:841–946.
3. Laney WR. Prosthodontics: a historical perspective. J Prosthodont 1997;6:2–6.
4. Brånemark P-I, Zarb GA, Albrektsson T. Tissue-integrated prosthesis: osseointegration in clinical dentistry. Chicago, IL: Quintesssence, 1985:350.
5. Sanders AE, Slade GD, Carter KD, Stewart JF. Trends in prevalence of tooth loss among Australians 1979–2002. Aust N Z J Public Health 2004;8:549–554.
6. Suominen-Taipole AL, Alanen P, Helenius H, Nordblad A, Utela A. Edentulism among Finnish adults of working age, 1978–1997. Community Dent Oral Epidemiol 1999;27: 353–365.
7. Zitzman NU, Hagman Z, Weiger R. What is the prevalence of various types of prosthetic dental restorations in Europe? Clin Oral Implant Res 2007;18(Suppl 3):20–33.
8. Caplan DJ, Weintraub JA. The oral health burden in the United States: a summary of recent epidemiologic studies. J Dent Educ 1993;57:853–862.
9. Douglas CW. The role of specialists and general practitioners in provision of prosthodontic services. J Prosthet Dent 1983;50:844–852.
10. Triplett RG. Current Issues Forum. CT-generated surgical guides and flapless surgery. Int J Oral Maxillofac Implants 2008;23:195.
11. Jensen OT. The Sinus Bone Graft, 2nd edn. Chicago, IL: Quintessence, 2006:366.
12. Jensen OT, Laster Z, Hibi H, Yamada Y, Ueda M. Alveolar distraction osteogenesis and tissue engineering. In: Lynch SE, Marx R, Nevins M, Wisner-Lynch L (eds). Tissue engineering 2nd edn, Ch. 14. Chicago, IL: Quintessence, 2008:296.
13. Brudvik JS. Advanced removable partial dentures. Chicago: Quintessence, 1999:164.
14. Mensor MG. Attachments for the overdenture. In: Brewer A, Morrow R (eds). Overdentures, 2nd edn. St Louis, MO: Mosby, 1980:162–190.
15. Preiskel HW. Overdentures Made Easy. London: Quintessence, 1996:248.
16. Krennmaier G, Krainhofer M, Piehslinger E. Implant supported maxillary overdentures retained with milled bars: maxillary anterior versus maxillary posterior concept. A retrospective study. Int J Oral Maxillofac Implants 2008; 23:343–352.
17. Chan W-YF, Nahri TO, de Baat C, Kalk W. Treatment of the atrophic maxilla with implant-supported overdentures: a review of the literature. Int J Prosthodont 1998;11:7–15.
18. Sillard R. Fixed removable dental implant system. US Patent No. 4, 921.016, June 5, 1990.
19. Toljanic JA, Antoniou D. Clark RS, Graham L. A longitudinal clinical assessment of spark erosion technology in implant retained overdenture prosthesis. A preliminary report. J Prosthet Dent 1997;78:490–495.
20. Van Roekel NB. Prosthesis fabrication using electrical discharge machining. Int J Oral Maxillofac Implants 1992; 7:56–61.
21. Douglas CW, Gammon MD, Atwood DA. Need and effective demand for prosthodontic treatment. J Prosthet Dent 1988;59:94–104.
22. Eckert SE, Wollan PC. Retrospective review of 1170 endosseous implants placed in partially edentulous jaws. J Prosthet Dent 1998;79:415–421.
23. State of the Science on Implant Dentistry Consensus Conference Proceedings, Section 3 Report. Int J Oral Maxillofac Implants 2007;22(Suppl):71–95.
24. State of the Science on Implant Dentistry Consensus Conference Proceedings, Section 1 Report. Int J Oral Maxillofac Implants 2007;22(Suppl):19–45.
25. Cronin RJ, Cagna DR. An update on fixed prosthodontics. J Am Dent Assoc 1997;128:425–436.
26. Lindquist E, Karlsson S. Success and failures for fixed partial dentures after 20 years service. Part 1. Int J Prosthodont 11; 2:133–138.
27. Laney WR. Restoration of acquired oral and paraoral defects. In: Laney WR, Gibilisco JA (eds). Diagnosis and Treatment in Prosthodontics, Ch. 15. Philadephia, PA: Lea and Febiger, 1983:377–446.
28. Laney WR. Restoration of congenital oral and paraoral defects. In: Laney WR, Gibilisco JA (eds). Diagnosis and Treatment in Prosthodontics, Ch. 16. Philadephia, PA: Lea and Febiger, 1983:447–505.
29. Toljanic JA, Eckert SE, Roumanas E, Beumer J, Huryn JM, Zlotlow IM et al. Osseointegrated craniofacial implants in the rehabilitation of orbital defects. An update of retrospective experiences in the United States. J Prosthet Dent 2005;94:177–182.
30. Kelly JR, Nishimura I, Campbell SD. Ceramics in dentistry: historical roots and current perspectives. J Prosthet Dent 1996;75:18–32.
31. McLean J. Evolution of dental ceramics in the twentieth century. J Prosthet Dent 2001;85:61–66.
32. Savitt ED, Malament KA, Socransky SS, Melcher AJ, Backman KJ. Effects on colonization of oral microbiota by a cast glass-ceramic restoration. Int J Periodontics Restorative Dent 1987;7:22–35.

33. Kelly JR, Campbell SD. Fracture surface analysis of dental ceramics. J Prosthet Dent 1989;62:536–541.
34. Rekow ED, Zhang Y, Thompson VP. Can materials properties predict survival of all-ceramic posterior crowns. Compend Contin Educ Dent 2007;28:352–369.
35. Lawn BR, Beng YD, Thompson VP. Use of contact testing in characterization of all-ceramic crown like layer structures. A review. J Prosthet Dent 2001;86:495–451.
36. Zhang Y, Lawn BR, Malament KA, Thompson VP, Rekow ED. Damage accumulation and fatigue life of particle abraded ceramics. Int J Prosthodont 2006; 19:442.
37. Witkowski S. CAD-CAM in dental technology. Quintessence. J Dent Technol 2005;28:169–184.
38. Dong JK, Luthy H, Wohlwend A, Sharer P. Heat-pressed. Int J Prosthodont 1992;4:9–16.
39. Fradeani M, Barducci G. Versatility of Empress restorations. Part 1: crowns. J Esthet Dent 1996;3:30–38.
40. Wohlwend A, Sharer P. Die-Empress-Technik. Quintessenz Z 1990:16:966.
41. Sadoun M. In Ceram: Zukenftige entwicklung mit In Ceram. In: Kappert HF (ed.) Volkeramik, Werkstoffkunde Zahntechnik, Klinische Erfahung. Berlin: Quintessenz, 1996:227–229.
42. Adair PJ, Grossman DG. The castable ceramic crown. Int J Periodontics Restorative Dent 1984;4:33–46.
43. Malament KA. The Dicor castable ceramic crown. In: Rhoads JE, Rudd KD, Morrow RM (eds). Dental Laboratory Procedures: Fixed Partial Dentures. St Louis, MO: Mosby, 1985:315–330.
44. Malament KA, Grossman DG. The cast glass-ceramic restoration. J Prosthet Dent 1987;57:674–683.
45. Fradeani M, Redemangi M. An 11-year clinical evaluation of leucite-reinforced glass ceramic crowns: a retrospective study. Quintessence Int 2002;33:503–510.
46. Haselton DR, Diaz-Arnold AM, Hillis SL. Clinical assessment of high strength all-ceramic crowns. J Prosthet Dent 83:397–404.
47. Malament KA, Socransky SS. Survival of Dicor glass-ceramic dental restorations over 14 years: Part 1. Survival of Dicor complete coverage restorations and effect of internal surface acid etching, tooth position, gender and age. J Prosthet Dent 1999;8:23–32.
48. Malament KA, Socransky SS. Survival of Dicor glass-ceramic dental restorations over 14 years: Part 2. Effect of thickness of Dicor material and design of tooth preparation. J Prosthet Dent 1999;81:662–667.
49. Malament KA, Socransky SS. Survival of Dicor glass-ceramic restorations over 16 years. Part 3. Effect of luting agent and tooth or tooth substrate core structure. J Prosthet Dent 2001;86:511–519.
50. McLaren EA. White SN. Survival of In Ceram crowns in private practice: a prospective clinical trial. J Prosthet Dent 2000;83:216–222.
51. Parks ED. Digital radiographic imaging. Is the dental practice ready? J Am Dent Assoc 2008;139:477–481.
52. Bauer JC, Brown WT. The digital transformation of oral health care. J Am Dent Assoc 2001;132:204–209.
53. Christensen GJ. The challenge to conventional impressions. J Am Dent Assoc 2008;139:347–349.
54. Dario DJ, Cucchiaro PJ, Deluzio AJ. Electronic monitoring of dental implant osseointegration. J Am Dent Assoc 2002;133:483–490.
55. Beumer J. Exploring the determinants of osseointegration: interview with Drs Ichiro Nishimura and Tahahiro Ogawa. Int J Prosthodont 2008;2:103–106.
56. Nishimura I, Huang Y, Butz F, Ogawa T, Lin A, Wang CJ. Discrete deposition of hydroxyapatite nanoparticles on a titanium implant with predisposing substrate microtopography accelerated osseointegration. Nanotechnology 2007;18:245101.
57. Preti G. Prosthetic Rehabilitation. London: Quintessence, 2008.
58. Carr AB, McGivney GP, Brown DT. McCraken's Removable Partial Prosthodontics. 11th edition. St Louis: Mosby, 2005.
59. Chaiyabutr Y, Brudvik J. Removable partial denture design using milled abutment surfaces and minimal soft tissue coverage for periodontally compromised teeth: a clinical report. J Prosthet Dent 2008;99:263-266.
60. Tjellstrom A. Other applications of osseointegrated implants. In: Brånemark P-I, Zarb GA, Albrektsson T. Tissue-integrated prosthesis: osseointegration in clinical dentistry. Chicago, IL: Quintesssence, 1985:350.

CHAPTER 6

Periodontology

Mariano Sanz

Definition

Periodontology is the science within dentistry that studies the tooth supporting tissues and implants in health and in disease.

Clinical periodontology involves the diagnosis, prevention and therapy of the diseases affecting the periodontium and procedures in the placements and maintenance of dental implants (Fig. 6-1).

The American Academy of Periodontology (AAP) in its glossary of terms[1] defines *periodontics* as the branch of dentistry that specializes in treating the supporting tissues of the teeth and in the placement, maintenance and treatment of dental implants. The AAP, therefore, differentiates between the science *(periodontology)* and practice *(periodontics)* of the specialty. In contrast, the European Federation of Periodontology (EFP) uses only the term periodontology, embracing both the study and the management of periodontal conditions and dental implants.

The AAP was founded in 1914 and has been the leading organization in periodontology, establishing, over the years, standards in periodontal education and practice that have shaped and facilitated the development of the specialty. The EFP was founded in 1990 as the umbrella organization embracing the national periodontal scientific societies from most European countries. Since its foundation, the EFP has successfully promoted

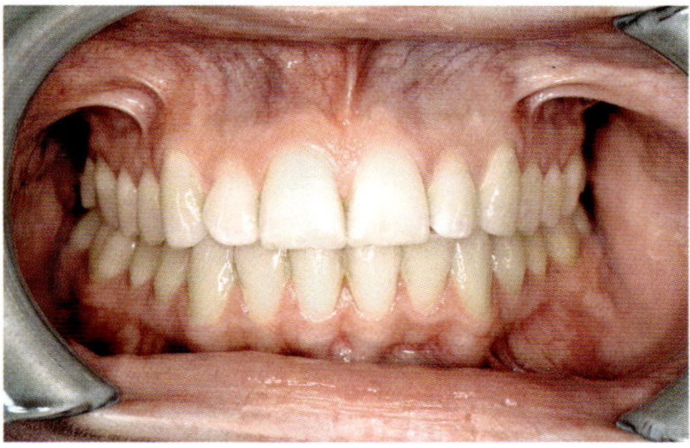

Fig. 6-1 Periodontology is the science within dentistry that studies the tooth supporting tissues and implants in health and in disease. The periodontium is the functional unit composed of the gingiva, the cementum, the periodontal ligament and the alveolar bone.

periodontal health and developed high standards of periodontal education in Europe.

Periodontology is one of the major oral health sciences. It was recognized as a dental specialty in the USA by the American Dental Association in 1947. In Europe, periodontology is also recognized as a specialty of dentistry in most of the countries of the European Union. As a distinct branch of dentistry, periodontology has achieved major developments both in education and research since the early 1970s. At the most recent international congresses on dental research (general sessions of the International Association for Dental Research, meetings of the Pan European Federation, and meetings of the American Association for Dental Research), almost 25% of the abstracts were related to periodontal research. Through sustained efforts in research, major breakthroughs have been made in different areas, including microbiology, identifying and sequencing the genome of specific periodontal pathogens as etiological factors in the initiation and progression of periodontal diseases, elucidating the inflammatory immune response and the mechanisms involved in tissue destruction, and describing the role of various risk factors in conferring individual periodontal disease susceptibility. Key advances have also been made in diagnosis and therapy, mostly in the field of tissue engineering and bone regeneration, with the development of therapeutic approaches intended to regenerate the tissues lost as a consequence of periodontitis. Also, the availability of osseointegrated implants since the early 1980s, with excellent long-term survival, has resulted in effective treatment options to restore the dentition in fully and partially edentulous patients, let alone in individuals in need of functional rehabilitation as a consequence of severe destructive periodontitis. Periodontology has played a key role in the expansion of the use of oral implants, from both a research and a clinical point of view. This may be appreciated when reviewing the expertise and interests of the major authors in the field and the membership of the editorial boards of the most prestigious scientific journals in implant dentistry.

Another major development in periodontology in recent years derives from information obtained from epidemiological population studies, which have demonstrated that periodontitis may increase the risk of various conditions, including osteoporosis, diabetes mellitus, pulmonary infections, preterm low birthweight, cardiovascular diseases, infections in various locations in the body and death. While the causal relationships between periodontitis and systemic conditions have not yet been proven in well-designed intervention trials, periodontitis has been shown to be associated with atherosclerosis, acute myocardial heart infarction, stroke and premature birth. These associations may pose an enormous challenge to public health systems, with priorities including reductions in cardiovascular disease and perinatal complications; specifically, there is a need to develop and train dental workforces further in preventing and managing existing levels of periodontal disease, notably in aging and disease-prone populations.

Historical milestones

Gingival and periodontal diseases, in their various forms, have afflicted humans since the dawn of history. Evidence of destructive periodontal disease, as indicated by bone loss, has been found in early humans in such diverse cultures as existed in ancient Egypt and early pre-Columbian America. Indeed, periodontal diseases were the most common of all diseases found in the embalmed bodies of the ancient Egyptians. Ancient Chinese and Indian medical scripts also considered periodontal diseases and possible remedies, recognizing, in particular, the importance of oral hygiene. In the classical world, Hippocrates discussed the etiology of periodontal disease, indicating that inflammation of the gums was caused by the accumulation of calculus.

In 1632, Anton van Leeuwenhoek in Holland was the first to describe the oral bacterial flora, based on microscopic examinations of scrapings from his own mouth. Modern dentistry did not begin to develop in Europe until the eighteenth century.

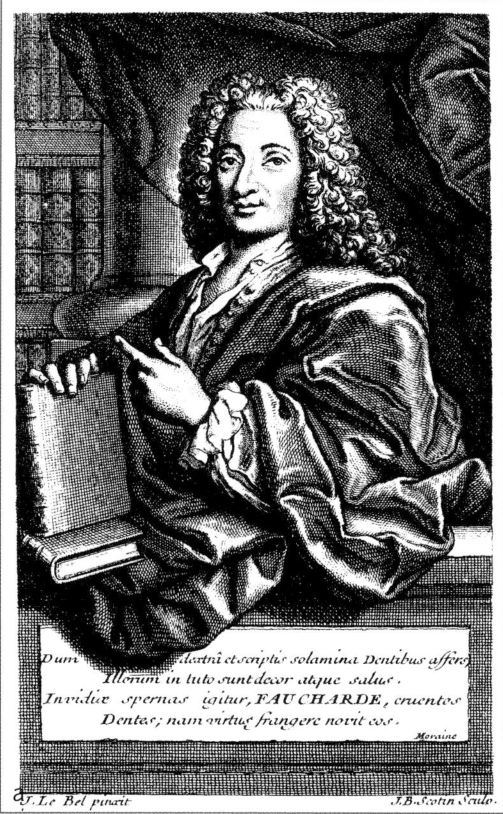

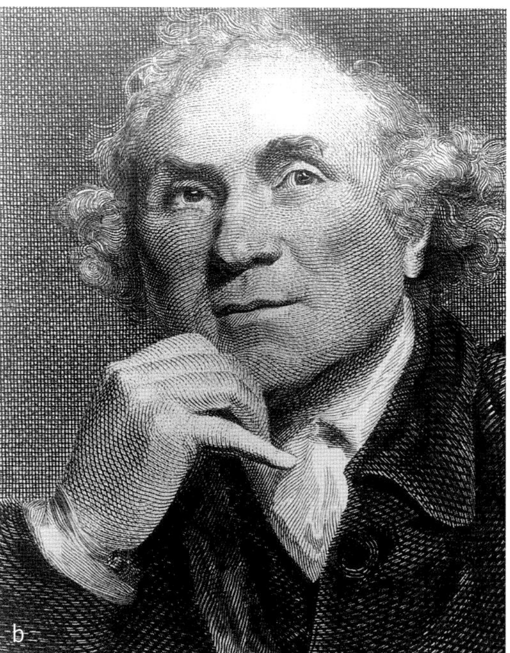

Fig. 6-2 (a and b) Pierre Fauchard (left) and John Hunter (right) are regarded as the founders of the dental profession. Their books established core knowledge in early dentistry by describing the features and treatments of known oral diseases, including periodontal diseases. (Reproduced from Carranza F, Shklar G (eds). History of Periodontology. Chicago, IL: Quintessence Publishing, 2003.)

Pierre Fauchard and John Hunter are regarded as the founders of the dental profession, being the authors, respectively, of 'Le Cirugien Dentiste' and 'The Natural History of the Human Teeth' (Fig. 6-2). These books established core knowledge in early dentistry by describing the features and treatments of known oral diseases, including periodontal diseases. It was not until the nineteenth century, however, that periodontology was established as a distinctive branch of dentistry. John Riggs, in the USA, was the leading authority in the field. As a consequence, certain conditions affecting the periodontium were, for many years, termed Rigg's disease. In the second half of the nineteenth century, three discoveries changed the practice of dentistry in general and of periodontology in particular: the discovery of anesthesia by Horace Wells, the description of the germ theory of disease by Louis Pasteur and the discovery of radiography by Wilhelm Röntgen. Together, these discoveries underpinned new understanding of oral diseases and the development of a rationale for their diagnosis and therapy.[2]

In the first third of the twentieth century, the Vienna school developed the histopathologic concepts of periodontal diseases that remain valid to this day. Bernhard Gottlieb and Balint Orban published extensive microscopic studies on periodontal conditions in humans, describing in detail periodontal tissues in health and disease. These authors emigrated to the USA in the 1940s, contributing greatly to the progress of periodontology in North America. An important group in Germany, led by Weski and Neumann, together with Widman in Sweden, developed and refined the surgical approach to periodontal therapy.[3]

The USA and Sweden led the field in basic and clinical periodontal research in the second half of the twentieth century. In the USA, Irving Glickman, Henry Goldman, Sigurd Ramfjord and Helmut Zander advanced understanding of the disease processes, together with evidence-based approaches to periodontal therapy.[2]

The modern era in studies of pathogenesis, prevention and treatment of periodontal diseases began in the mid-1960s, with human and animal experimental evidence demonstrating the critical role of bacteria in the initiation of gingivitis and periodontitis. In Scandinavia, Jens Waerhaugh, followed by Harald Löe and Jan Lindhe, showed that bacteria in dental plaque and the immunological response to these microorganisms were the key factors in periodontal disease pathogenesis. This work, together with related clinical studies, formed the basis of modern periodontal therapy. The classical experimental gingivitis study by Löe et al. (1967)[4] clearly demonstrated a cause–effect relationship between plaque accumulation and the development of gingivitis. The longitudinal clinical studies conducted in Sweden by Jan Lindhe and colleagues[3] and in Michigan by Sigurd Ramfjord and colleagues[5] clearly demonstrated that periodontitis progression can be arrested by therapy and the results of therapy can be maintained long term, provided the patient complies with effective preventive and related therapeutic measures. These workers also showed that gingivitis may be prevented by effective plaque control, which, in turn, prevents the initiation of periodontitis.

During the twentieth century, periodontal microbiology was studied in depth. In the first part of the century, microbiologists, relying on the culture methods available at that time, believed that certain microorganisms, including amoebae and streptococci, were the primary etiologic agents of periodontal disease. The concept of specific causative bacteria was soon discarded. Subsequent research, conducted in the 1970s and early 1980s, implicated bacterial plaque deposits as the primary causation of gingivitis and periodontitis. Socransky in the USA and Slots in Europe undertook pioneering studies, demonstrating that bacteria isolated from periodontal pockets in different periodontal conditions were distinct. Subsequently, longitudinal studies in the 1980s provided further evidence that specific bacteria were associated with sites of active disease progression. At the 1996 World Workshop in Periodontics, the leaders in the field at the time agreed that only a few of the more than 500 different bacteria present in the oral flora were significantly associated with the etiology of periodontitis. These included *Aggregatibacter actinomycetemcomitans* (previously *Actinobacillus actinomycetemcomitans*), *Porphyromonas gingivalis*, *Tannerella forsythia* (previously *Tannerella forsythensis*) and *Treponema denticola* (Fig. 6-3).[6] In recent years, periodontal microbiology has focused on studying the ways in which these pathogenic microorganisms are organized within the subgingival microflora. These bacterial species adhere to the tooth surfaces and are organized in a complex structure – the dental plaque – which is considered now as an example of a biofilm.[7] Bacteria within these highly organized communities live adhered to dental surfaces, in close juxtaposition to periodontal tissues and well protected from the natural antibacterial defense mechanisms. These bacterial communities behave differently to individual bacteria and bacteria in a planktonic state. This behavior accentuates their pathogenicity and self-protection. The biofilm concept has prompted a change in the classical approach to diagnosis and antimicrobial therapy in periodontology (Fig. 6-4).[8]

The twentieth century also brought major advances in the understanding of the role of the susceptible host in the pathogenesis of periodontitis. For most of the century, periodontal investigators focused primarily on periodontal pockets in an attempt to understand how and why these defects form. This knowledge, derived mostly

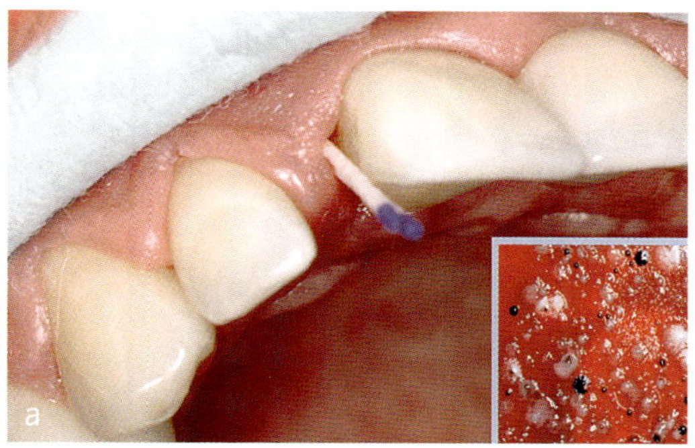
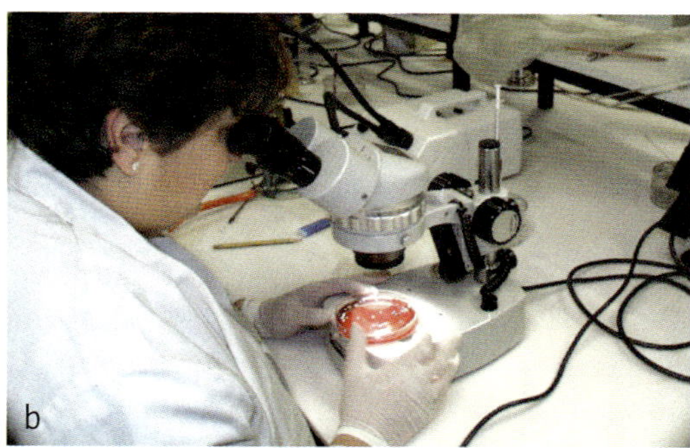
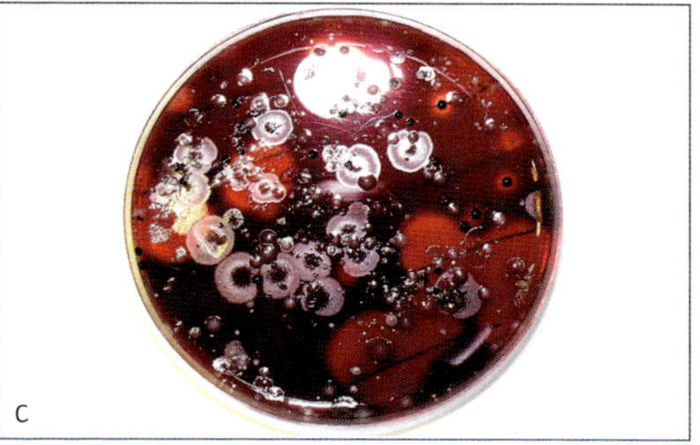

Fig. 6-3 (a to c) Anaerobic culture of a subgingival plaque sample showing specific periodontal pathogens, including *Porphyromona gingivalis*, *Prevotella intermedia*, *Peptostreptococcus micros* and *Fusobacterium nucleatum*.

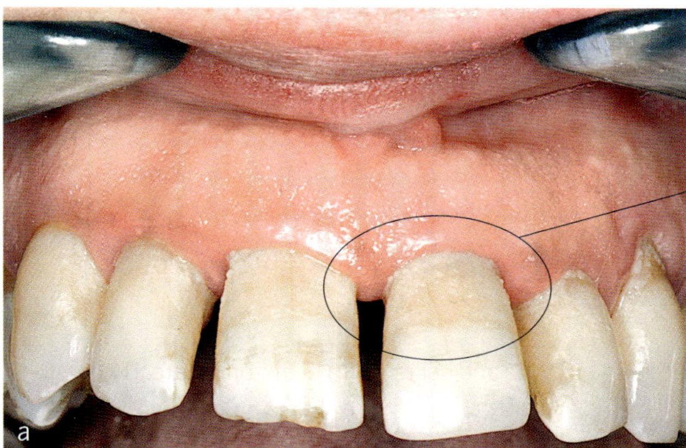
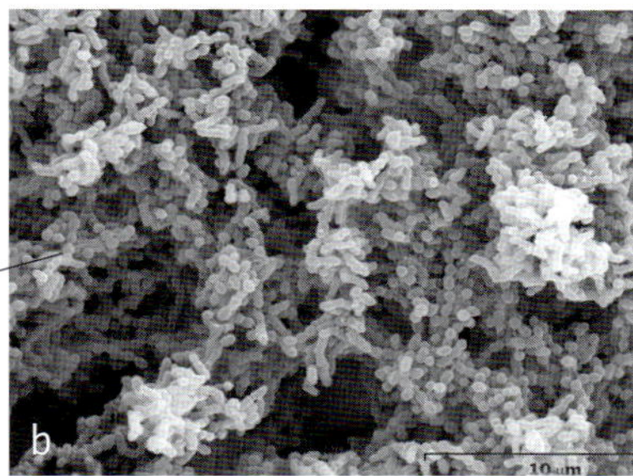

Fig. 6-4 Bacteria within biofilms are structured in organized communities that adhere to dental surfaces, in close juxtaposition to periodontal tissues and well protected from natural antibacterial defenses. The behavior of these bacteria differs from that of individual bacteria, accentuating their pathogenicity and self-protection.

from descriptive studies of animal and human biopsy material, lacked the understanding of the dynamics of the initiation and progression of periodontal disease. Around the 1970s, a major shift in emphasis occurred when researchers began to study the cells, enzymes and mediators involved in the host response against the microbial challenge. The critical role of the innate response to plaque, mainly mediated by the polymorphonuclear neutrophils, became more widely recognized as a direct cause of periodontal tissue destruction.[9] Combined research in microbiology and immunology revealed that some clinical disease patterns, or phenotypes, were associated with both characteristic bacteria and a distinct host response. For example, different microbiologic and immunologic characteristics were described for localized juvenile periodontitis and chronic adult periodontitis. Concurrently, the initiation and progression of periodontitis were described in terms of distinct histopathological patterns. These provided insights into the pathogenic processes.

The extensive research undertaken through the mid-1980s led to critical refinements to the pathogenesis model, describing specific bacteria initiating the disease process by activating host responses, which could be either protective or destructive. Bacteria elicit an inflammatory and immune response in the tissues – the key factor in disease expression. In the 1990s, immunologic and molecular techniques improved, and the roles of cytokines and inflammatory cell mediators came to the forefront of the periodontal literature. Cytokines, including tumor necrosis factor-α and interleukins 1α, 1ß, 6 and 8, were studied extensively. The effects of these agents on gene expression, cell signaling and downstream actions, such as promoting the release of enzymes, prostaglandins and matrix metalloproteinases (MMPs), confirmed their role in the alterations of the connective tissue and bone metabolism characteristic of periodontitis.[9,10] Although the model describing a simple relationship between the microbial challenge and the immunologic responses may have held true when mean data were considered, remarkable variations were observed in host responses and in the clinical expression of disease from individual to individual. This individual variation was clearly demonstrated in a key longitudinal study published by Harald Löe and colleagues[11] reporting the incidence of periodontitis in a population in Sri Lanka with no plaque control. Although extensive gingivitis and progressive periodontitis developed in most individuals, only a subset of the population developed severe periodontitis in response to massive bacterial accumulations.

To add further complexity to these early conceptual models, there was a growing appreciation of the importance of genetic variation in determining the development and severity of periodontal disease. This was apparent from studies in twins; genetic influences accounted for as much as 30–60% in the clinical expression of periodontitis.[12]

The realization of the impact of genetic inheritance and the demonstrated individual variations in disease expression changed the concept that periodontal disease is a major global public health problem, affecting the majority of people over 35 years of age in a similar manner. Currently, there is a new understanding that not all subjects are equally susceptible to periodontal disease. The focus has, therefore, shifted to the study of the risk of disease, examining the role of various environmentally, acquired and inherited risk factors for periodontal disease. These factors include diabetes mellitus, use of tobacco, poor oral hygiene, specific microflora and stress.[13,14]

A key factor in periodontal disease pathogenesis is the ability of specific bacteria to evade the inflammatory and immune response, while at the same time releasing potent factors, such as lipopolysaccharides, that cause chronic inflammation and tissue destruction. This chronic inflammatory state not only affects the periodontal tissues but is also able to elicit a systemic response. This results in the release of acute phase proteins and cytokines in the serum, leading to a systemic inflammatory state that may influence other complex chronic conditions, including cardiovascular disease. The study of the association between periodontitis and systemic diseases has developed into a new field of research: periodontal medicine. This research includes epidemiological association studies, animal and laboratory investigations and intervention clinical trials designed to provide evidence that periodontitis is an independent risk factor in the development and progression of some complex systemic conditions, including diabetes, cardiovascular disease and complications in pregnancy.[15]

Treatment concepts

Current treatment concepts in the management of destructive periodontal diseases are based on existing knowledge of the etiology and pathogenesis of these conditions. There are three key elements that have clear implications in therapy.

- *Pathogenic bacteria in biofilm communities.* Periodontitis is caused by pathogenic bacterial species located in the subgingival environment. These bacterial species are organized in complex communities within a biofilm, which adheres to the tooth surfaces in close vicitinity to the periodontal tissues. Not all bacteria within the biofilm have the same pathogenic potential. There is a specific set of microbial pathogens that are endowed with potent virulence factors which enable them to colonize the subgingival microflora, to circumvent the local host defenses and to elicit a strong inflammatory response, leading to tissue destruction.[16]
- *Host response mechanisms.* Periodontal pathogens do not cause direct tissue destruction; their pathogenicity relies on the activation of host immune inflammatory mechanisms, leading to alterations in the bone and connective tissue homeostasis. This results in the destructive changes that define the periodontitis phenotype.[9]
- *Disease modifiers.* A small group of disease modifiers strongly influence the susceptibility of individual patients to periodontitis; these include smoking, genotype, obesity, stress and diabetes.[13]

The importance of the presence of known periodontal pathogens in well-organized bacterial communities, adherent to the root surface in the subgingival microenvironment, lies in the specific defense strategies that these biofilms have evolved to overcome both the natural defensive mechanisms and standard antibacterial therapies. These strategies compromise the efficacy of treatment regimens based solely on the use of chemical antibacterial compounds. These agents lack the capacity to penetrate the bacterial communities and, as a consequence, do not exert their antibacterial activity where it is required.[7]

Another important factor in pathogenesis is the host immune inflammatory response, leading to chronic inflammation. This is responsible for both tissue destruction and any systemic inflammatory state. Anti-inflammatory medication is, therefore, a valid adjunctive to periodontal therapy.[17]

Risk assessment has become a key element of periodontal diagnosis, given that individual susceptibility will eventually modulate how the host is able to control the bacterial challenge. Of the known risk factors, there are some, such as the genome, that cannot be modified and, as a consequence, are not influenced by therapeutic intervention. The control of others, however, has become a key component in modern periodontal therapy, including strategies aimed at smoking cessation, weight loss and achieving a well-controlled systemic condition.[14]

An important factor in current approaches to the treatment of destructive periodontal diseases is not only the arrest of the disease process through control of the infective and inflammatory components, but also the aim of restoring the anatomy and function of the periodontium. This approach has two main objectives: first, the regeneration of lost periodontal tissues, including cementum, connective tissue, bone and gingival attachment, mostly in interdental locations; second, the reconstruction of soft tissues, primarily where there has been localized buccal gingival recession, with the goal of restoring root coverage and obtaining a favorable esthetic outcome.

These three strategies - anti-infective, anti-inflammatory and reconstructive - will be dealt with separately in this chapter, although they must always be considered together in the treatment of a patient suffering periodontitis. The treatment plan must be based on a thorough diagnosis, including detailed examination of the patient's periodontal status, through careful probing and radiographic assessments; risk assessment, taking account of the history of tobacco use, systemic state and, in specific situations, examination of the microbial composition of the subgingival biofilm; a genotype profile; and/or a nutritional assessment and dietary analysis.

Modern epidemiological data, derived from well-designed population studies, have clearly shown that slight to moderate chronic periodontitis is prevalent in older patients, affecting more than 30% of the population over 60 years of age. Periodontitis in older patients, however, responds very well to conventional anti-infective therapy, resulting excellent long-term prognoses. The management of older patients usually does not need sophisticated diagnostic methods, surgical interventions or reconstructive techniques. In contrast, the management of severe chronic periodontitis and aggressive periodontitis, affecting a minority of the adult population (< 10%),[18] usually requires a complex diagnostic and therapeutic approach. In these patients, it is of great importance to control the etiological component: periodontal pathogens. It is, therefore, recommended that microbial diagnosis is undertaken to identify and quantify putative periodontal pathogens in the subgingival biofilm, and a careful risk assessment is carried out to assess any factors that may enhance the patient's susceptibility and influence the therapeutic interventions. In patients with periodontitis, the presence of all infrabony defects and mandibular furcations must be recorded through careful periodontal and radiographic evaluation, with the aim of considering periodontal regenerative therapy as part of the overall treatment plan.

Cause-related therapy and anti-infective strategies

The main goal of cause-related periodontal therapy is to establish proper infection control through reduction in the bacterial load to below the patient's threshold for disease. Achieving this goal involves various treatment phases:

- the establishment of an optimal self-performed plaque control regimen by means of effective oral hygiene measures
- the reduction of living bacteria in the biofilm, together with the removal of calcified deposits adhering to tooth surfaces and other retentive areas that may facilitate further biofilm accumulation
- the prevention of recurrences of periodontal disease by regular monitoring and supportive periodontal treatment.

The preventive phase is based on compliance with self-performed plaque control, mainly through the use of either a manual or a powered toothbrush, together with flossing or other methods of effective

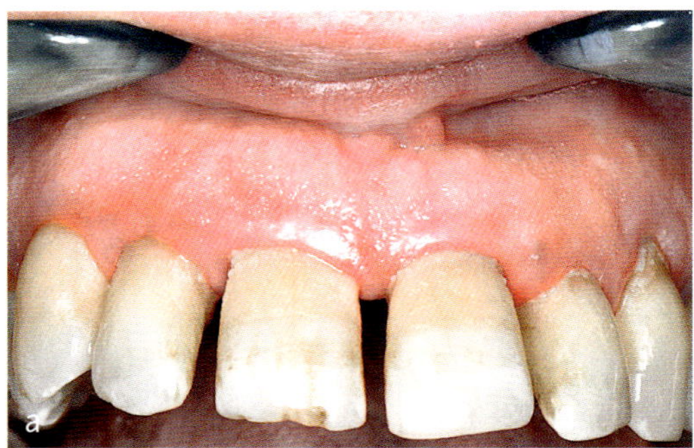

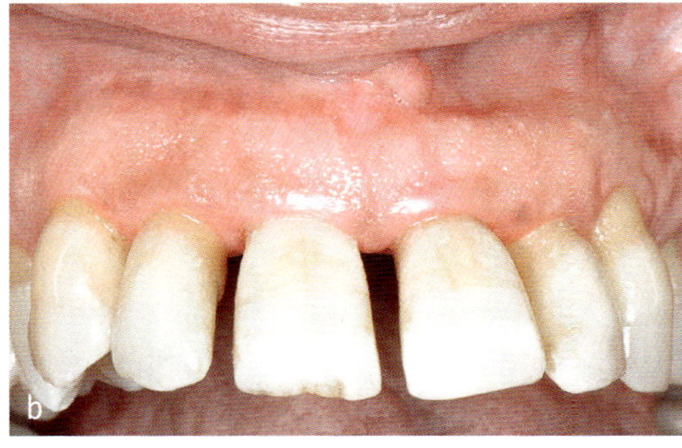

Fig. 6-5 (a and b) Cause-related therapy involves mechanical disruption of plaque and calculus deposits using various instruments and techniques. This patient, diagnosed as having advanced chronic periodontitis, was treated by scaling and root planing, and subsequently demonstrated significant reductions in probing pocket depths, reduced gingival inflammation and increased gingival recession.

interdental cleaning.[19] Despite the simplicity of these plaque control measures, the majority of the population are not able to comply effectively and, as a result, develop gingivitis. Various antimicrobial and anti-inflammatory substances have been included in dentifrices (tryclosan and stannous fluoride) and mouthwashes (chlorhexidine and essential oils) to improve the efficacy of plaque control, resulting in significant reductions in gingivitis and thereby helping to prevent the recurrence of periodontitis.[20]

Cause-related therapy, therefore, involves mechanical disruption of plaque and calculus deposits, using various instruments and techniques, sometimes coupled with the administration of adjunctive antimicrobial drug therapy. The effects of this therapeutic approach are measured by comparing attachment levels and pocket depths before and after treatment (Fig. 6-5).

A number of systematic reviews on the efficacy of mechanical non-surgical periodontal therapy have been published during the last decade.[8,21] There is a consensus among these reviews that subgingival debridement, combined with proper supragingival plaque control, is an effective treatment modality in reducing pocket depth and improving attachment levels. The effectiveness of these procedures decreases with increasing pocket depth, especially when probing depths exceed 5 mm.

The traditional approach to root debridement involves the use of hand instruments, available in various designs and described as curettes, hoes or scalers. They all have a sharp working tip, which is used to mechanically break the bond between the deposit and the tooth substrate. The process is time consuming and physically demanding, with deposits on root surfaces ranging typically from simple biofilms to hard tenacious calculus that requires attention to detail, manual dexterity and a thorough knowledge of tooth anatomy to eliminate. This treatment is termed scaling and root planing (SRP) since it involves the removal of plaque and the calculus deposits and 'contaminated root cementum' to render a root surface biocompatible for soft tissue healing. This concept has been challenged by investigations demonstrating that endotoxins are loosely rather than firmly adherent to the surface of root cementum and, as such, may be readily removed without the need to plane away root surface. Moreover, different scientific reports have demonstrated that 'smooth' root surfaces are not a prerequisite for periodontal healing.[8] Consequently, root instrumentation is preferably carried out with instruments that cause minimal root substance removal but are effective in disrupting the biofilm and removing calculus. With this goal, new approaches have been proposed as alternatives to traditional SRP. The technologies have ranged from the use of power scalers to ultrasonics and lasers.

Power-driven instruments differ from hand instrumentation in that they are relatively blunt and rely on the action of a vibrating tip, driven by sonic or ultrasonic technologies, to disrupt the plaque and calculus. Compared with SRP, power-driven instruments have the advantage of being easier to use and may take significantly less time than hand instruments to complete the task. The disadvantage is that the clinician has little, if any, tactile control and the powered instrument may have the potential to damage the root surface, producing indentations and unwanted scratches in the hard tissue surface. Although the implications of such damage to the outcome of therapy have not been demonstrated, root surface damage is undesirable. Systematic reviews assessing the efficacy of power instrumentation in the treatment of periodontitis have found that clinical outcomes are similar in terms of pocket reduction and attachment gain to those achieved with hand instrumentation.[22] Each method of instrumentation, if used appropriately, appears to yield the same degree of subgingival calculus removal, control of subgingival plaque and healing response. Given that power-driven instrumentation completes subgingival debridement quicker, this may justify the trend amongst clinicians to select power-driven, ergonomically advantageous scalers over hand instruments.

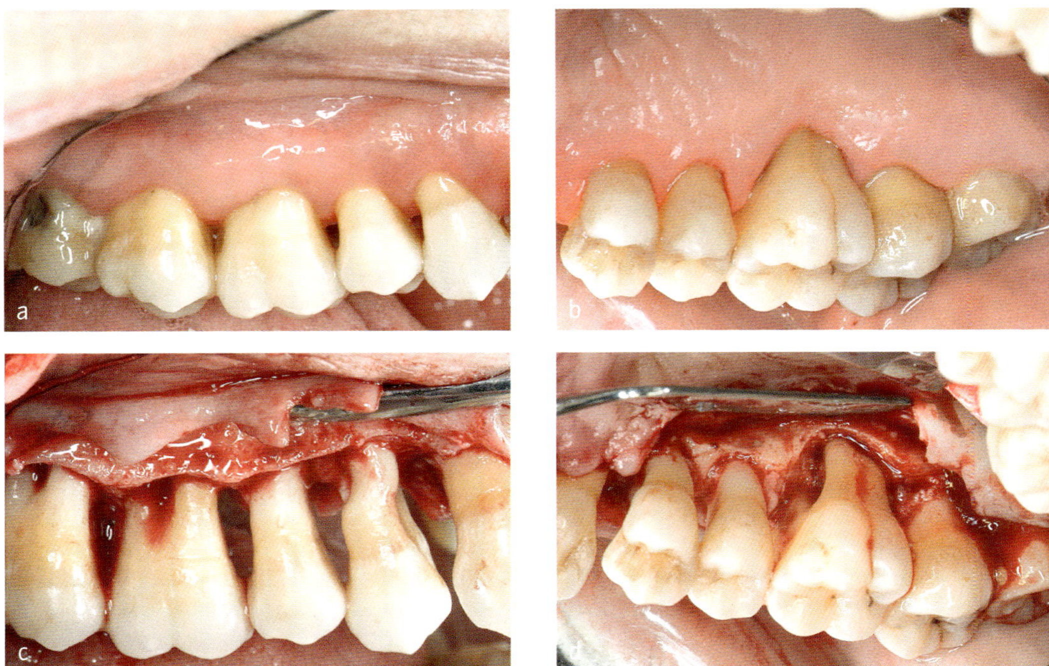

Fig. 6-6 (a to d) This patient, diagnosed as having advanced chronic periodontitis, was treated by scaling and root planing in combination with flap surgery to facilitate access for root debridement. The presence of deep probing depths, complex root anatomy, furcation involvement and intrabony osseous defects decreases the efficacy of non-surgical root instrumentation.

Non-surgical cause-related therapy has limitations in the treatment of deep pockets and sites difficult to reach, such as furcations and intrabony defects. In these situations, the treatment goal is to reduce probing depths, maintain or improve attachment levels and reduce the incidence of bleeding on probing. Resolution, in some cases, may be attained only if SRP is provided in combination with flap surgery that facilitates access to root debridement. Indeed, a number of systematic reviews comparing the efficacy of mechanical non-surgical periodontal therapy with access flap surgery have shown improved periodontal outcomes with surgery in pockets deeper than 5 mm (Fig. 6-6).[23]

In recent years, the use of laser radiation has been introduced as an alternative, or as an adjunctive, treatment to conventional, mechanical periodontal therapy. Lasers commonly used in dentistry use wavelengths ranging from 600 to 11000 nm including semiconductor diode lasers, the Nd:YAG laser (neodymium-doped yttrium, aluminum and garnet), the Er:YAG laser (erbium-doped yttrium, aluminum and garnet) and the CO_2 (carbon dioxide) laser. A recently published systematic review on the efficacy of different laser radiations as an alternative to non-surgical mechanical therapy has shown that most laser radiations of different diode laser wavelengths have inferior outcomes compared with SRP.[24] Only the use of the Er:YAG laser resulted in similar clinical outcomes to SRP, both in the short and the long term (< 24 months). This may be related to the specific characteristics of the Er:YAG laser radiation, including selective calculus ablation, hemostasis and bactericidal effects against periodontopathic pathogens (Fig. 6-7). This systematic review also highlighted the scarcity of well-controlled clinical studies with sufficient power to allow valid conclusions to be drawn. There is therefore, limited

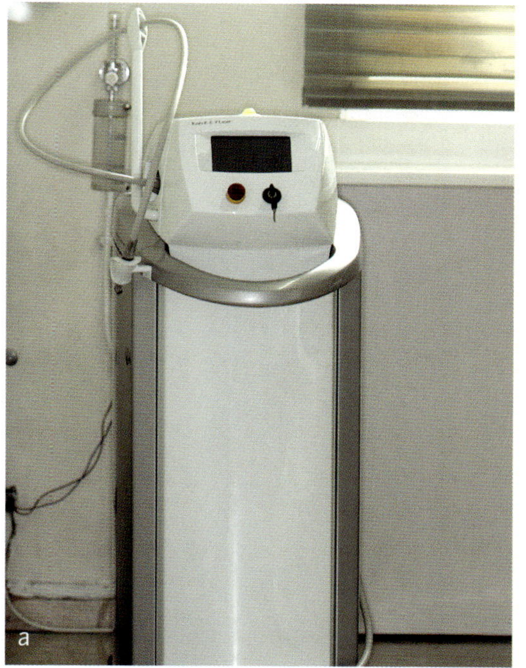

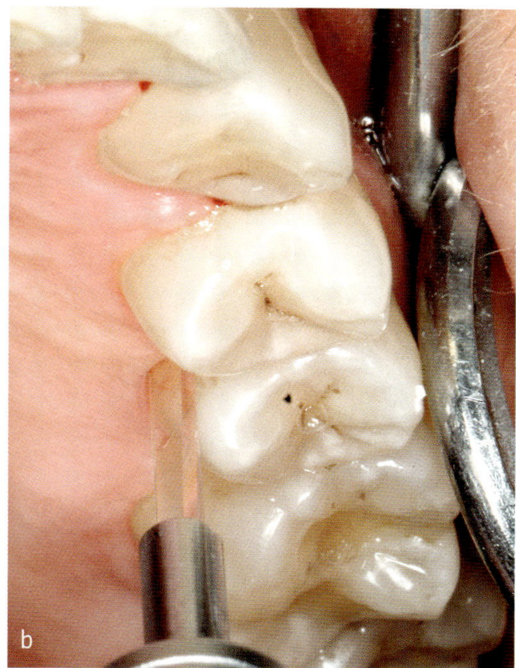

Fig. 6-7 (a and b) Only the use of the Er:YAG (erbium-doped yttrium aluminum garnet) laser has resulted in similar clinical outcomes to scaling and root planing, probably because of the specific characteristics of the laser radiation; effects include selective calculus ablation, hemostasis and bactericidal effects against periodontopathic pathogens.

available information, let alone good evidence, to recommend the use of laser technologies in the treatment of periodontitis.[24]

One traditional SRP is usually carried out on one jaw quadrant at a time in a series of appointments. This treatment regimen has been challenged by Quirynen and co-workers,[25] who argued that the presence of untreated periodontal pockets during treatment may represent a significant reservoir for the reinfection of adjacent treated sites, with the intraoral transmission of periodontal pathogens from periodontal pockets to recently instrumented and healing periodontal sites being highly likely. To avoid this, Quirynen et al [25]have proposed a treatment approach termed 'full mouth disinfection,' advocating the disinfection of the entire oral cavity within a period of 24 h. This involves mechanical root debridement, together with disinfection of bacterial reservoirs in the tongue and tonsils by means of tongue scraping and the extensive use of antimicrobial agents, including chlorhexidine. This treatment approach, despite having a clear biological rationale, has not been shown clinically to have advantages over the conventional quadrant by quadrant debridement (SRP).[26]

Since periodontitis is an infectious disease, the use of systemic antimicrobial drugs as part of the treatment of periodontal disease has been debated for decades. Given the limited capacity of currently used antimicrobial drugs to penetrate subgingival biofilms, it is suggested that the use of such drugs in the treatment of periodontitis should be as an adjunct to mechanical debridement, not an alternative therapy. This possible adjunctive benefit of using systemic antimicrobial drugs in the treatment of periodontitis has been reported in two systematic reviews presented at international workshops,[27,28] which concluded that the overall additive effect of antibiotics on clinical parameters was limited. Adjunctive antimicrobial therapy resulted in a significant improvement in clinical outcomes only in specific clinical situations, including patients with very deep pockets, progressive or 'active' disease or with specific microbiological profiles. Given the inherent problems associated with the use of antibiotics, the application of systemic antimicrobial drugs in periodontitis should be restricted to certain patients and specific periodontal conditions.[29]

An alternative approach to the systemic administration of antimicrobial drugs is to apply the drug directly into the diseased pocket. In this way, locally delivered drugs may provide an effective concentration at the site of infection, with minimal systemic load and low risk of bacterial resistance. Systematic reviews of clinical outcomes with the adjunctive use of locally delivered antimicrobial drugs compared with SRP alone have demonstrated a statistically significant added benefit, but concluded by questioning the clinical significance of such adjunctive therapy.[20] Concerns are based largely on cost–benefit considerations, suggesting that the use of locally delivered antimicrobial drugs should be restricted to sites that do not respond adequately to mechanical instrumentation.

Anti-inflammatory strategy

Although the primary etiologic basis of periodontal disease is the accumulation of bacteria at the biofilm–gingiva interface, the excessive host inflammatory response and/or inadequate resolution of inflammation is critical to the pathogenesis of the tissue destruction that occurs in periodontitis. Since major drivers of tissue destruction are MMPs, cathepsins and other osteoclast-related mediators, agents that directly or indirectly block the activity of osteoclasts may represent potential 'bone-sparing' therapies to be used as an adjunct to traditional periodontal therapy. Research that demonstrated the protective effects of common non-steroidal anti-inflammatory drugs (NSAIDs) and tetracyclines led to the concept of host modulation as a means of limiting the progression of periodontitis. The first attempts at using NSAIDs as an adjunct to standard periodontal therapy were not very successful; enhanced clinical outcomes being countered by secondary effects linked to long-term anti-inflammatory medication. The discovery of the potential inhibitory effects of the MMP-8 and MMP-13 protease mechanisms associated with low-dose tetracyclines and tetracycline analogs have renewed interest in previously discredited treatment regimens.[10,17] Indeed, recent systematic reviews have shown that subantimicrobial-dose doxycycline therapy is an effective adjunctive systemic therapy to the traditional mechanical therapies in the management of periodontitis. Improved outcomes persist for approximately 9 months in adults with chronic periodontitis, as observed in gains in clinical attachment levels and reductions in probing depth.[10]

Although questions remain regarding optimizing treatment efficacy, the evidence clearly suggests a strong potential for the modulation of the host response in aiding disease management, including traditional mechanical therapy.[30]

As the understanding of the pathways of inflammation has matured, a better understanding has emerged regarding the molecular basis of the resolution of inflammation. Resolution is an active, agonist-mediated, well-orchestrated return of tissue homeostasis. A growing body of research suggests that chronic inflammatory periodontal disease involves a failure of resolution pathways to restore homeostasis. The isolation and characterization of resolving agonist molecules has opened a new area of research, which is investigating endogenous lipid mediators of resolution as potential therapeutic agents for the management of inflammatory periodontitis. Work in animal models of periodontitis has revealed the potential of this therapeutic approach, based on the use of proresolvin lipid mediators that contribute to the restoration of tissue homeostasis.[31] Such proresolvin molecules include lipoxins, which are endogenously produced from the metabolism of arachidonic acid, and other exogenous proresolvin molecules, including resolvins and protectins derived from omega-3 polyunsaturated fatty acids. These newly identified lipid mediators represent a potentially powerful intervention that stimulates resolution pathways, leading to the restoration of homeostasis, possibly without the multiple side effects ascribed to traditional anti-inflammatory antagonist-based treatments. Clinical studies in humans will be required to elucidate the efficacy of this therapeutic approach.

Regenerative strategy

Reconstructive procedures have been used with varying degrees of success during the past decades to realize the regeneration of the lost attachment apparatus in different types of periodontal lesions, including intraosseous, furcation (inter-radicular) and recession defects. The most investigated reconstructive methods reported in the literature are based on the use of autogenous bone, bone substitutes, membranes for guided tissue regeneration (GTR), growth factors and combinations of the above.

Regeneration of the periodontium is a major goal in the treatment of teeth affected by periodontitis. Regenerative periodontal therapy aims for a predictable restoration of supporting periodontal tissues (new periodontal ligament, new cementum with inserted connective tissue fibers and new bone) that had been lost as a consequence of periodontal disease. Although in some cases a nonsurgical or a conventional surgical periodontal therapy may result in bone regrowth, histological studies have demonstrated that an epithelial lining is often interposed between the root surface and the newly formed bone, leading to repair rather than regeneration.[32] Considerable histologic and clinical evidence has been gathered since the 1980s indicating that periodontal regeneration can be achieved in humans for the successful management of certain specific periodontal lesions. In particular, three clinical approaches have been widely employed with considerable success: GTR with barrier membranes, bone grafting and the use of enamel matrix derivatives (EMDs).

The placement of a barrier membrane (GTR) over denuded root surfaces and debrided periodontal defects has been shown to exclude epithelial downgrowth and allow periodontal ligament and alveolar bone cells to repopulate the isolated space selectively, resulting in new cementum, connective tissue attachment and bone formation. Recent systematic reviews on the efficacy of this regenerative procedure in the treatment of periodontal intra-osseous defects have demonstrated statistically significant tissue attachment gains compared with those achieved with access flaps alone.[33,34] The amount of tissue regenerated is limited by the available space under the membrane, suggesting that the space provision and wound-stabilizing effects of the barrier membrane may substantially influence the healing process. In addition, these studies have shown a high degree of variability in terms of clinical attachment level gains, which is dependent on a variety of patient, defect and surgical factors. Patient factors include cigarette smoking, residual periodontal infection and oral hygiene. An ideal protocol for regenerative surgery should include a thorough nonsurgical periodontal regimen to avoid residual infection and inflammation in the defect area, together with a high degree of patient compliance, including smoking cessation and excellent plaque control.[35]

The depth of the intrabony component of the defect, the number of residual walls and the initial probing depth are important anatomic factors influencing the final outcome. Among the technical and surgical factors, membrane exposure and contamination have been associated with less-favorable outcomes. To avoid this occurrence, different flap designs have been proposed, aiming to maintain primary closure of the flaps in the critical interdental area. These modified flap designs allow access to the defect area while preserving the interdental papilla.[35]

One widely employed technique in reconstructive periodontal surgery, as an alternative to the use of barrier membranes, is the use of various types of grafting material to fill the periodontal defects. Data from recent systematic reviews summarizing clinical outcomes following the application of

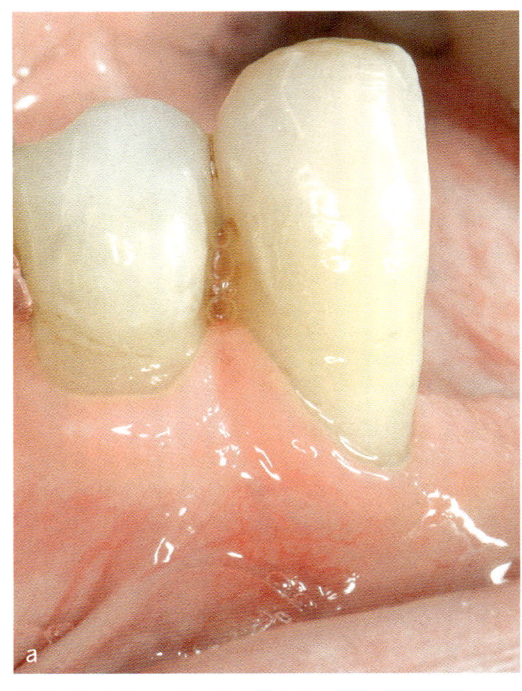
a

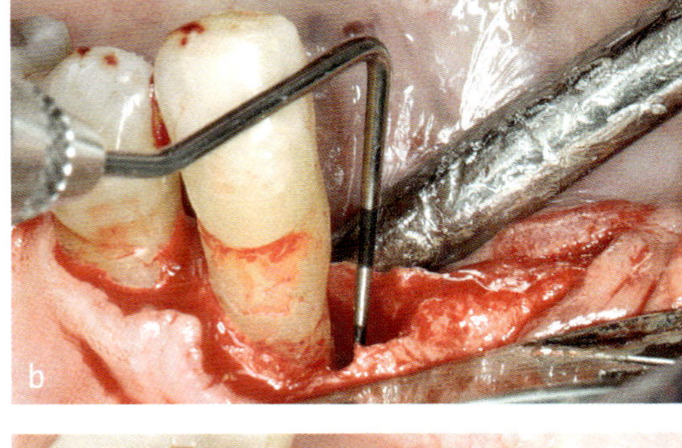
b

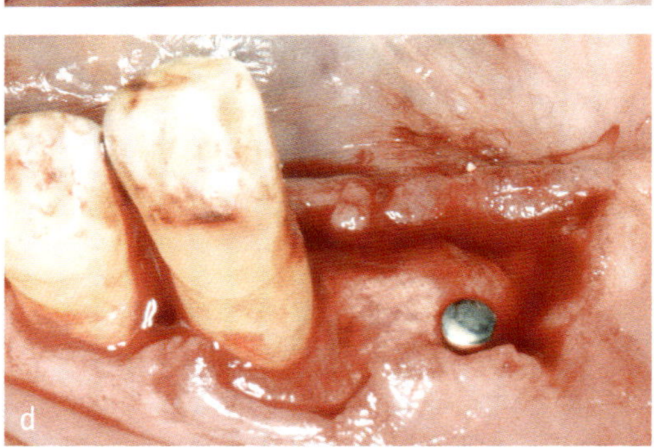
d

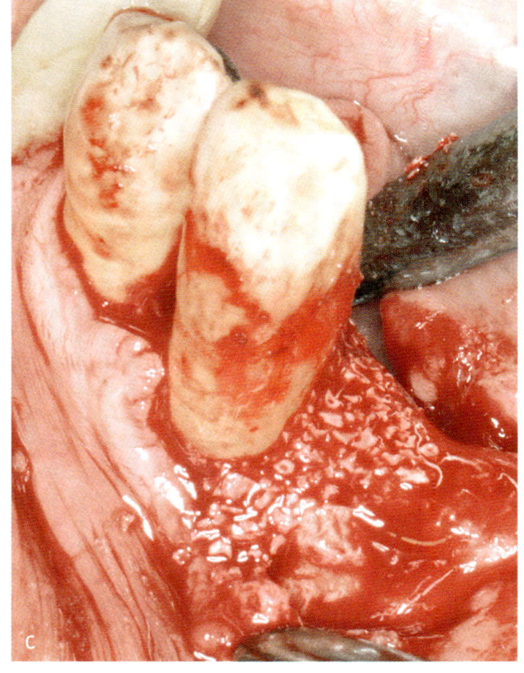
c

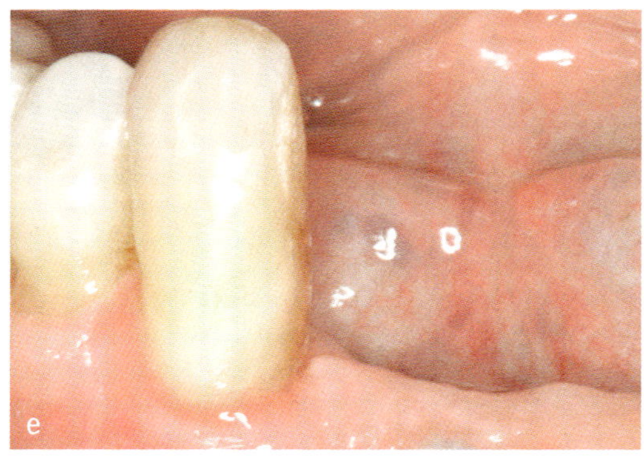
e

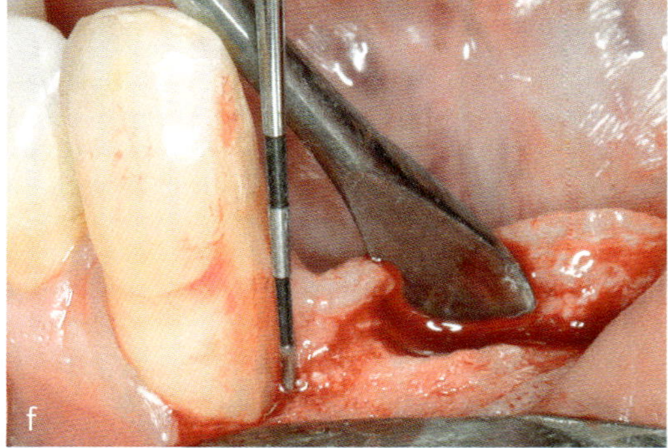
f

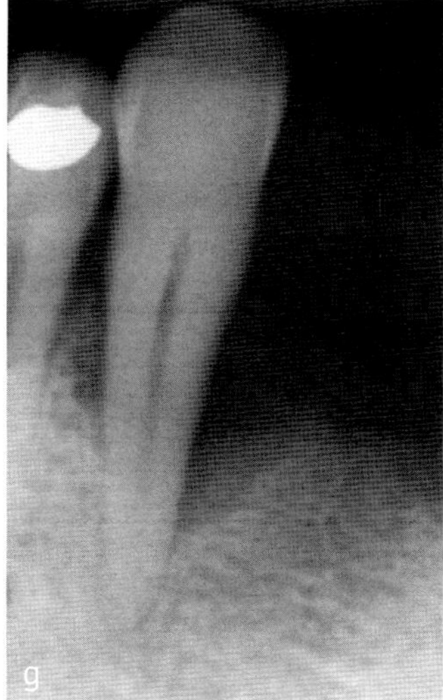

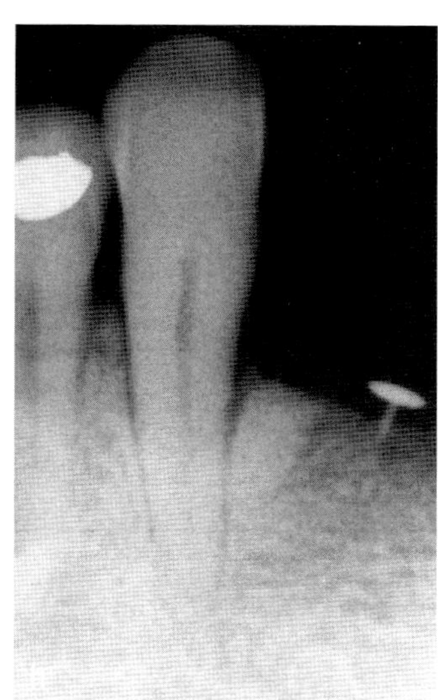

Fig. 6-8 (a to g) The combination of barrier membranes and grafting materials has been used in the treatment of periodontal osseous defects to overcome problems related to the collapse of the barrier membrane, specifically in defects with a complicated, non-contained morphology. **(h)** At a one year re-examination, complete regeneration of the defect is seen.

specific biomaterials as bone replacement grafts have indicated that both bone grafts and bone substitutes are significantly more effective than open flap debridement in improving attachment levels and reducing probing depths. Differences in clinical attachment level gains, however, vary considerably according to the biomaterials used. It is, therefore, difficult to draw conclusions on the use of specific graft biomaterials.[36]

The combination of barrier membranes and grafting materials has been used to overcome problems related to the collapse of the barrier membrane. Specifically, the treatment of intra-osseus defects with complicated, non-contained morphology using a combination of barrier membranes and grafting materials results in superior clinical outcomes compared with treatment with barrier membranes alone (Fig. 6-8).[35,37]

The biologic rationale for using grafting materials is based on the assumption that such materials may facilitate formation of alveolar bone, periodontal ligament and root cementum by serving as a scaffold and, when combined with barrier membranes, provide space under the membrane for the accumulation and retention of bone forming osteogenic cells.[36]

The third most used regenerative material is EMD, which has been available since 1997. Clinically, EMD is used for periodontal regeneration in teeth affected by periodontitis, root coverage procedures and replantation. The material used consists of the EMD, water and a carrier (propylene glycol alginate). EMDs are naturally derived proteins from porcine tooth buds that have the capacity to attract and stimulate differentiation of connective tissue cells into cementoblasts, thereby stimulating the formation of new cementum, connective tissue attachment and bone. The biologic rationale for using EMDs is to replicate the embryologic events that occur during the formation of the root in tooth development: biomimetic regeneration. EMDs have a wide variety of biologic activities, stimulating different cell types, both directly and indirectly, by increasing cell attachment of gingival and periodontal ligament fibroblasts; favoring cell proliferation of periodontal ligament fibroblasts; down-regulating expression of genes involved in early inflammatory events of wound healing; and

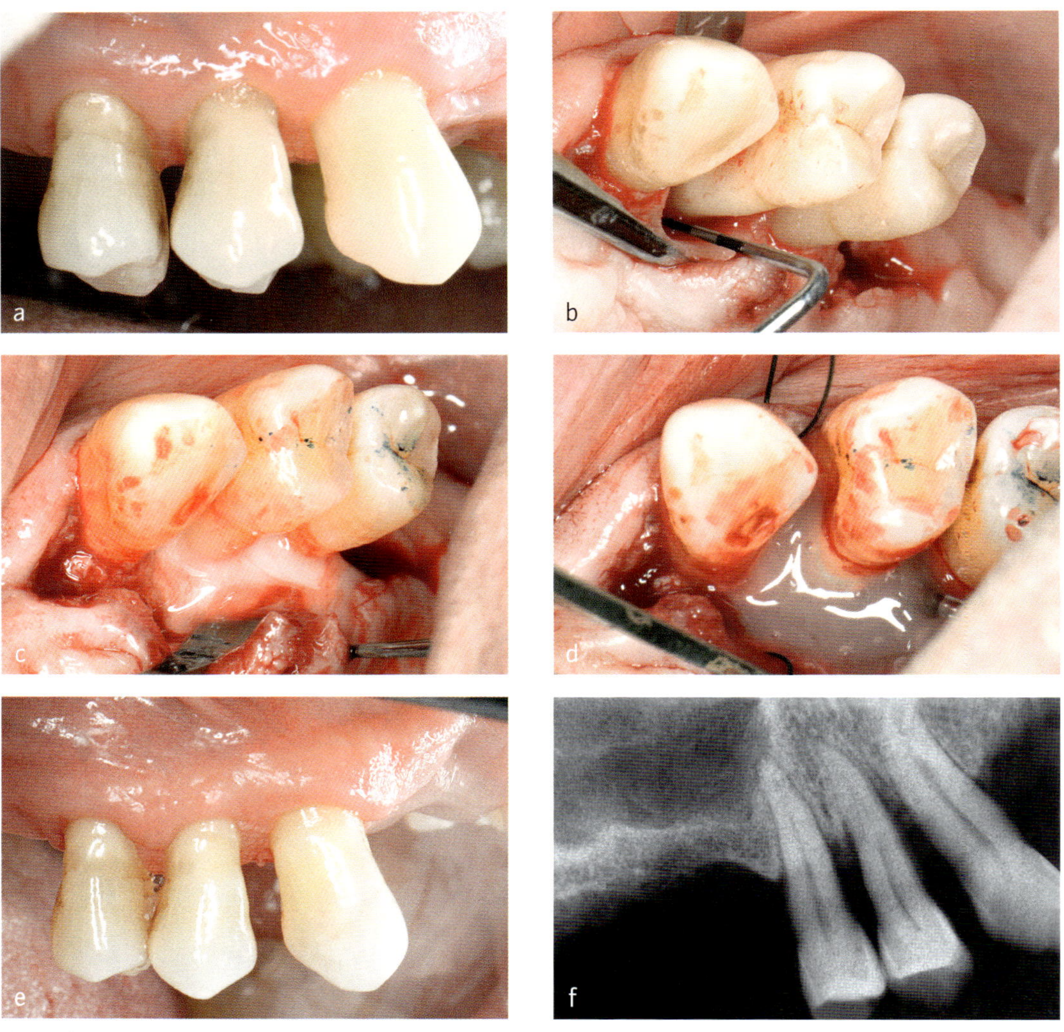

Fig. 6-9 (a to e) Application of enamel matrix derivatives (EMDs) on surgically exposed denuded root surfaces in the treatment of a deep periodontal osseous defect. **(f)** The radiograph one year later shows regeneration of the defect. EMD has been shown to be easier to handle clinically and results in fewer undesirable postsurgical effects than the guided tissue regeneration technique.

upregulating expression of genes encoding growth- and repair-promoting molecules. The end result is that EMDs stimulate wound healing, connective tissue repair and bone apposition.

Considerable histologic and clinical evidence gathered since the 1980s indicates that the application of EMDs on surgically exposed denuded root surfaces previously affected by periodontal destruction results in periodontal regeneration with significant clinical attachment gains.[38] Systematic reviews assessing the efficacy of this regenerative procedure have demonstrated statistically significant clinical gains,[39,40] indicating significant differences between EMD and open flap debridement in the postsurgical changes of clinical attachment levels, pocket depth and radiographic marginal bone levels. In comparative studies between EMD and GTR, although the clinical outcomes are similar with the use of both procedures, EMD has been found to be easier to handle clinically and result in fewer undesirable postsurgical effects (Fig. 6-9).[41]

The existing evidence does not provide clinicians with a clear indication for choosing a single or combined regenerative approach that would work in all clinical situations. Cortellini and Tonetti, in 2005,[35] made an attempt to build an evidence-based regenerative strategy to guide clinicians through a decision process to optimize the clinical outcomes of periodontal regeneration in intrabony defects. Their strategy stated that wide and non-supportive defects should be treated by the use of bioabsorbable barriers, supported with a bone substitute graft material, thus avoiding the collapse of the barriers and overlying soft tissues into the coronal part of the defect. When defects are narrow and present with a predominantly two–three wall morphology, a bioabsorbable barrier or EMDs may be used successfully.

Mucogingival therapy is a general term used to describe periodontal surgical procedures aimed at the correction of defects in morphology, position and/or the amount of soft tissue and underlying for bone support teeth and implants.[1] In 1993, Miller proposed the term periodontal plastic surgery,[42] considering that mucogingival surgery had moved beyond the traditional treatment of problems associated with the amount of gingivae and recession type defects to include correction of ridge form and soft tissue esthetics. These treatments, therefore, have a main reconstructive esthetic purpose and may include soft tissues and bone. Treatments include gingival augmentation, root coverage, correction of mucosal defects around implants, crown lengthening, gingival preservation with ectopic tooth eruption, removal of aberrant frenums, prevention of ridge collapse associated with tooth extraction and augmentation of the edentulous ridge. Of all these procedures, marginal tissue recession (the displacement of the soft tissue margin apical to the cementoenamel junction with exposure of the root surface) typically found at buccal sites is the most common esthetic concern. These lesions are usually caused by tissue trauma through vigorous tooth brushing, in particular in young individuals. The lesions are self-limited provided the etiology is controlled. There are, however, indications for the surgical reconstruction of the soft tissues, with the goal of covering the exposed roots. These indications are primarily based on esthetic demands and to reduce root sensitivity. In addition, in some cases the change in the topography of the marginal soft tissue will facilitate plaque control and reduce localized chronic inflammation.

Root coverage procedures are surgical interventions aimed to treat recession type defects. They are classified as pedicle soft tissue graft procedures and free soft tissue graft procedures. Depending on the direction of the transfer of the flap, the pedicle graft procedures are termed rotational flap procedures (e.g. laterally sliding flap, double papilla flap) or advanced flap procedures (e.g. coronally advanced flap [CAF], semilunar coronally advanced flap). These procedures may include the placement of a barrier or the application of EMDs between the graft and the root surface to encourage full regeneration of the connective tissue attachment.

The autogenous free soft tissue graft procedures may be performed as an epithelialized graft or as a subepithelial connective tissue graft (CTG), both usually taken from the masticatory mucosa in the palate (Fig. 6-10).

The ultimate goal of a root coverage procedure is the complete coverage of the recession defect with good appearance related to adjacent soft tissues and minimal probing depth. Recent systematic reviews confirm that the CAF procedure is a safe and reliable approach, associated with consistent recession reduction, if not complete coverage of the recession (Fig. 6-11). The results of meta-analyses show that only two combinations (CAF plus CTG and CAF plus EMD) provide better results than CAF alone. CAF plus CTG results in better clinical outcomes for both coverage of the recession defect (odds ratio, 2.49) and reduced recession (+0.49 mm) compared with CAF alone. The best results may be obtained with CAF plus CTG.[43,44]

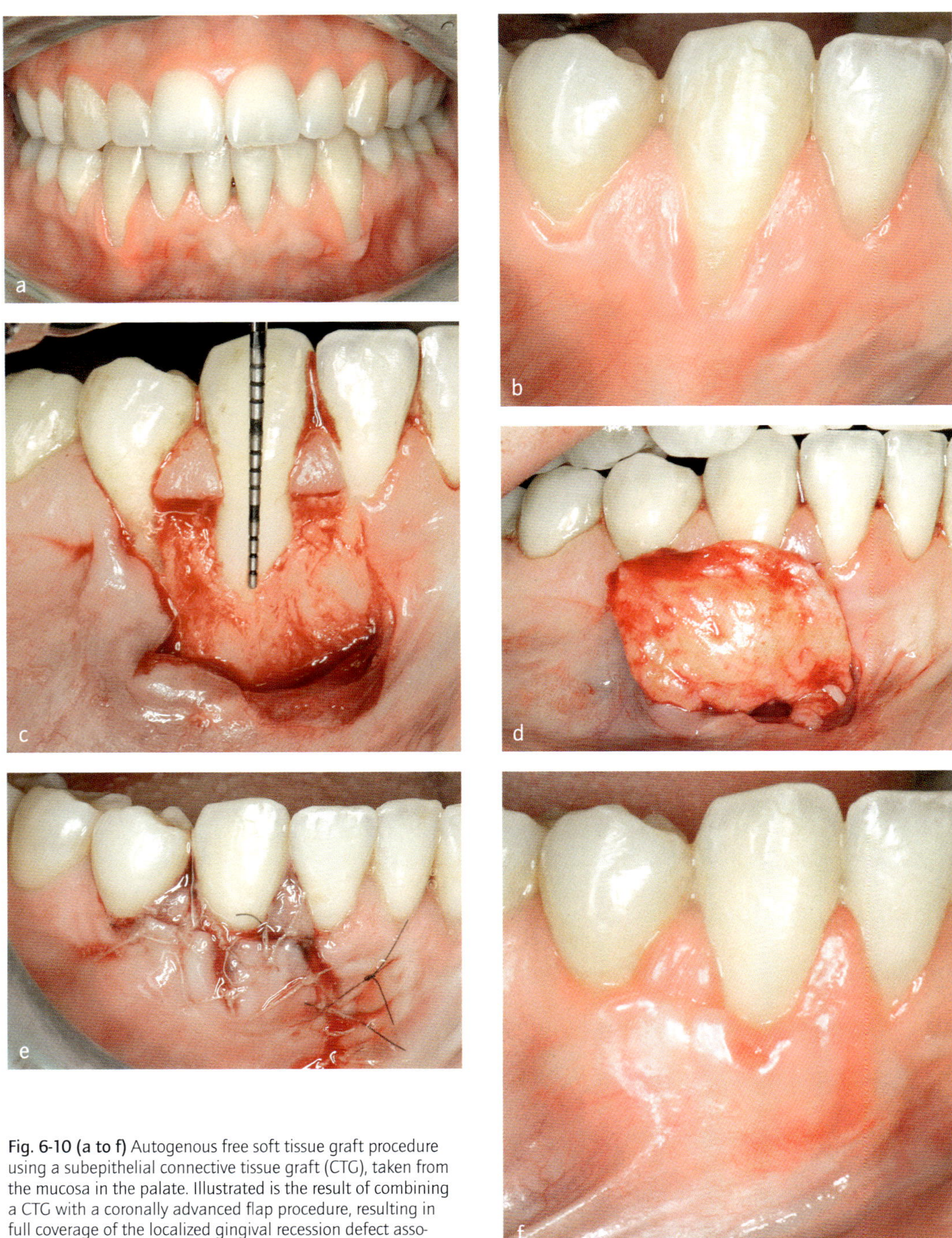

Fig. 6-10 (a to f) Autogenous free soft tissue graft procedure using a subepithelial connective tissue graft (CTG), taken from the mucosa in the palate. Illustrated is the result of combining a CTG with a coronally advanced flap procedure, resulting in full coverage of the localized gingival recession defect associated with the mandibular right canine.

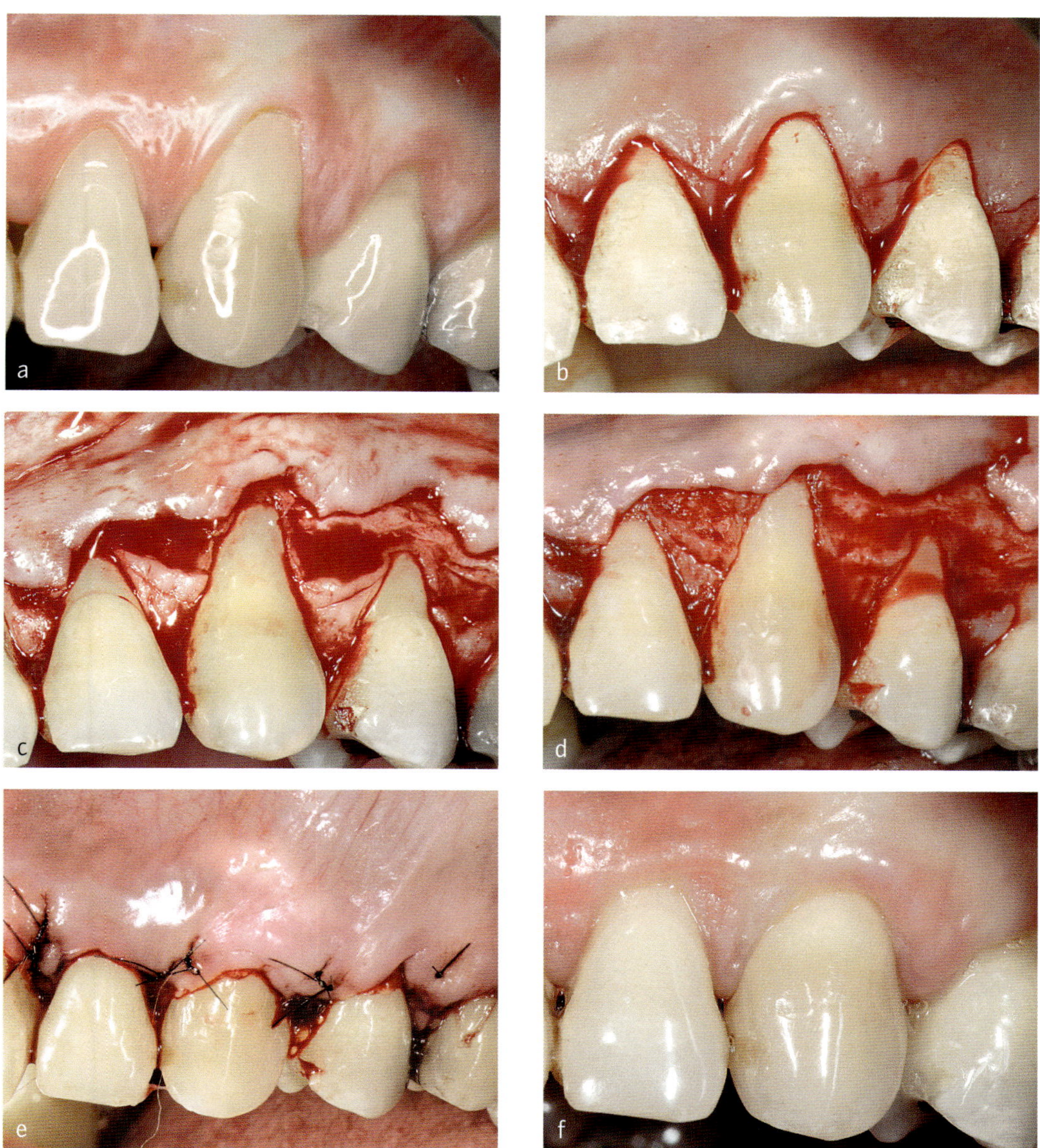

Fig. 6-11 (a to f) Localized gingival recessions can be treated effectively using the coronally advanced flap procedure. The result of applying this surgical procedure in the treatment of multiple localized gingival recessions is typically a complete coverage.

The decision as to whether to select CTG or EMD should depend on the specific objectives of the surgery. The CAF plus CTG procedure has been shown to be superior in terms of increasing keratinized tissue and, therefore, this approach should be used when keratinized tissue augmentation with recession reduction is the treatment goal.[43] On the contrary, CAF plus EMD appears to be an easier procedure than CAF plus CTG and does not require a donor area for CTG harvesting, which generally results in greater postoperative discomfort in the first month following therapy.[44] In addition, the cost–benefit ratio of CAF plus EMD should be carefully evaluated, since there are no differences between the two procedures in terms of coverage of the recession and recurrence of defects. Both systematic reviews also revealed that the use of barrier membranes in conjunction with CAF did enhance the clinical outcome. Therefore, the use of barrier membranes for the root coverage procedure appears to be inadvisable, especially considering the high incidence of complications, including membrane exposure.[43,44]

Vision 2020

Advances in research and relevant technologies will bring major breakthroughs in the diagnosis, prevention and treatment of destructive periodontal diseases.

New understanding of periodontal disease pathogenesis will include knowledge on the subgingival biofilm organization and composition. It has been estimated that about one third of the bacteria present in the subgingival biofilm has yet to be identified, based on studies assessing differential DNA fractions from pooled subgingival plaque samples. Advances in molecular genetics will provide key information to describe and otherwise characterize the bacteria of the subgingival biofilm and, in turn, identify the real periodontal pathogens. Although the genomes of certain specific bacteria implicated in periodontitis, such as *P. gingivalis*, are known, there is a lack of information in respect of the genetic variability of such pathogens. Future knowledge will allow the diagnosis of the presence of the pathogens and pathogenic clones actually responsible for disease expression. The use of these pathogenic clones may lead to the development of vaccines that will protect against periodontal infection.

New understanding of periodontal disease pathogenesis will also include knowledge of the dynamic biologic networks that intervene in the host immune inflammatory response against bacteria of the biofilm. This knowledge will lead to the incorporation of gene, protein and metabolite data into periodontal diagnosis algorithms, creating opportunity for new classification systems that will define individuals who are disease prone, resistant to therapy, good responders, etc. The combination of diagnosis based on the subgingival microbial composition, clinical features, systemic risk factors, inflammatory molecule profiles and genetic background will allow effective targeting of preventive and therapeutic strategies specific to individuals. In addition, the monitoring of specific metabolites in saliva and gingival tissue fluids, such as MMP-8 in saliva and fragments of bone collagen in tissue fluids, will enable the progression of periodontitis and its response to therapy to be monitored effectively.

The treatment of periodontitis will have two definite phases: first, the treatment of the disease by eliminating the infection and the inflammatory response; and second, the regeneration of the lost periodontium.

Advances in microbiology and antimicrobial technologies will lead to more effective antimicrobial drugs able to permeate the biofilm and effectively destroy the subgingival flora. Moreover, the development of new classes of anti-inflammatory drugs such as endogenous resolvins and protectins, will treat inflammation by an active, agonist-mediated return to tissue homeostasis. This will probably be coupled with the introduction of specific diets and the application of nutragenomics. Current information links diets rich in omega-3-fatty acids with a reduction in the genetic predilection to metabolic syndrome.

Recently, advances in the areas of cellular and molecular biology have allowed the elucidation of functions of growth factors and morphogens and their participation in the different phases of periodontal wound healing. Bioactive molecules have been experimentally tested to treat periodontal defects, including bone morphogenetic proteins, transforming growth factor, basic fibroblast growth factor, insulin-like growth factor 1, cementum-derived growth factor, neurotrophins, vascular endothelial growth factor and parathormone-related protein. Although the only clinical information available at present indicates that these factors can be safely and effectively used for treating periodontal defects, randomized controlled clinical trials are required to investigate their clinical efficacy and cost-effectiveness. Future knowledge on these and other yet-to-be-identified molecules, together with the development of advanced surgical techniques, will allow the development of sophisticated regenerative approaches. These new treatment modalities will herald a new era in the reconstruction of intrabony periodontal defects, together with supra-crestal regeneration, achieving, in this manner, the 'restituito and integrum' of the periodontium.

Advances in the prevention and therapy of periodontal infections should reduce the prevalence of periodontal diseases, and as a consequence, periodontal treatment needs should diminish. This will be balanced by higher reconstructive treatment demands generated by esthetic and patient demands in current and future societies. The focus on health and health-related behaviors will also stimulate desire to maintain the natural dentition and, thus, will increase demand for regenerative periodontal procedures.

Acknowledgements

I appreciate the contribution of Drs Elena Figuero, Marta Escribano, Ignacio Sanz and Fabio Vignoletti to the material included in this chapter.

References

1. American Academy of Periodontology. Glossary of Terms. Chicago, IL: American Academy of Periodontology, 1991 (http://www.perio.org/consumer/glossary.htm).
2. Carranza F, Shklar G. History of Periodontology. Chicago, IL: Quintessence, 2003.
3. Lindhe J, Westfelt E, Nyman S, Socransky SS, Haffajee AD. Long-term effect of surgical/non-surgical treatment of periodontal disease. J Clin Periodontol 1984;11:448–458.
4. Löe, H, Theilade E, Jensen SB, Schiott CR. Experimental gingivitis in man. J Periodont Res 1967;2:282–289.
5. Ramfjord SP, Caffesse RG, Morrison EC, Hill RW, Kerry GJ, Appleberry EA et al. 4 modalities of periodontal treatment compared over 5 years. J Clin Periodontol 1987;14:445–452.
6. Sigmund S, Socransky ADH. Periodontal microbial ecology. Periodontol 2000 2005;38:135–187.
7. Marsh PD. Dental plaque: biological significance of a biofilm and community life-style. J Clin Periodontol 2005; 32(Suppl 6):7–15.
8. van der Weijden GA, Timmerman MF. A systematic review on the clinical efficacy of subgingival debridement in the treatment of chronic periodontitis. J Clin Periodontol 2002;29(Suppl 3):55–71.
9. van Dyke TE. Cellular and molecular susceptibility determinants for periodontitis. Periodontol 2000 2007;45: 10–13.
10. Giannobile WV. Host-response therapeutics for periodontal diseases. J Periodontol 2008;79(Suppl 8): 1592–1600.
11. Löe H, Anerud A, Boysen AH, Morrison E. Natural history of periodontal disease in man. J Clin Periodontol 1986; 13:431–440.
12. Michalowicz BS, Diehl SR, Gunsolley JC, Sparkes B, Brooks CN, Koertge TE et al. Evidence of a substantial genetic basis for risk of adult periodontitis. J Periodontol 2000; 71:1699–1707.
13. Kornman KS. Mapping the pathogenesis of periodontitis: a new look. J Periodontol 2008;79(Suppl 8):1560–1568.
14. Bergstrom J. Periodontitis and smoking: an evidence-based appraisal. J Evid Based Dent Pract 2006;6:33–41.
15. Williams RC. Understanding and managing periodontal diseases: a notable past, a promising future. J Periodontol 2008;79(suppl 8):1552–1559.
16. Offenbacher, S, Barros SP, Beck JD. Rethinking periodontal inflammation. J Periodontol 2008;79(Suppl 8): 1577–1584.
17. Salvi GE, Lang NP. Host response modulation in the management of periodontal diseases. J Clin Periodontol 2005; 32(Suppl 6):108–129.
18. Papapanou PN, Tonetti MS. Diagnosis and epidemiology of periodontal osseous lesions. Periodontol 2000 2000; 22:8–21.
19. Nicholas CC. Current concepts in toothbrushing and interdental cleaning. Periodontol 2000 2008;48:10–22.
20. Hanes PJ, Purvis JP. Local anti-infective therapy: pharmacological agents. A Systematic Review. Ann Periodontol 2003;8:79–98.
21. Hallmon WW, Rees TD. Local anti-infective therapy: mechanical and physical approaches. A systematic review. Ann Periodontol 2003;8:99–114.
22. Tunkel J, Heinecke A, Flemmig TF. A systematic review of efficacy of machine-driven and manual subgingival debridement in the treatment of chronic periodontitis. J Clin Periodontol 2002;29(Suppl 3):72–81.
23. Heitz-Mayfield LJA, Trombelli L, Heitz F, Needleman I. Moles DR. A systematic review of the effect of surgical debridement vs. non-surgical debridement for the treatment of chronic periodontitis. J Clin Periodontol 2002;29 (Suppl 3):92–102.

24. Schwarz F, Aoki A, Becker J, Sculean A. Laser application in non-surgical periodontal therapy: a systematic review. J Clin Periodontol 2008;35(Suppl 8):29–44.
25. Quirynen M, De Soete M, Boschmans G, Pauwels M, Coucke W, Teughels W et al. Benefit of one-stage full-mouth disinfection is explained by disinfection and root planing within 24 hours: a randomized controlled trial. J Clin Periodontol 2006;33:639–647.
26. Lang NP, Tan WC, Krähenmann MA, Zwahlen M. A systematic review of the effects of full-mouth debridement with and without antiseptics in patients with chronic periodontitis. J Clin Periodontol 2008;35(Suppl 8):8–21.
27. Haffajee AD, Socransky SS, Gunsolley JC. Systemic anti-infective periodontal therapy. A systematic review. Ann Periodontol 2003;8:115–181.
28. Herrera D, Alonso B, León R, Roldán S, Sanz M. Antimicrobial therapy in periodontitis: the use of systemic antimicrobials against the subgingival biofilm. J Clin Periodontol 2008;35(Suppl 8):45–66.
29. Herrera D, Sanz M, Jepsen S, Needleman I, Roldan S. A systematic review on the effect of systemic antimicrobials as an adjunct to scaling and root planing in periodontitis patients. J Clin Periodontol 2002;29(Suppl 3):136–159.
30. Preshaw PM. Host response modulation in periodontics. Periodontol 2000 2008;48:92–110.
31. van Dyke TE. The management of inflammation in periodontal disease. J Periodontol 2008;79(Suppl 8):1601–1608.
32. Caton JG, Greenstein G. Factors related to periodontal regeneration. Periodontol 2000 1993;1:9–15.
33. Murphy KG, Gunsolley JC. Guided tissue regeneration for the treatment of periodontal intrabony and furcation defects. A systematic review. Ann Periodontol 2003;8:266–302.
34. Needleman IG, Worthington HV, Giedrys-Leeper E, Tucker R. Guided tissue regeneration for periodontal infra-bony defects. Cochrane Database Syst Rev 2006;(2):CD001724.
35. Cortellini P, Tonetti MS. Clinical performance of a regenerative strategy for intrabony defects: scientific evidence and clinical experience. J Periodontol 2005;76:341–350.
36. Trombelli L, Farina F. Clinical outcomes with bioactive agents alone or in combination with grafting or guided tissue regeneration. J Clin Periodontol 2008;35(Suppl 8):117–135.
37. Sculean A, Nikolidakis D, Schwarz F. Regeneration of periodontal tissues: combinations of barrier membranes and grafting materials – biological foundation and preclinical evidence. A systematic review. J Clin Periodontol 2008;35 (Suppl 8):106–116.
38. Dieter DB. Biological mediators and periodontal regeneration: a review of enamel matrix proteins at the cellular and molecular levels. J Clin Periodontol 2008;35(Suppl 8):87–105.
39. Esposito M, Grusovin MG, Coulthard P, Worthington HV. Enamel matrix derivative (Emdogain) for periodontal tissue regeneration in intrabony defects. Cochrane Database Syst Rev 2005;(4):CD003875.
40. Giannobile WV, Somerman MJ. Growth and amelogenin-like factors in periodontal wound healing. A systematic review. Ann Periodontol 2003;8:193–204.
41. Sanz M, Tonetti MS, Zabalegui I, Sicilia A, Blanco J, Rebelo H et al. Treatment of intrabony defects with enamel matrix proteins or barrier membranes: results from a multicenter practice-based clinical trial. J Periodontol 2004;75:726–733.
42. Miller PD Jr. Periodontal plastic surgery. Curr Opin Periodontol 1993:136–143.
43. Roccuzzo M, Bunino M, Needleman I, Sanz M. Periodontal plastic surgery for treatment of localized gingival recessions: a systematic review. J Clin Periodontol 2002;29 (Suppl 3):178–194.
44. Cairo F, Pagliaro U, Nieri M. Treatment of gingival recession with coronally advanced flap procedures: a systematic review. J Clin Periodontol 2008;35(Suppl 8):136–162.

CHAPTER 7

Endodontology

Kishor Gulabivala and Yuan-Ling Ng

Definition

Endodontology is concerned with the study of the form, function and health, injuries to and diseases of the dental pulp and periradicular tissues. The principal disease is apical periodontitis or inflammation of the periodontal ligament and supporting tissues, which is usually preceded by pulpitis or inflammation of the dental pulp (Fig. 7-1). The primary etiology of persistent pulpitis and apical periodontitis is infection, although they may also be transiently manifested after chemical, mechanical or thermal injuries. The principal goals of management are prevention or treatment of inflammation and its associated pain. Prevention consists of protecting the integrity of teeth, and treatment consists of controlling the source of inflammation, namely infection or further injuries. The principal procedures are tooth structure restoration, pulp dressing to allow its healing or regeneration, root canal treatment to help to eliminate intraradicular infection and promote periapical healing and regeneration, and surgical procedures to facilitate access to tissues not readily reached through the tooth.[1]

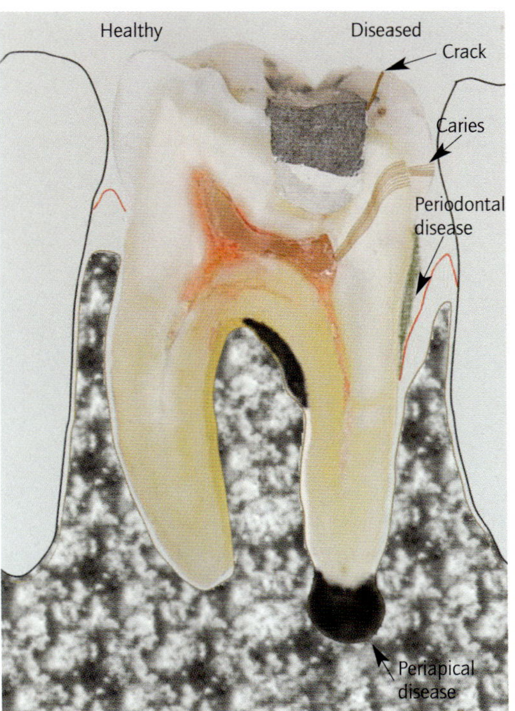

Fig. 7-1 A tooth in health and disease.

Historical milestones

A reconstruction of the historical development of endodontology is hampered, as in any discipline, by the incomplete threads of information recovered from different parts of the world and belonging to different time periods. The challenge is to piece together the thread fragments by correct time and space location, a science and an art in itself, to enable the synthesis of a coherent story. This demands accurate facts, considerable imagination and intuitive skill, as well as an understanding of the local cultures, lifestyles and contemporary demands of those times. Fortunately, a few authors[2–9] have already attempted such a synthesis.

Historical basis for concepts of bacterial infection, pulp diagnosis and therapy

Historically, dental treatment was mostly carried out for pain relief. As early as 2700 BC, the Chinese had recorded arsenic placement near the tooth to cure dental pain. Around 500–300 BC, the recommended treatments by Hippocrates for a painful tooth included cauterization using acids or hot wires, Greek physicians applied saffron and cedar gum, and the Chinese used acupuncture. Recognition of the origin of toothache as lying within the tooth, caused by nerve stimulation and inflammation, came later and led to the use of small trephines to open and drain the tooth.

The concept of worm-like infestation as a cause of dental disease appeared in China in the Ying Dynasty, around 1400 BC and was later reported in the Mediterranean area, around 1300 BC. Antony van Leeuwenhoek is credited as the first to identify oral bacteria using an embryonic microscope in 1683; being widely regarded as the 'father of modern microscopy.' It was, therefore, natural that the formulation of a bacteriological rationale for endodontic treatment would follow; and it came with a bacteriopathologic study of over 200 pulps by Willoughby Dayton Miller working in Robert Koch's laboratory in Berlin. Miller used a microscope to observe the presence of a variety of organisms in samples obtained from root canals of diseased teeth. He also noted that cultivation of the samples revealed a much simpler flora, leading him to predict that the sampled root canal bacteria would be difficult to cultivate in the laboratory. The concept that antibacterial materials might be used to treat carious dentin became established with the use of antiseptics such as oxysulfate of zinc and materials based on zinc oxide-eugenol. Unfortunately, the results of pulp capping at that time were unpredictable, with the condition of the dental pulp being diagnosed with a rudimentary electric pulp tester or hot water at various temperatures.

The development of the biologic basis of endodontics is interesting for the range of concepts explored and the strength of feeling with which debates raged about their merits or faults; few writers on either side of the controversy were altogether consistent. An example of this type of debate was centered around the issue of 'vitality' of teeth. Academic thinkers and writers lined up on opposite sides, as 'vitalists' or 'non-vitalists'. The 'vitalists' believed that blood flowed into the pulp through the apical foramen and out through the dentinal wall and periodontal membrane. Therefore, the whole dentin core of a tooth 'died' immediately after the pulp was destroyed by disease or surgical intervention. The 'dead tooth' was then putatively considered to be a foreign body by the adjacent living tissues, leading to inflammation, suppuration and ultimately death of these tissues. Therefore, pulp capping rather than pulp extirpation was preferred and popularized. The main opponents to the 'vitalistic' theory were scientists studying anatomy and physiology of teeth in England over a time frame preceding the establishment of the great debate. They collectively established the idea that teeth were fastened at the base of the alveolus through their neurovascular bundles as well as by the membrane of bone, but that neither the blood vessels nor the nerves from the pulp or the alveolus entered the tooth. They propagated the practice of pulp extirpation.

The 'vitalistic' theory held sway until it was challenged by the new 'septic' theory. General surgeons, realizing the importance of pathogenic organisms in various diseases, eventually adopted the aseptic surgical techniques introduced by Lister in 1867. The recovery of a parasite, *Leptothrix buccalis*, from tooth surfaces, caries lesions and dentinal tubules lent credence to this notion. The proponents of the 'septic' theory suggested that the pathogenic organisms were the cause of pulp disease and treatment failure. Successful pulp and root canal treatment were, therefore, deemed to require the destruction of these organisms using powerful and penetrating antiseptic agents. Through this process of tension and competition between concepts emerged the development of both pulp and root canal treatments: a progressive synthesis of growing knowledge of anatomy, physiology and pathology of the diseases, together with adventurous developments in equipment, chemical agents and technical skills.

Historical origin of root canal treatment

Once the dental pulp was considered compromised, the idea of removing it became established. Pulp extirpation evolved slowly from what was surely an extremely painful experience, involving the use of hot instruments or corrosive acids (sulfuric or nitric), to a relatively painless process, involving the prior application of arsenic trioxide. The use of arsenic trioxide was introduced into Europe by Spooner in 1863, although it had already been used by the Chinese since 200 AD for treatment of pulpitis. The potential of leakage of arsenic through the root canal, destroying adjacent vital supporting tissues, was recognized. Topical cocaine was subsequently adopted for anesthetizing the pulp by Freud in 1884. The progressive evolution of methods for pulp extirpation and root canal treatment continued through the refinement of the procedures and materials used, by trial and error. The first reference to materials being inserted into a tooth was found in the Ebers Papyrus, dated about 1500 BC, a concoction of fruit, onion, cake dough and plant material being used.

The term 'root canal treatment' did not appear until 1520 AD, when the first reference to any formn of canal preparation ('trephining') and filling was made by Benedictus of Faenza. The technical problem of reaching the root apex was recognized as a consequence of being intentional root canal treatment and replantation being practiced in France by Bourdet in 1757 and by Hunter in London in 1771. These embryonic endodontic procedures were taken to the USA from England by Wooffendale in 1783.

Curiously, the concept of packing the root canal system evolved earlier than the notion of cleaning the canal system thoroughly. Materials and techniques were developed from the concepts of packing gold foil into cavities using specially designed instruments. The compaction of gutta-percha (as points, chloro-percha or thermoplastized material) into canals appears to have originated at or around the same time of the work by Bourdet and Hunter. Many other root-filling materials, such as gold wire, oxychloride of zinc cement, wood or cotton with carbolic or creosote and iodoform- or paraform-containing materials, were also documented. An early form of tooth isolation using rubber dam was introduced by Barnum in 1864, while root canal broaches for pulp extirpation and hoe-like instruments for canal shaping were invented by Maynard in 1838, in the USA.

Based on the 'septic' theory, Witzel applied Lister's antiseptic technique in 1873 to pulp and root canal treatment using phenol as the antiseptic agent. Other root canal sterilizing agents and techniques included chlorophenol, sodium dioxide, a mixture of metallic sodium and potassium (Schrier's paste), 20–40% sulfuric acid and electromedication. The last procedure, which was subsequently called electrosterilization, was further refined, developed and popularized by a number of dental clinicians. The electrolytes were zinc or sodium chloride, the active agent being chlorine, which also happens to be the active part of sodium hypochlorite, still the first-choice canal irrigant in the twenty-first century. As the focus on 'sterilization' of the root canal grew, so examination of the root canal for bacteria prior to root filling was advocated.

The discovery of X-rays by Röntgen in 1895 had a almost immediate direct impact on endodontics, as the procedure that had been 'blind' up to then included a means of imaging the hidden tissues. Such images were used for canal length determination during root canal treatment only three years later by Kells (1899). Most importantly, the merit of preserving natural teeth either by pulp capping or root filling became established.

The focal infection era

The promising foundations for modern endodontics were shaken in 1904 when Billings brought the apparent relationship between oral sepsis and bacterial endocarditis to the attention of dentistry and medicine. This concept was not new, having been raised as early as 700 BC in Assyria; even Hippocrates talked about the link in 40 BC. Much later, WD Miller coined the term 'focus of infection' and highlighted a possible link between 'mouth germs' and systemic disease. Rosenow, a student of Billings, having introduced the 'theory of focal infection', claimed that streptococci were found in many diseased organs and were capable of spreading through the bloodstream to establish other foci of infection at distant sites. The disastrous consequences that this theory highlighted were only fully realised when a lecture delivered to the faculty of McGill University in Montreal, Canada, by an English surgeon, W Hunter was published in the *Lancet*.[10] He criticized private dental clinicians who ignored sepsis in and around teeth, by accusing them of creating a 'mausoleum of gold over a mass of sepsis', to which he claimed there was no parallel in the whole realm of medicine or surgery. He specifically targeted conservative dental clinicians working in London, who had adopted American methods and skills to rebuild broken dentitions with gold fillings, caps, fixed partial dentures and dentures. Although his intention was probably to encourage dental clinicians to identify poor hygiene and correct it through antiseptic dressings and oral health education, his message was misconstrued. It resulted in the dental and medical profession focusing on pulpless teeth, as well as other putative foci of infection (tonsils, nasal sinuses, gastrointestinal tract, appendix, cervix, uterus, ovaries, prostate, vas deferens). Extraction of teeth was considered the quickest, easiest and surest means of eliminating oral sepsis.

The clinical practice of endodontics at the time was largely determined through sheer force of opinion by the putative seniority of the medical fraternity, which many dental clinicians aspired to join. The sentiment was clearly expressed by Shandalow in 1928,[11] '...coincident with the realisation of the intimate interrelationship between medical and dental science, there is soon to be bestowed upon the younger profession, a new dignity, a sort of accolade in the form of elevation to the standard of a medical specialty'. The focal infection theory reigned for approximately 50 years until around 1940. During this era, 'evidence' supporting the theory continued to be presented by its major proponents. Fears of fatal oral sepsis from deficient root canal treatments led to widespread extraction of pulpless teeth. Endodontics virtually disappeared from many dental schools, except for the teaching of pulp biology. In some areas, treatment was restricted to anterior teeth, as it was believed to be too difficult to eradicate the infection from posterior teeth. Dentists who advocated extraction of all teeth were known as the 'one hundred percenters'. Curiously, the 'focal infection theory' did not influence the practice of dentistry in continental Europe.

The leading opponents of the focal infection theory challenged the validity of supporting evidence for the theory, on the grounds of poor study design, lack of controls and confounding factors. Johnson in 1926[12] advocated retention of pulpless teeth, whenever they were amenable to successful treatment, and he encouraged dental clinicians to take a more rational approach to making decisions about the management of pulpless teeth. Fortunately, these opponents, together with a group of conscientious and skilful root canal therapists, promoted good-quality root canal treatment and followed principles still used today.[13–24] They adopted diagnostic radiography and aseptic techniques, as well as bacteriological and histological methods to assess their treatment. Some of them analyzed the clinical outcome of their treatment systematically and reported favorable success rates. Rhein in 1912[25] advocated the use of rubber dam, good access to canals, cleansers such as Schreier's paste to dissolve organic tissue and chloro-percha to fill the root canal system. He also emphasized the importance of the coronal seal. Thus, this group of highly skilled and visionary clinicians acted as custodians of the art of endodontics. Gradually, the pendulum swung back to the conservation of teeth, so that, by the 1950s, root canal treatment was accepted by both the medical and the dental professions, and endodontics was recognized as a distinct branch of dentistry.

Historical basis for modern endodontics

The principles of contemporary pulp and root canal treatment were soon established, with those presented by Hall in 1928[26] still holding true in the twenty-first century. He suggested that endodontic treatment should never destroy a vital pulp; heed surgical asepsis; use measurement to control instrument trauma; not be performed without radiographs; not enlarge the apical foramen or go beyond the cementodentinal junction; not pump, push, or expel septic matter through the apical foramen; not employ tissue-destroying drugs; and never leave a tooth unsealed. He also advocated the performance of proper outcome studies and counseled against drawing conclusions from a few special cases under observation for only a short time.

Recognition of the role of bacteria in the pathogenesis of periapical disease was interrupted by many digressions and problems, both scientific and political. The importance of this heritage is that the 'cultural' attitudes amongst members of this discipline have shaped modern endodontics. Fashions continue to dominate the cycles of change, which have seen either biomechanical or biological styles alternate in importance. Overall, dental clinicians have identified more closely with biomechanical reasoning and, as a consequence, the biological rationale has been neglected.[27,28] Nowhere is this more evident than in the shift from an approach that demanded a sample and culture test to detect residual bacteria prior to root canal filling to one that hardly considers bacterial involvement but emphasizes the esthetic quality of canal preparation and obturation. Debate centers around how to negotiate canals to greater diameters, in the hope of eliminating more bacteria, removing more organic tissue and filling more lateral canals in the quest for cleanliness. The potential effect on dentin strength has largely gone unnoticed.

Treatment concepts

The principles of contemporary endodontics have changed little since the paper by Hall in 1928.[26] While the teaching of endodontics today is underpinned by biological rationale, with a considerable body of supportive evidence, its practice by dental clinicians remains driven by procedural protocol. In some ways, this is hardly surprising, given that the treatment itself is very practical and very dependent on technical skill. The discipline, therefore, attracts practitioners who have a penchant for precise attention to detail and fine skills. The expectations of satisfaction with the procedures are marked by the radiographic 'look' of the root filling. The debate about 'biological' versus 'technical' approaches remains relevant even today, more than 80 years after the issue was flagged up by Noyes.[27] The current drive towards evidence-based dentistry and medicine has seen the publication of systematic reviews on outcomes of root canal treatment, which show with clarity that the probability of radiographic evidence of periapical healing has not increased within this time frame. For a discipline to survive and thrive, a suitable blend of efficacy, efficiency, utility and cost-effectiveness must be achieved by its principal therapies. This requires a deep understanding of the problem and solution designs from first principles based on this understanding, as well as the skills necessary to deliver these designs. It is for this reason that the clinical academics who lead this field must retain both academic and clinical credibility, maintaining a foot in both camps and demonstrating first-hand knowledge. Individuals with such a broad spectrum of skills are a rarity today and recruitment to such academic positions is a problem. It is these individuals who will sustain and develop endodontics and act as the custodians of its science and art for the future, much in the way that Johnson and co-workers did at the beginning of the last century.

A description of the biological foundation of the discipline must, therefore, form a starting point for understanding 'contemporary treatment concepts'.

Anatomy and physiology of teeth and surrounding support tissues

The dental pulp is a minute piece of connective tissue (approximately 25 mm^3) akin to any other in the body, consisting of cells, nerve fibers and blood vessels embedded in a gel-like ground substance. Its unique characteristics are conferred by its encasement in the relatively rigid but resilient dentin, which it secretes and with which it is intimately linked, anatomically and physiologically, by a layer of specialized cells called odontoblasts. The entire structure is, therefore, called the pulp–dentin complex and forms the bulk of the tooth. The genetically determined, three-dimensional distribution of the odontoblasts maps out the final shape of the tooth at an early stage. Given the small size of the odontoblasts compared with the bulk of dentin, it is evident that the laying down of dentin must be a co-ordinated process, beginning from the outermost periphery of the tooth and progressing to the final resting position of the odontoblasts, lining the junction between pulp and dentin. The implication is that as dentin is laid down by the odontoblasts, these cells must migrate towards the center of the pulp, but in doing so leave an extension of their cell body around which the mineralization takes place. The cell extension is the odontoblastic process and its surrounding dentin effectively forms a channel, the dentinal tubule. The advancing front of organic dentin matrix remains unmineralized and is called predentin. The net effect is that as each of the millions of odontoblasts lay down dentin matrix and withdraw towards the center of the pulp tissue, a hard shell of dentin permeated by millions of tubules (with an approximately radial distribution), each containing a cellular process, is created. The dentin is covered and protected by enamel in the crown and cementum in the root. The diameter of the tubules is approximately 3 μm near the pulp and > 1 μm peripherally, accounting for 45% of the pulp surface and 1% of the outer surface, which junctions with enamel. The dentinal tubules make up 20–30% of the volume of dentin and are filled with a unique protein-rich fluid under positive pressure. Fluid exchange may take place from the pulp outwards or in the reverse direction.

Dentin formed during tooth development is called primary and that laid down after tooth development is called secondary. Both are physiological and are deposited evenly at 4 μm and 0.8 μm per day, respectively. Irregular secondary dentin is laid down unevenly at a rate of 3 μm per day as a defensive response to noxious external stimuli such as dental caries, attrition, abrasion and abfraction. Dentin matrix is a composite of organic (20%) and inorganic (70%) materials and water (10%); far from being inert, it has embedded within it various growth factors that are released when the matrix is damaged. The physical properties of the teeth are determined by the major inorganic component and, significantly, by the organic and water components.

Odontoblasts are specialized cells incapable of further division once fully mature; if damaged, they may be replaced from undifferentiated mesenchymal cells. The potential to stimulate such cells for controlled regeneration is the subject of much therapeutic interest for the future.

Although the three-dimensional distribution of the resting position of the odontoblasts after the formation of primary dentin must, by definition, follow the general outline of the outer form, or starting position, the presence of major neurovascular bundles supplying the pulp tissue, together with local variations in three-dimensional topography, lead to interesting and important variations in the complexity of the root canal anatomy.[29-32]

The remainder of the pulp consists of ground substance into which are embedded fibroblasts and inflammatory cells, collagen fibers and a complex network of blood vessels (Fig. 7-2) and nerve fibers. The fibroblasts are responsible for producing the proteins and carbohydrates that form the viscous substance of the matrix, which accommodates humoral and immune cellular infiltrates produced during inflammatory responses. Lymphatic vessels help to clear away exuded fluid and macromolecules and return the tissue to the status quo. Biological or chronological aging may reduce the cellular and neurovascular elements and thereby reduce the ability of the aged pulp to respond to injury. The pulp tissue has a rich neurovascular supply that reaches it via arterioles and nerve bundles through the root end (apical foramina) and lesser lateral accessory supplies (lateral canals). These allow an exchange of tissue fluid between the periodontal and pulpal tissues; otherwise, the cementum forms an impervious barrier to macromolecules, making root canal treatment feasible.

The vascular system in the pulp, consisting of arterioles, capillaries and venules, is uniquely designed to help to overcome the problems of its non-compliant encapsulation within dentin. Its uniqueness lies in the arteriovenous shunts, which allow blood to be shunted directly from arterioles to venules to prevent a build-up of unsustainable pressure. Tissue pressure changes are also buffered by the barrier effect of the ground matrix. Inflammation caused by local injuries may, therefore, be localized, including pulp abscesses surrounded by normal tissue. These insights have changed the perception of the pulp from being fragile to relatively resilient.

The nervous system in the pulp consists of a rich innervation of sensory (A-fibers and C-fibers serving pain and proprioception) and autonomic nerves (serving the vasculature). The true contribution of the nerve supply to the functions of the pulp are probably more complicated than originally thought, considering the diversity of the neuropeptides they produce and their role in neurogenic inflammation. The faster-conducting, larger diameter myelinated A-delta(δ)-fibers relay sharp,

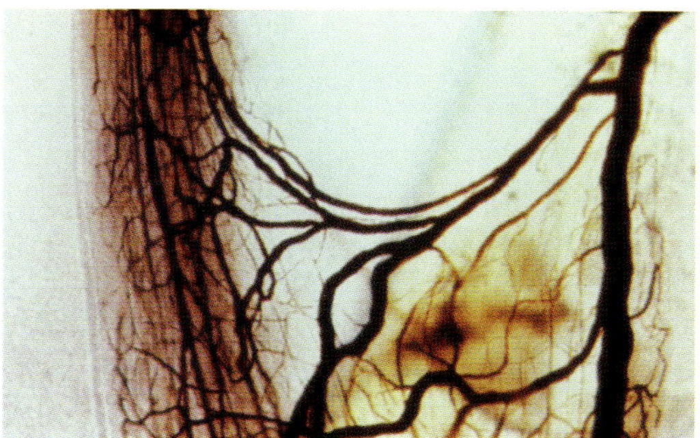

Fig. 7-2 Network of blood vessels in a section of dental pulp.

localized dentinal pain, while the slower-conducting, smaller diameter unmyelinated C-fibers conduct the duller throbbing, poorly localized pain. Aδ-fibers are stimulated by drilling, probing, air drying, heating/cooling the tooth and osmotically active fluids. Dentin sensitivity is explained by the hydrodynamic theory, in which stimuli cause a rapid movement of fluid in the dentinal tubules, mechanically stimulating the Aδ-fibers. Dentin sensitivity may, therefore, be controlled by blocking the tubules. C-fibers are stimulated by noxious stimuli, that is, those that incur tissue damage. The fast-conducting, larger diameter myelinated Aδ-fibers respond to non-noxious mechanical stimulation of the intact crown and may be important in the regulation of mastication and loading of teeth, but they also respond to dentin stimulation. Variations in the thresholds of nerve fiber stimulation and patients' perception and tolerance of pain contribute to the wide range of pain descriptors, making diagnosis of the pulp condition unreliable on the basis of pain history alone.

Beyond the formative function of the pulp, its continued existence is unlikely to be vestigial. The definite change in the rate at which primary and secondary dentin are deposited suggest a designed lifetime role. By inference, the *raison d'être* of the pulp and dentin must be to provide the tooth with the resilient characteristics necessary for withstanding masticatory load. The slight, but evident, viscoelastic deformation of the tooth must be detectable by proprioceptors in the pulp. There is indirect evidence for proprioceptive mechanisms in the pulp, which may partly explain the greater susceptibility of pulpless teeth to fracture.

The pulp has been thought of as a sensory organ, serving to forewarn of damage or impending damage, although this is not always foolproof.

In addition to sensory defenses, the inflammatory response of the pulp contributes to recruitment of the full array of non-specific and specific immunologic responses. At early stages of pulp infection, there is a non-specific inflammatory response dominated by polymorphonuclear leukocytes (PMNs) and macrophages. A specific antibacterial immune response follows and consists of lymphocytes, macrophages and plasma cells. This system protects the pulp against external molecular and microbial stimuli. An extremely important function of the pulp-dentin complex, working in concert with inflammation, is secondary and tertiary (reactionary and reparative) dentin formation, together with dentinal tubule sclerosis (calcification) to block off further ingress of noxious factors. Such reparative mechanisms in the pulp-dentin complex mimic developmental processes. During tooth formation, molecular signals between epithelial and mesenchymal cells control the induction of odontoblast differentiation. Such molecular signals, involving growth factors, have a profound effect on various cellular activities and are found throughout the body. A subclass of these molecules, the transforming growth factor-ß, (TGFß) family, is responsible for signaling odontoblast differentiation. The differentiated odontoblasts synthesize and secrete TFGß together with other growth factors and sequester them into the calcified dentin matrix, probably amongst the organic components; the precise location is unknown. The subsequent dissolution of the dentin matrix as a result of caries or tooth surface loss releases these molecules to exert their influence on healing. The TGFß molecules released by mild dentin-pulp injury diffuse along a concentration gradient down the dentinal tubules, against the outward flow of dentinal fluid, to stimulate viable odontoblasts to lay down reactionary dentin. Injury sufficient to damage odontoblasts irreversibly results in replacement from the mesenchymal cell pool. This is a lengthy process, requiring the migration and differentiation of new cells, followed by secretion of a new matrix. The resulting dentin is, therefore, less well organized and is known as reparative dentin. An important factor interfering with the reparative process is continuing microbial challenge from coronal leakage.

The tissues surrounding the root (periradicular) consist of cementum, the periodontal ligament and alveolar bone. Cementum covers the radicular dentin, abutting the enamel in 70%, overlapping it in 20% and separated from it by a gap in 10% of teeth. The cementum is principally an inorganic tissue that is more impervious than dentin. It is because of this property of cementum that root canal treatment is at all possible. Cementum provides attachment for the periodontal ligament fibers, which suspend the tooth from the alveolar bone. It is laid down throughout life in compensation for loss of occlusal tooth substance and plays a most important physiologic role in the repair of resorbed cementum and dentin. The breakdown in this normal mechanism may result in external root resorption. Cementum formation around the apical foramina is the desirable end result of successful healing following root canal treatment.

The periodontal ligament is a dense fibrous connective tissue that supports and attaches the tooth to its alveolar socket. Its principal component is collagen, in a gel-like matrix. The fibers are arranged in specific groups, each with individual functions, including gingival, transseptal, alveolar crest, horizontal, oblique and apical. Functional adaptation occurs in the intermediate plexus. Although the main cell types found are fibroblasts and occasional defense cells, the root sheath of Hertwig (contributes to the root formation) does not involute completely after root formation but degenerates into a 'perforated bag of epithelial cells,' called the rests of Malassez. These cells proliferate when stimulated by inflammation and may form a cyst. They also produce cytokines and participate in the apical defense response. Blood supply to the periodontal ligament originates from the inferior dental artery. Nerve bundles enter the periodontal ligament through numerous foramina in the alveolar bone and end in small rounded bodies near the cementum. The nerves carry pain, touch and pressure sensations and form an important part of the feedback mechanism of the masticatory apparatus. The ligament has a proprioceptive function and acts as a viscoelastic cushion by virtue of its fibers and hydraulic fluid systems. The ligament responds to functional overloading by widening to relieve the load on the tooth. The periodontal ligament also plays an important role in the eruption of teeth and healing after surgery or trauma. Vascular communications between the pulp and periodontium form pathways for transmission of inflammation and microorganisms between the tissues.

Alveolar bone is the part of the maxilla and mandible that supports teeth by forming the *other* attachment for the periodontal ligament. The shape and structure of the bony trabeculae reflect the stress-bearing requirements of the site. The inorganic surfaces of bone are lined by osteoblasts, which are responsible for bone formation; those that become incorporated within mineral tissue are called osteocytes and maintain contact with each other via canaliculi. Osteoclasts are responsible for bone resorption and may be seen in Howship's lacunae. Bone is a dynamic and labile tissue, continually forming and resorbing in response to functional requirements and under the influence of inflammatory mediators at either the periapex or the marginal attachment. In health, the crest of the alveolus lies approximately 2 mm apical to the cemento-enamel junction, but in periodontal disease it may lie further towards the root apex.

Pathology of pulpal and periapical disease

Pulp injury: pathology and diagnosis

The pulp may be injured either by interference with its blood supply or by damage to the pulp-dentin complex. Direct interference with the blood supply may occur in acute (impact) or chronic (occlusal) traumatic injuries. Injuries through the pulp-dentin complex may occur by induction of cracks or fractures in tooth structure, again through acute or chronic traumatic injuries, or by exposure of dentin through natural (attrition, abfraction), dietary (attrition, erosion), parafunctional (attrition, abrasion), habitual (abrasion), pathologic (caries) or iatrogenic (operative or cosmetic) processes.

Exposure of dentin causes direct physical injury to odontoblastic processes and, more importantly, exposes the pulp to microorganisms. The degree of exposure is dependent on the surface area and depth of dentin involved. The physiopathologic mechanisms in place – namely inflammation, outflow of dentinal fluid, temporary blockage of tubules by protein molecules, followed later by mineralization (dentinal sclerosis) and formation of reactionary dentin – help to close off the avenues of direct pulp exposure. If such closure is not possible because the pulp is compromised and unable to generate the reparative response, then the unabated inflow of microbial stimulants causes chronic inflammation and pulpal demise. The rate of damage to the dentin, whether carious or non-carious, may also influence the ability of the pulp to defend itself.

Protection of the pulp-dentin complex is dependent on exposed dentin being covered using restorative materials. Such coverage may simply aim to provide a protective layer or may simultaneously replace the missing tissue, restoring form, function and esthetics. The complexity and invasiveness of the restorative procedures may, in turn, induce further damage to the pulp, but this may be seen as a necessary risk to afford protection. It is important to appreciate the damaging effect of the restorative procedures. A key issue is the manner by which the material is attached to the tooth structure: whether this involves mechanical or chemical retention, each has advantages and limitations.

The relative importance of the different factors causing pulp injury when restorative procedures are employed has been debated at length. In the

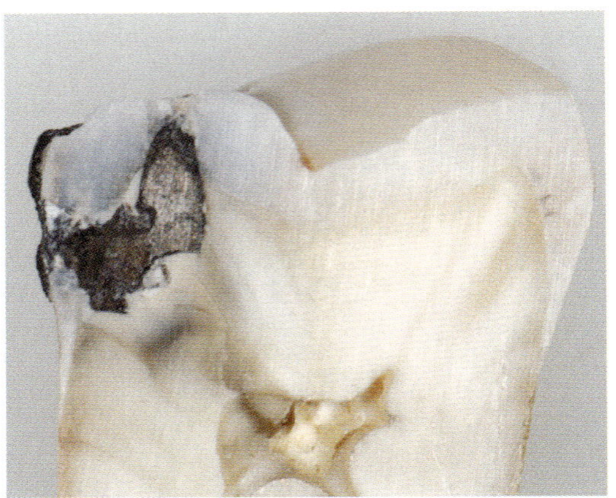

Fig. 7-3 Leakage around a restoration.

past (pre-1960s), the effects of restorative procedures and materials dominated thinking in respect of etiologic factors. Controlled animal and human histologic studies (during the 1960s and early 1970s) showed that the effects of restorative procedures and restorative materials were reversible, provided microbial leakage at the interface between restorative material and dentin was controlled using, typically, a barrier of zinc oxide-eugenol cement.

Current understanding is that pulp injury is multifactorial; the emphasis is placed on the complex interplay between size of cavity, remaining dentin thickness, restorative material, microbial leakage and pulpal inflammation. The relationships remain unclear. The degree of injury to the pulp and its ability to survive is dictated, in large part, by the amount of remaining dentin and the number of viable odontoblasts. It is, therefore, important to preserve as much dentin as possible, as it provides a natural buffer to further injury. Cutting deep cavities or crown preparations increases the number of dentinal tubules involved, reduces the survival of odontoblasts and increases the degree of pulp inflammation. This inflammation may be aggravated by dehydration, heat generation and microbial and chemical factors reaching the pulp. Heat generation may be influenced by bur type (diamond or tungsten, large or small), rotation speed (type of handpiece), duration and nature of bur contact (intermittent or continuous, high or low interfacial pressure, bur stalling), cutting technique (slot versus surface removal), vibration and adequacy of coolant spray. Although it is difficult to quantify the threshold of dentin thickness critical to pulp survival, < 0.25 mm appears to result in severe inflammation. Additionally, pulpal inflammation tends to be most severe in teeth with cavities contaminated by microflora.

Localized dentinal injury may induce a localized zone of pulpal inflammation. The process of spread of inflammation from a localized site to the rest of the pulp is not fully understood. It may be related to the ability of the pulp to close off dentinal tubules by the action of replacement odontoblasts formed from undifferentiated mesenchymal cells. If this fails to 'wall off' the source of inflammation, then the inflammation becomes persistent and chronic. The greater the number of dentinal tubules involved and the greater the degree of odontoblast injury, the larger the volume of pulp tissue affected by inflammation. The localized response may, or may not, progress to more severe inflammation, depending on the provoking factors. The notion of accumulative pulp damage became established with the idea that the process begins with caries, tooth surface loss or trauma, is aggravated by a series of restorative procedures and then is worsened by bacterial leakage (Fig. 7-3). The persistent injury from leakage suppresses healing and promotes inflammation, which becomes chronic and spreads through the tissue leading to 'total pulpitis'. Such pulpitis is asymptomatic in 50% of cases. In clinical practice, teeth undergoing treatment may have a history of previous treatment and pulp inflammation, which may go undiagnosed if asymptomatic.

It is, therefore, possible that restorative intervention, however minimal, superimposed upon pre-existing asymptomatic pulp inflammation may be sufficient to tip the balance and cause a sudden flare-up with symptoms or cause silent necrosis. The pulp space and tissue may then rapidly become infected if exposed to bacteria, progressing to possible abscess formation.

If the injury is limited, the pulp may be able to survive and recover, albeit remaining 'fibrosed,' less cellular and more susceptible to necrosis with further insults. The dynamics of pulpal inflammation may produce a range of histologic pictures including areas of chronic inflammation coexisting with micro-abscesses and partial necrosis. Clinical signs and symptoms of pulp disease have a poor correlation with the state of the pulp. This makes clinical diagnosis and treatment planning extremely difficult. Added to this picture of uncertainty, there may be radiographic periapical changes associated with inflammation of the coronal pulp. A reasonably clear distinction can only be made between vital (albeit inflamed) and necrotic pulps using currently available pulp tests. Following traumatic impact injuries, sudden severance of the blood supply can result in total necrosis of the pulp, without any subsequent radiographic periapical change. Such change may become evident only in the event of infection of the necrotic pulp.

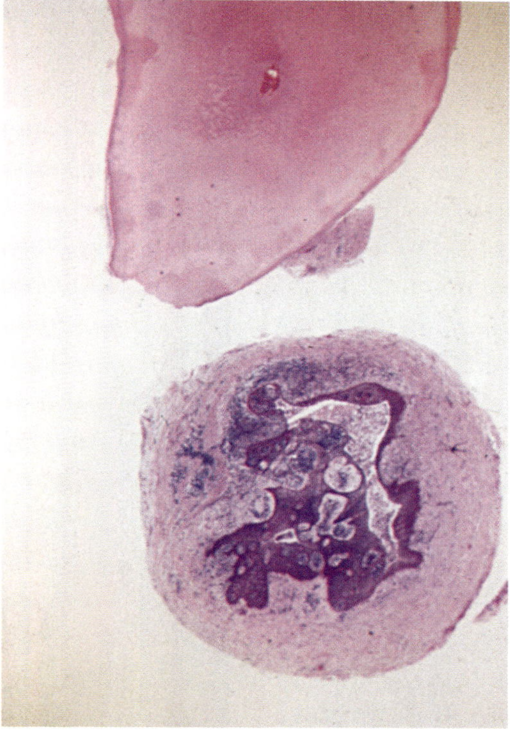

Fig. 7-4 Root apex with chronic inflammatory lesion containing a central cystic cavity.

Periapical disease: etiopathogenesis and diagnosis

Periapical disease is a sequel of pulpal disease, but it often becomes evident before complete necrosis of the pulp. Conversely, sterile necrosis of the pulp can be accompanied by an absence of periapical disease; early theories suggested the possible involvement of stagnant tissue fluid and necrotic pulp tissue, but both theories were disproved. Bacterial products have been implicated in the initiation of periapical disease, which further develops only in the presence of progressive bacterial colonization of the root canal system. The role of viruses in the initiation and subsequent development of periapical disease has not been proven, but they may enhance the pathogenic potential of bacteria. Periapical disease is, therefore, the result of interaction between bacteria and bacterial products and the host defenses. Both non-specific and specific host defense mechanisms are recruited to defend against the potential invasion of the body by bacteria. The periapical lesion is the retreat of the bone tissue away from the source of infection, creating space for body defense processes in the immediate vicinity to counter the infection. The full range of immune mechanisms is implicated in the development of the periapical lesion. The clinical course of the periapical lesion is variable, resulting in diverse presentations, which have been classified into: acute apical periodontitis, chronic apical periodontitis, acute periapical abscess or suppuration (without sinus tract), chronic periapical abscess or suppuration (with sinus tract) and radicular cysts. The relative contribution of the normal inflammatory and immune responses varies in these clinical variants. The nature of the lesion (except in the incipient lesion) is primarily chronic inflammatory (granulomatous) tissue (Fig. 7-4),

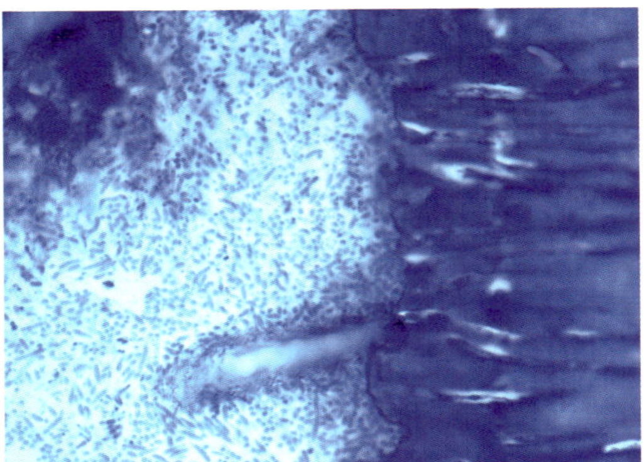

Fig. 7-5 Bacterial biofilm on root canal dentin wall.

indicating that inflammation and attempts at healing are coexistent. Depending on the state of the lesion, there may be a variable degree of tissue destruction, with the consequent concentration of acute inflammation cells, PMNs and macrophages in the vicinity of the apical foramina, including the root canal.

Bacteria gain access to the root canal system through open dentinal tubules, caries or mechanical exposures of the pulp, lateral canals or cracks in the tooth. The point of entry of the bacteria is likely to dictate the subsequent development of the infection and its distribution. Bacterial invasion usually begins in the coronal part of the tooth and root, notably along the dentin wall, though dying pulp tissue may also become colonized by bacteria. The pattern of bacterial colonization varies from tooth to tooth. In some teeth, bacteria may appear in small numbers in the root canals near the apical foramen, in particular in teeth with intact pulp chambers. Where vital pulp tissue is present apically, the intensity of the infection tapers off towards it. In other teeth, the bacterial colonization becomes scant at the mid-root level, only to become heavy in the apical portion, where it is associated with a well-developed periapical lesion. In teeth exposed by caries, the canals are usually evenly coated with a thick bacterial biofilm. A description of the variation and nature of the bacterial types in different parts of the canal system may convey important insights about the infection, but the available information is presently limited and more in situ observational studies are required.

The bulk of the microbial flora in root canals exists in the form of a biofilm, rather than as a loose collection of a variety of morphologically distinct bacterial forms (cocci, rods, filaments) (Fig.7-5). The filamentous forms may be found adhering perpendicular to the canal wall, with coccoid forms arranged in parallel chains. Cocci occasionally attach to the filaments to give a 'corncob' appearance. The interbacterial spaces are filled with an amorphous extracellular matrix. This biofilm may be continuous or broken. Different clusters of bacteria may communicate with each other through fluid films or columns by means of molecular messengers. Individual cells within this 'cooperative' may respond to their immediate surroundings and neighbors by switching on or off relevant genes for survival. The bacterial community is influenced by, as yet undiscovered, ecological factors in the root canal system, including positive and negative associations between species. Such associations may be a consequence of nutritional interactions, local physiological conditions (Eh, pH), bacteriocins and bacterial coaggregation. The overall ecological picture is one of a complex polymicrobial community that may 'function as one', rather like a multicellular organism, in response to its environment. Nutrition depletion may slow bacterial metabolism and allow some bacteria to enter a starvation or dormant state, which may make them impossible to culture if sampled. In certain situations, only the presence of adequate numbers of bacteria enables the expression of certain virulence genes, a condition communicated amongst the bacteria by 'quorum-sensing' molecules.

Some of the flora of the root canal may appear to be suspended in a moist canal lumen among vast numbers of PMNs. The apparent planktonic suspension of bacteria may be an illusion created by the inability to visualize the intercellular matrix, but this needs in situ clarification. The PMNs may be seen to form a distinct wall separating the bacterial

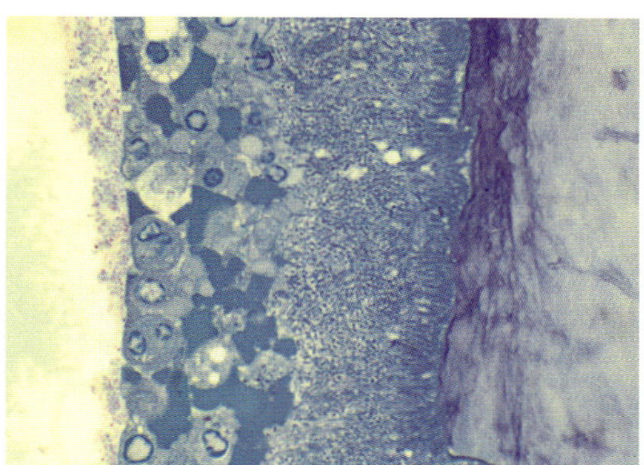

Fig. 7-6 Polymorphonuclear leukocytes attempting to wall-off bacterial biofilm on the root canal wall.

biofilm on the canal wall from the canal lumen, notably in apical locations (Fig. 7-6). Morphological studies do not reveal the identity of bacteria and must, therefore, be supplemented either by cultivation studies or in situ hybridization studies.

Cultures of root canal bacteria show the presence of *Actinomyces*, black-pigmented and non-pigmented *Bacteroides*, *Enterococcus*, *Fusobacterium*, *Lactobacillus*, *Peptostreptococcus*, *Streptococcus* and *Veillonella* species. Supplementing these data by culture-independent techniques for bacterial detection and identification has shown that the bacterial flora is dominated by strains represented by the phyla Firmicutes and Actinobacteria; some strains also represent the phyla Bacteroidetes and Proteobacteria. The mean number of taxa reported using both cultivation and molecular approaches is 20 per sample. These are dominated by anaerobes, in particular Gram-positive species. Statistical estimates of undetected bacteria reach 80 taxa per root canal sample. The Gram-negative bacteria probably dominate the canal lumen and surface, especially apically, while Gram-positive bacteria may dominate dentin infection. The reason for desiring accurate identification of bacteria in root canals is to disclose those bacteria or combinations of bacteria playing key roles in disease progression, its acute exacerbation, resistance to treatment or treatment failure.

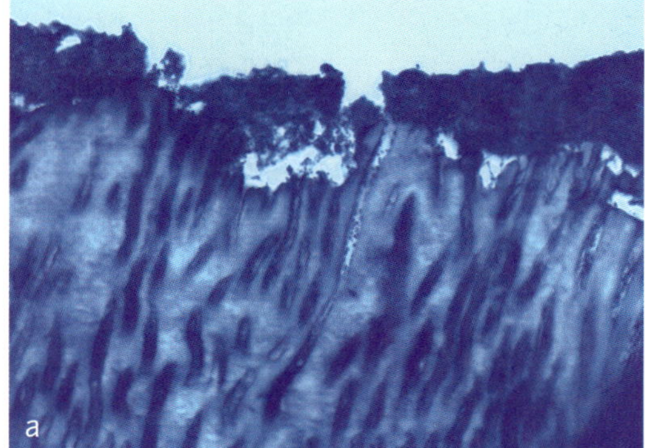

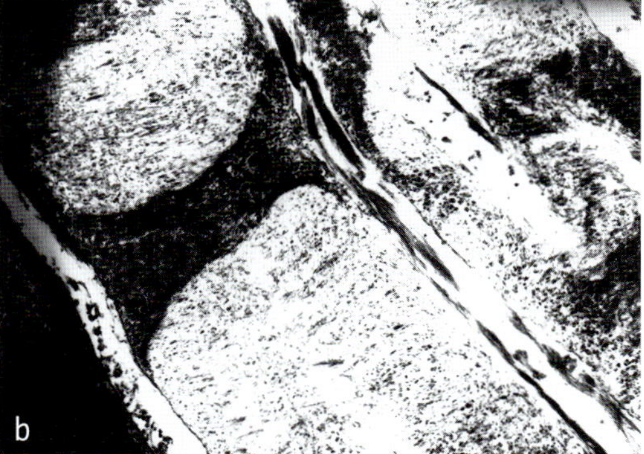

Fig. 7-7 Bacterial penetration of dentinal tubules. (a) Bacterial biofilm on the root canal wall with penetration of bacteria into dentinal tubules. (b) Bacterial cells in dentinal tubules shown by transmission electron microscopy.

Bacterial penetration into dentin is evident when infection has spread along the dentinal wall following pulp necrosis. The predentin is readily and commonly infected, but the calcified dentin less so. Bacterial penetration into dentin around the root canal is limited, sometimes penetrating a third to half the depth of dentin containing tubules that end in a vital periodontal membrane (Fig. 7-7). Only where tubules end in necrotic periodontal tissue can bacteria be observed along the entire length of the tubules. Dentin tubule infection is deeper apically, in particular in teeth exposed by caries. The bacteria invading deep (0.5–2.0 mm) layers of dentin in the root canals of carious teeth are mostly strict anaerobes (80%), with a predominance of

Gram-positive rods (68%) and Gram-positive cocci (27%). *Lactobacillus* (30%), *Streptococcus* (13%) and *Propionibacterium* species (9%) dominate dentin infection. The presence of Gram-negative bacteria in root canal dentin is confirmed by the presence of lipopolysaccharide to a depth of 300 μm.

The mean number of cells in infected teeth is estimated at 10^8 colony-forming units (CFU) per mL sample (range 10^1–10^8 CFU/mL). The number of genera per tooth ranges from 1 to 16 (mean range, 6–9), and the number of species per tooth ranges from 1 to 12 (mean range, 2–6). The density of cells, 10^5 cells/mL sample, is consistent with other infections, though at the lower end of the spectrum.

Epithelial cells or PMNs often plug the apical foramen, but where the microbial front extends into the periapical lesion, there may be variable tissue necrosis and a PMN response. In the latter instance, the tissue immediately around the tooth apex may be lyzed and occupied by an apparently young apical plaque. Scalloped root resorption may be found, with multilayered bacteria embedded in an extracellular matrix. The bacteria in this plaque have been observed to be mainly cocci and rods, but fibrillar forms may also be present. Such extraradicular extension of bacteria is rare. Mainly anaerobic bacteria occur in the periapical tissues, perhaps associated with foreign or dead (cellular or dentinal) material, to which the defense cells have no access. The main species implicated in periapical tissue invasion include *Actinomyces* species and *Propionibacterium propionica*. Many other species in the root canal flora have been implicated, but their presence in the periapical tissues remains controversial given the difficulties of proving that samples tested are not contaminated. The majority of chronic periapical lesions do not contain bacteria, although bacterial invasion of the periapical tissues is common in acute exacerbation, where for reasons yet unknown, the root canal bacteria overwhelm local periapical defenses. The fact that the majority of periapical lesions heal following tooth extraction suggests that true extraradicular infections are rare. Cementum is rarely infected except in extraradicular infection (usually by *Prevotella*, *Fusobacterium*, *Peptostreptococcus*, *Eubacterium* and *Campylobacter* species); these species can be reconciled with teeth associated with sinus tracts.

The host reaction, in the form of the developing periapical lesion, is dependent upon the nature of the mixed infection. Periapical disease is caused by a polymicrobial infection of the root canal system, with a direct relationship between the size of the periapical lesion and the number and type of bacterial strains. The periapical host response is essentially chronic inflammation, indicating persistence of the irritant stimulus (bacteria), given the protective sanctuary of the root canal system from host defenses. Therefore, the cell profile, in addition to the ubiquitous PMNs and macrophages, contains a small population of eosinophils and mast cells and various proportions of immune (lymphocytes and plasma) cells. Epithelial cells may be present in up to 50% of lesions. Other tissue elements in the periapical lesion include endothelial cells and fibroblasts, both common where there are attempts at healing. The periapical lesion is T lymphocyte dominated, although B lymphocytes may also be present. The relative proportion of T and B lymphocytes is dependent on the nature and activity of the lesion; the T/B cell ratio being significantly higher in lesions containing radicular cysts than in granulomas and apical scar lesions. Plasma cells may actively produce local antibodies.

The neural and immune systems interact in controlling the non-specific and specific defensive responses. Microorganisms may also participate in this regulatory function. A conceptual model describing the entire sequence of interactions between the cellular (microbial and host) and neural components, leading to the progressive development of the periapical lesion, is far from complete. Synthesis of the model requires integration of information from human and animal studies at cellular and molecular levels, as described below.

As root canal infection matures and progresses apically, certain bacterial products and bacteria are able to stimulate the periapical tissues via the apical foramina. In a previously unexposed host, the initial response may be non-specific acute inflammation, consisting of a fluid exudate followed by a cellular exudate; PMNs are attracted to the site by a number of bacteria-derived chemoattractants. In a previously exposed host, this initial exudate brings with it circulating antibodies; the resultant antigen–antibody complexes cause further PMN migration by activation of complements C3b and C5a. The effect of preexisting immunity helps to confine bacteria to the apical foramina, requiring only a sparse cellular infiltrate, with fibroencapsulation of the rich granulation tissue. In contrast, lack of preexisting immunity results in poor bacterial confinement and a more diffuse cellular infiltrate, which spreads within the trabecular system. These histologic pictures translate into radiographic views of small, well-circumscribed, periapical radiolucencies and extensive diffuse lesions, respectively. The acute response may be accompanied by the usual clinical signs of pain, tenderness on percussion and tooth elevation, but it may also be too transient and minimal to be noticed. Little bone resorption may have taken place and no radiographic changes may be discernible.

Since bacteria and their products may remain in the root canal system, both a delayed and a specific immune response are mounted. These responses are mediated by direct stimulation by the bacteria and their products of the host cells and cascade triggers from subsequent responses. Depending on the nature of the stimulus and host susceptibility, a whole range of effects may be manifested, including types 1–4 hypersensitivity reactions. The magnitude of the response varies from individual to individual, depending upon both the stimulus and the host characteristics. In some cases, the host response may be exaggerated, causing greater damage than the bacterial assault. The clinical progression of the lesion may take one of several paths, including acute apical abscess formation, chronic suppuration with sinus tract formation, or conversion to a chronic, stable but dynamic state. In the event that bacteria enter the periapical tissues, they are normally removed rapidly by PMNs and macrophages, the latter releasing leukotrienes and prostaglandins. The leukotrienes attract more macrophages to the site, contributing to bone resorption and creating space for invasion by more immune cells. Cytokines intensify the local vascular response and osteoclastic bone resorption, and can provoke a general alert by endocrine stimulation of fever and output of acute phase proteins and other serum factors. Death of bacteria, PMNs and macrophages in this encounter can result in suppuration, which may follow an acute or a chronic course. In the latter, cytokines and lipopolysaccharide from bacterial breakdown products may stimulate the epithelial cells in the rests of Malassez to proliferate and line a tissue path for pus to escape to a body surface (usually intraoral). The prevalence of various clinical presentations in the disease process is unknown. It is likely that the majority follow an asymptomatic chronic progression.

Chronic lesions may undergo acute exacerbations as a result of changes in the balance between the bacteria and host responses subsequent to a proliferation of specific bacteria. Such acute phases, accompanied by invasion of the periapical lesion by viable bacteria (many of which will die there), may also result in increase in the size of the periapical lesion. The change in the relative balance between the bacteria and the host defenses causes variations both in the histologic and clinical picture, although there is no strong correlation between these pictures.

The proliferation of epithelial rests of Malassez is evident in about half of all periapical lesions. The pattern of proliferation includes formation of strands, arcades and rings of cells at the junction between adjacent connective tissue and the granulation tissue. Proliferation may also occur within the body of the granuloma, possibly plugging the apical foramen, limiting egress of bacteria and their toxins. In some instances, these epithelial plugs bulge out into the periapical lesion, forming a sac connected to the root and continuous with the root canal, termed a bay or pocket cyst. In such circumstances, microorganisms in the root canal have direct access to the 'cyst' cavity and may invade it. A true cyst has been defined as a separate pathologic, epithelium-lined cavity, usually containing fluid or semi-solid material. It does not communicate with the root canal or any other opening; it develops in periapical lesions with a prevalence of approximately 9%. The proliferating epithelium surrounds an abscess, isolating it from nutrients and causing degeneration. The bay cyst, by inference, heals by elimination of the bacterial contamination of the root canal, whereas successful treatment of the true cyst may require surgery. Persistent periapical lesions may represent chronic inflammation caused by residual infection (intra/ extraradicular), a foreign body response or a radicular cyst.

Diagnosis of apical periodontitis is based on the presenting symptoms and the results of both clinical and radiographic examinations. The presence of acute inflammation or an abscess in the periodontal ligament causes local tenderness to pressure and percussion, which may spread and intensify during peripheral sensitization. Spreading apical infection may be intensely painful and associated with systemic signs of malaise, fever and lymph node involvement. The presence of intra- or extraoral swellings and sinuses signal the periapical problem, but an asymptomatic chronic periapical lesion may only be detected by radiographic imaging.

Radiographically, teeth with apical periodontitis may be associated with a range of presentations from mere alteration in the architecture and width of the periodontal ligament space to frank periapical radiolucency. Unfortunately, the sensitivity (35–88%) of conventional radiography to detect periapical disease is far from ideal. Cone beam computerized tomography, requiring only 8% of the effective dose of conventional computerized tomography, is capable of producing three-dimensional images with accurate recording of lesion size and no superimposition of anatomical structures. This technique has rapidly gained popularity amongst endodontists, despite an absence of evidence in respect of sensitivity or specificity. It has been shown that 34% of periapical lesions associated with posterior teeth may only be diagnosed by cone beam tomography.

Concepts of pulp-dentin protection, repair and regeneration

Prevention of pulp-dentin injury

Ideally, perfectly formed natural teeth, well aligned in a Class 1 occlusion, with canine guidance and absence of parafunction would retain their intact outer covering throughout life, and if they are maintained free of plaque, would not be subject to the two most common dental diseases: caries and periodontal disease. Add to this the absence of acute and chronic traumatic injuries and, in theory, there should be no need for endodontic care. The reality is that teeth may be malformed, malaligned, poorly occluded, poorly maintained, subject to the common dental diseases and subjected to stresses and strains, resulting in the need for endodontic care. This is evidenced by the fact that half of all adults have suffered apical periodontitis by 50 years of age. Prevention of injury to the pulp-dentin complex, therefore, requires good personal and professional maintenance of the dentition, the elimination of damaging habits and, where necessary, only minimally invasive dental intervention. The principal causes of damage to the dental hard tissues include caries, tooth surface loss (wear), traumatic injuries and, increasingly, cosmetic interventions by dental clinicians. Whatever the source of injury, the guiding principle should always be minimal intervention and maximal preservation of dentin. Malformed teeth should be diagnosed early and preventive measures instituted to protect the pulp when possible. Caries, periodontal diseases and tooth surface loss should be prevented and, if present, controlled and treated.

An intact and functional pulp-dentin complex is considered crucial to the long-term survival and function of teeth. A physiologically intact and functional pulp-dentin complex will maintain its ability to remain vital. The pulp only becomes compromised when the pulp-dentin complex is damaged beyond functional repair or is anatomically breached, causing severe inflammation, which compromises the chances of recovery. Clinical management of pulp-dentin problems may, therefore, be divided into those with and those without a breach of the pulp chamber. Procedures designed to preserve the pulp have traditionally been labeled as indirect pulp capping, direct pulp capping and pulpotomy. The rationale for, and consequences of, these procedures need to be understood. Indirect pulp capping is intended to facilitate formation of reparative dentin to consolidate the defensive barrier. Direct pulp capping and pulpotomy are intended to regenerate the lost tissue, close the breach and achieve an intact pulp chamber, followed by an increase in dentin thickness through reparative dentin formation. This requires responsive and vital odontoblasts capable of laying down protective secondary and tertiary (reparative and reactionary) dentin and inducing dentinal sclerosis.

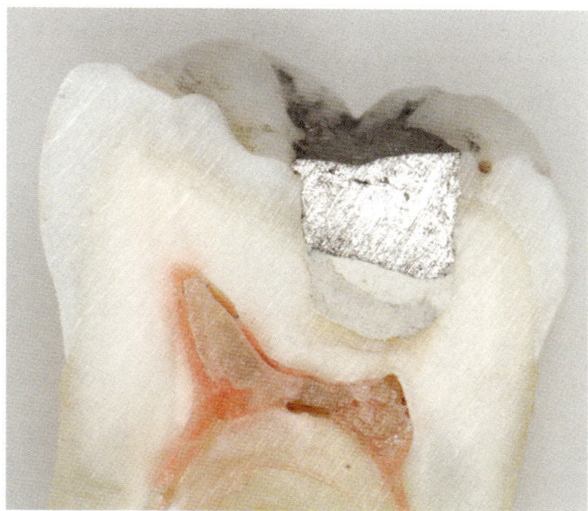

Fig. 7-8 Tooth with indirect pulp cap.

Protection of injured pulp-dentin complex and prevention of microbial leakage

In treating caries, a conservative cavity should be cut to access and remove softened, carious dentin. In relatively deep cavities, a lining of hard-setting calcium hydroxide cement may be placed to facilitate repair through solubilization and release of growth factors to stimulate odontoblasts into action and the killing of residual bacteria within the dentin. A base, typically of zinc oxide-eugenol or resin-reinforced glass-ionomer cement may be placed over the calcium hydroxide to help prevent microbial leakage prior to placing the restoration.

In very deep preparations, additional considerations come into play, as there may be microbreaches in the integrity of the pulp chamber. Under these circumstances, indirect pulp therapy may be considered. The technique is used when excavation of all the carious dentin might risk a traumatic breach of the pulpal space (Fig. 7-8). In such circumstances, some softened, unstained carious dentin may be left in the base of the preparations. Following the placement of a lining of a hard-setting, calcium hydroxide cement, the tooth may be restored by means of a definitive restorative material or, if re-entry is considered to be indicated, a transitional restoration. This latter approach is not considered to be supported by the rate of secondary dentin formation. At 3 μm per day, only 0.27 mm of dentin would be formed in three months, perhaps an inadequate thickness to prevent a traumatic exposure. Furthermore, the practical problem with re-entry techniques is that it is difficult to gauge the depth of the residual caries. As a consequence an unacceptably thick layer of carious dentin may be left, together with necrotic pulp tissue subjacent to the lesion. Further, the accepted guideline that dentin softening and staining precede bacterial invasion may not be completely valid; bacterial invasion of hard dentin is a distinct possibility. Indirect pulp capping may, therefore, be an unpredictable procedure. Success relies on correct diagnosis of the pulp condition, leaving only a small amount of carious dentin, and controlling microbial leakage.

When dentin is cut or ground with a metal instrument during restorative procedures, a smear is formed over its surface. Although the smear layer prevents good adaptation and adhesion of restorative materials in the cavity, it may plug the dentinal tubules to help to protect the pulp from microbial leakage. The use of newer generations of dentin adhesives involves complete removal of the smear layer to facilitate the formation of an effective hybrid layer. The restorative or bonding material causes transient pulp inflammation, but long-term protection from exposure to bacteria and their products should enable the inflammation to subside.

Many restorations fail as a consequence of microbial leakage. Microbial leakage tends to be greater in association with larger restorations with long cavosurface margins and greater potential for tooth deformation under loading, causing marginal percolation.

The approaches to the prevention of microbial leakage may be divided into those seeking to reduce gaps between restoration and cavity and those relying on the antibacterial properties of materials. Predictable reduction in marginal gaps is dependent upon the properties of the material and optimal manipulation, taking account of interfacial relationships between restorative material and tooth tissue. For long-term success, the interface between restoration and tooth must be durable, in particular under loading. Unfortunately, no material is yet able to meet such demands; consequently, all adhesive materials fail some time after placement and allow microbial leakage. While much emphasis has been placed on gap reduction or elimination, little emphasis has been placed on the reduction of microbial leakage. Irrespective of the strategy adopted for the protection of operatively exposed dentin, whether by the traditional use of liners and bases or the so-called etch and bond techniques, the inability to seal cavity margins effectively and block-off all dentinal tubules is the weak link in respect of pulp survival in perpetuity. Open dentinal tubules provide a potential pathway for bacteria and their products to invade and cause persistent chronic pulp inflammation, with the inevitable risk of pulp death. Open dentinal tubules associated with a healthy pulp do, however, offer resistance to bacterial invasion compared with non-vital pulp. The time taken for a chronically inflamed pulp to die has not been defined, but depending on the initial condition, nature of the continuing stimulus and the pulp response, it may take weeks to many years.

The desirable outcome of any operative intervention is that the physiologically responsive pulp–dentin complex generates reactionary dentin and closes dentinal tubules through sclerosis. Reactionary dentin response increases dentin thickness and is positively related to the size of the cavity, remaining dentin thickness, the response to acid etching and microbial leakage. The greatest reactionary dentin response is evident in cavities with remaining dentin thickness between 0.25 and 0.5 mm, especially in the presence of microbial leakage. It may be that this depth is optimal for the stimulation effects of solubilized growth factors released from dentin during restorative procedures. Further reduction of dentin thickness increases odontoblast damage and reduces the reactionary dentin response. Restorative materials play a minor role in stimulating reactionary dentin, but the effects are enhanced by reduced dentin thickness, especially to < 0.5 mm. A calcium hydroxide liner produces the maximum response, and zinc polycarboxylate cement no response. This effect is probably mediated via the direct stimulation of odontoblasts.

Regeneration after pulp chamber breaches

The pulp may be breached or nearly breached through caries, tooth surface loss, acute traumatic injury or cavity preparation. In each case, the operator must estimate the preexisting pulpal status: the extent of injury and degree of microbial contamination. In the case of an acute or chronic (tooth surface loss) traumatic injury, the hard tissue wound is clearly seen and its history will give an indication of the extent of the damage to the pulp. The nature of an acute injury will give an indication of the probable damage to the pulp and its chances of successful regeneration. When dealing with a deep lesion of caries, the picture is less clear as the proximity of the caries to the pulp is unclear. Its acute or chronic nature provides some insight into the degree of pulp injury. Estimation of damage must, by definition, be clinical in nature, yet the desired assessment is judgement of the histologic state of the pulp. This judgement can only be made on the basis of the history of pain, examination findings, pulp tests and radiographs. Unfortunately, the poor correlation between histopathology and clinical signs and symptoms leave the operator with an educated guess. Despite this, it is often stated that teeth exhibiting a history of no pain or signs of periapical disease stand a good chance of successful pulp therapy. Estimation of the proximity of caries to the pulp and the extent to which the superficial pulp may be necrotic and contaminated by bacteria is intuitive and based on experience. The aim of the treatment is to remove all infected hard or soft tissue and to restore the tooth with a bacteria-excluding tight restoration to preserve the health of the residual pulp tissue.

Successful treatment of pulp exposures by direct pulp capping is guided by the same prerequisites as for healthy pulp: low bacterial contamination and absence of subsequent microbial leakage. When excavation of deep caries leads to a traumatic exposure of the pulp, at least minor bacterial contamination of the pulp tissue is assumed. Pulps exposed to salivary contamination for several hours following traumatic injury may still be successfully pulp capped. Minor contamination of the exposure by saliva during operative procedures is unlikely to affect the outcome. The most important factor is a healthy pulp. The pulp is likely to be healthier in younger teeth; however, age is not always a good prognostic indicator.

Direct pulp capping requires good tooth isolation, preferably by rubber dam. The cavity should be caries free and the pulp wound fresh and exuding a limited amount of blood or serum. The wound is gently washed with sterile water or saline to remove contaminants, debris and dentin chips and then decontaminated by washing with sodium hypochlorite (0.5%). This helps to achieve hemostasis. If persistent bleeding is encountered, hemostasis may be achieved with wet cotton pellets. Profuse, prolonged (> 5min) bleeding indicates severe pulp inflammation and the need for a more radical approach to treatment. Once hemostasis is achieved, the wound surface is dressed with setting or non-setting calcium hydroxide.

Pulpotomy is the term applied to removal of coronal pulp tissue when the exposed pulp is believed to be too severely contaminated by bacteria or too inflamed to give a satisfactory prognosis. The extent to which pulp tissue should be removed is not strictly defined. In fractured teeth with exposed pulps, the pulp surface may exhibit one of two reactions: proliferation with an epithelium-covered surface (pulp polyp), where pulpal inflammation is limited to a depth of 2 mm, or ulcerative necrosis with inflammation of the pulp penetrating several millimeters. The aim of the procedure is to expose healthy tissue. The success of the procedure depends upon removal of necrotic and inflamed tissue. This is best achieved with a water-cooled abrasive diamond bur used at high speed in an intermittent light stroking motion to minimize implantation of dentin chips into the exposure. All debris must be removed to achieve a clean wound. The principles of therapy are identical to direct pulp capping, except that the exposure is larger and the calcium hydroxide is applied deeper into the root. After hemostasis is achieved, calcium hydroxide is gently applied without pressure and covered with a layer of zinc oxide-eugenol mixed to a thin consistency to eliminate microbial leakage to the exposure. Some advocate cutting a step in the cavity to support a plastic or Teflon disc to resist the packing of zinc oxide-eugenol dressing. If a composite restorative material is to be used, a resin-modified glass ionomer may be used to cover the calcium hydroxide. The restoration is then placed (Fig. 7-9).

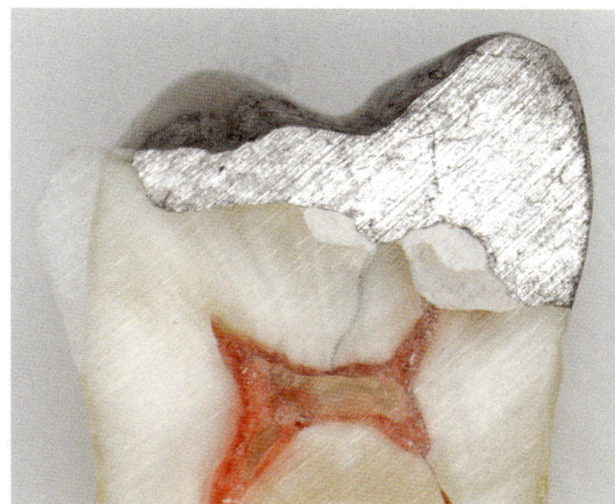

Fig. 7-9 Tooth with direct pulp cap.

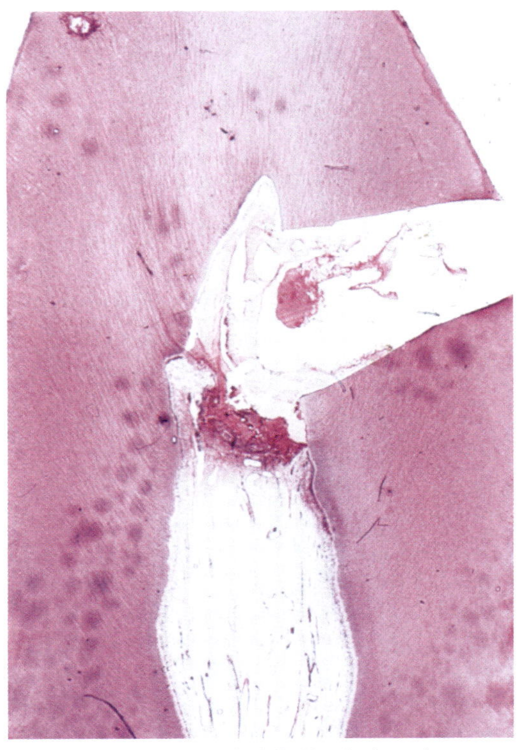

Fig. 7-10 Histologic image of calcified barrier formation following direct pulp capping.

There is no obvious relationship between size of exposure and success rate. It might be expected that exposures from caries lesions would have a lower success rate, but, in the absence of previous pulpal symptoms, success rates may be similar to those of traumatic exposures. The key factors for a successful outcome are good preexisting potential for the replacement of odontoblasts, a good reactionary dentin response and the absence of inflammation-causing microbial leakage. All pulp therapy should be followed up to determine outcome. An initial assessment is recommended at 6–12 weeks, followed by review at six months and thereafter annually. Vitality tests should be judged with caution in pulpotomized teeth because of the distance of the pulp from the surface. In pulp capping and pulpotomy, additional tests include radiographic and manual checking for the presence and integrity of the calcified barrier bridge by removing the dressing and direct probing (Fig. 7-10). In the absence of complete fixed bridge formation, the treatment is considered failed and root canal treatment should be initiated without delay. In addition, where there are incompletely formed roots, there should be radiographic

Table 7-1 Success rates of pulp therapy

Studies	Teeth (T)/cases (C)	Follow-up (years)	Success rate (%)
Shovelton et al. 1971[33]	412 (T)	2	69–78 (NP)
			50–80 (P)
Haskell et al. 1978[34]	149 (C)	5	87
Cvek 1978[35]	60 (T)	3	96
Baum and Holz 1981[36]	110 (C)	4	90
Santini 1983[37]	481 (C)	0.5	75
Horsted et al. 1985[38]	510 (T)	5	82
Mejàre and Cvek 1993[39]	31 (T)	4	93 (NP)
	6 (T)	4	66 (P)
Caliskan 1995[40]	26 (T) (pulpotomy)	1-6	92 (NP)
Barthel et al. 2000[41]	64 (T)	5	56 (NP)
	69 (T)	10	13 (NP)
Al-Hiyasat et al. 2006[42]	204 (T)	3	59

NP, no preexisting pain; P, preexisting pain.

evidence of progressive root formation. Once root formation is complete, some believe that it is desirable to perform elective root canal treatment to avoid complications of continued root canal calcification. This is not a universally accepted axiom. Outcomes of pulp therapy are summarized in Table 7-1.[33-42]

Treatment of the compromised pulp need not always involve regenerative therapy; the options include either pulp therapy to preserve the pulp or pulpectomy and root canal treatment to sacrifice it. The choice is based on the operator's perception of the long-term prognoses associated with the options. The decision is also likely to be significantly influenced by overall treatment planning considerations. A single tooth in an otherwise intact arch lends itself to a conservative approach. For a tooth scheduled for a cast restoration, possibly an abutment, elective root canal treatment may be more pragmatic. This option must be balanced against the potentially poor survival of root-treated abutments. Where there are no overriding restorative considerations, the choice between preservation of the pulp or its extirpation is often guided by the clinician's views in respect of pulp therapy, derived from their teachers and previous clinical experience. Two schools of thought have arisen: one believes in pulp preservation; the other in inherent susceptibility to long-term failure. The latter school of thought offers high success rates (95%) for the root canal treatment on teeth with vital pulps compared with late intervention (85% success) given complications including irregular pulp calcification and internal resorption. The only exception is pulp therapy in the treatment of incompletely formed roots.

Root canal treatment

Root canal treatment is a procedure used to treat two biologically distinct disease processes. In both cases, the technical aspects of the procedures are virtually identical and consist of removing either diseased and dying pulp tissue or dead pulp tissue and established bacterial infection. The principal challenges are to access the intraradicular pulp space and its walls. To achieve this goal, when the surfaces and spaces concerned are small and hidden from direct view, is technically challenging. Contemporary root canal treatment procedures are, conceptually, age old. They consist of a series of interdependent steps, starting with coronal access involving removal of the roof of the pulp chamber under aseptic conditions. Next, the root canals are located and negotiated, in preparation for their mechanical enlargement and sculpting (shaping) by controlled intraradicular dentin removal to give a tapering cavity that follows the shape and curvature of the roots and extends to the canal terminus (Fig. 7-11). This process, by inference, generates dentin particles and organic debris that must be flushed out to maintain access and patency to the apical canal anatomy. The ability to maintain patency is enhanced by the use of fluids capable of dissolving and digesting both organic and inorganic diseased tissues. During this flushing process, the irrigants simultaneously disrupt the bacterial biofilm. The intraradicular canal preparation facilitates irrigation of the more complex root canal system, preferably with antiseptic or antibacterial solutions. Chemical debridement of organic tissue and antibacterial activity is continued between visits by sealing a chemical agent (preferably in solution) in the canal system. The coronal access is then temporarily sealed and the tooth left for at least a week; after which, the tooth is re-entered under similar aseptic conditions and the canal system re-irrigated to remove the antibacterial dressing and any residual bacteria. If obvious clinical signs and symptoms of disease have subsided, the root canal system is considered ready for root filling. The stages prior to root filling are usually sufficient to achieve periapical healing.

The purpose of root filling is to fill the root canal system with an inert material to seal off the periapical tissues from the canal system and the oral environment. It also helps to incarcerate residual infection in the root canal system. Permanent restoration of the access cavity provides coronal seal, preventing reinfection of the root canal system.

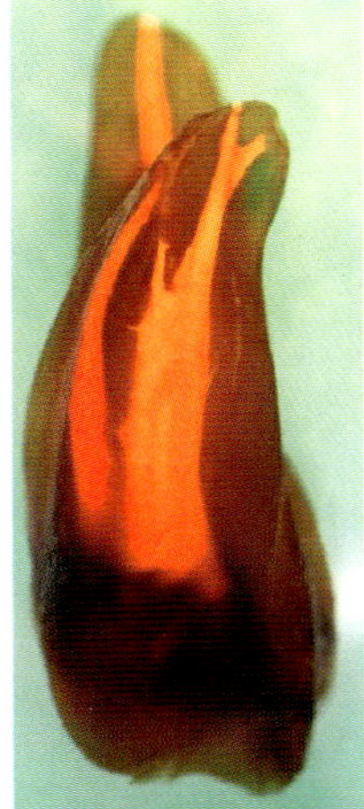

Fig. 7-11 Cleared tooth showing tapering prepared and filled root canals, uninstrumented and filled root canals and uninstrumented and unfilled canal.

The culture test during root canal treatment has fallen out of favor for a variety of reasons. The issue though remains controversial and there are still some who practice it. The immediate outcome measure of root canal treatment is the radiographic appearance of the root filling. Good radiographic appearance does not, however, necessarily predict successful root canal treatment, judged by periapical healing and resolution of the periapical tissues. For this, the criteria are an absence of clinical signs and symptoms and reduction in the size of the periapical radiolucency until normal architecture is restored. This can take up to three years or longer.

In summary, root canal treatment is a chemomechanical procedure, involving technical, mechanical and irrigation steps that non-specifically aim to eliminate or reduce the intraradicular bacterial flora to within host tolerance.

Mechanical intraradicular preparation

The purpose of mechanical preparation of the root canal system is to create access to it. The aim of this extension of the coronal (radicular) access cavity is to obtain and maintain 'patency' to the apical part of the root canal system. The ideal shape of the radicular access cavity is a general tapering form, which may have a circular or slightly eccentric cross-section. The final form depends on the instruments used and the manner in which they are manipulated. The mechanical preparation involves using metal instruments of graded sizes to negotiate to the apical terminus without losing patency, a process which enables the existing canal to be subtly modified at the points of contact with the instrument. By doing so, the apical part of the canal is enlarged to the size of the last used instrument. Once the apical enlargement is complete, the rest of the canal is then shaped or sculpted into a predefined taper, using sequentially larger instruments (stainless steel) at shorter distances or sequentially more tapered instruments (nickel-titanium) to the full length. The exact dimensions of the taper and apical size are determined by the need to allow antibacterial fluids and later root-filling materials to be delivered to the full extent of the root canal system in a controlled manner. It is considered convenient to have preshaped the coronal part of the canal to the final taper at the outset, because it:

- allows easier canal location for each instrument
- reduces change in length of the canal during preparation
- allows a larger reservoir of irrigant for apical replenishment
- allows better apical tactile sense
- reduces potential for apical blockage
- reduces potential for apical transportation.

This goal of producing a regularly tapering canal shape is achieved by controlled removal of intracanal dentin such that the original shape and curvature of the main root canal(s) are retained. This together with a relatively conservative final preparation size helps to ensure that the root is neither weakened nor perforated. It is this phase of the procedure that is renowned for the tactile surgical skill required for root canal treatment, and the reason for the high proportion of technically poor root canal treatment performed in general dental practice worldwide. The sequential use of stainless steel instruments of graded sizes to achieve the required taper gradually demands immense tactile skill. The development of nickel-titanium instruments, manipulated by handpieces in continuous rotational motion, has considerably eased this aspect of the procedure, simplifying it and making it less fatiguing and more predictable. The catch, however, is that the instruments cannot be used to negotiate calcified and acutely curved canals without risk of fracture. Furthermore, their sole use results in the clinician losing the essential tactile skills required for root canal treatment. The adept and astute clinician will, therefore, retain the use of stainless steel instruments for negotiation and enlargement in order to maintain tactile skills, while using the instruments of greater taper to produce the final shape efficiently.

In narrow uncomplicated canal systems, the mechanical preparation may be sufficient to effect the almost complete removal of the microbial biofilm. This, however, is a rare achievement even in anterior, single-rooted teeth. The truth is that there is always a variable proportion (30–50%) of non-instrumented surface in the root canal system.

The effect of mechanical preparation on the bacterial flora has been tested. Taking the studies together, negative cultures were achieved in 4.6–53% of teeth (mean, 25%).

Chemical intraradicular preparation

From the above, it is evident that it is necessary to use chemically active fluid agents delivered through the radicular access cavity to kill remaining bacteria on the instrumented surfaces and, even more importantly, to disrupt the residual microbial biofilm on the uninstrumented surfaces. Wider and larger radicular access cavities may allow better delivery of chemical agents to the uninstrumented surfaces, especially the all-important apical anatomy. A balance has to be struck, however, between the desire to improve delivery of chemical agents and the maintenance of the strength of the tooth. The rationale for mechanical preparation infers that minimal mechanical preparation should be required in wide straight canals.

The process of bacterial biofilm disruption by antibacterial fluids and dressings is fraught with problems. The problems are three-fold: first, the irrigant fails to reach, in sufficient concentration, the narrow and 'distant' apical anatomy, let alone the ramifications branching off the main root canal system; second, despite effective irrigant delivery, the multilayered, three-dimensional microbial biofilm structure with its polysaccharide matrix protects the deeper layers of slowly metabolizing organisms; and, third, the biologically responsive biofilm senses the environmental changes and alters its gene expression to adapt to new conditions.

The problem of irrigant delivery into the root canal environment is immense and has not been adequately studied. The major problem is one of inadequate mixing of initial and replenishing fluids in the canal. As far as current understanding allows, the problem may be reduced by enlarging and shaping the radicular access cavity sufficiently to allow the irrigant to reach the apical anatomy using appropriately sized narrow-gauge hypodermic needles. The fluids may then be mixed by agitation using a reasonably well-fitting gutta-percha cone, commercial devices or ultrasonic agitation.

The second problem may be overcome, at least in the coronal two thirds of the root canal system, by using a relatively large volume and high concentration of irrigant to give longer-lasting chemical potency. Again, the problem is one of sufficient mixing of spent and fresh irrigant to allow adequate action on the 'distant' bacterial cells, in particular in the apical and accessory anatomy.

The combined action of mechanical and chemical cleaning is more efficient than either method alone, and agitation of the irrigant enhances its action further. Chemical action without mechanical preparation is impossible except in naturally wide canals. This is unfortunate because the ideal method would allow delivery of the irrigant without preparation. A chemically active irrigant would allow more conservative canal preparation, as reliance on dentin removal for decontamination – a forlorn hope – would be reduced. This is the so-called chemo-mechanical method of root canal system preparation.

The use of higher concentrations or frequent replenishment of antibacterial agents may allow inhibitory doses to reach at least some of the distant bacteria along a diffusion gradient. Killing some of the bacterial constituents of the biofilm may allow the physiological chain of interreliance between bacteria to be broken, so that the more fastidious species are killed by a 'domino' effect, subsequent to deprivation of nutrients and stimulants from their neighbors.

Root canal treatment probably works by a combination of direct and indirect killing effects; the importance of the latter is probably hugely underestimated in modern endodontics.

Ineffective treatment techniques allow survival of deep-seated, usually Gram-positive, bacteria, which may then recolonize the root canal system. Such survivors may, by definition, be hardier adaptable strains capable of living independently of other species in the unique nutrition-depleted conditions prevailing in the treated canal. This would make their further eradication at the next visit more difficult. A poor first attempt at root canal treatment may result in a more resistant infection at the next step; consequently, it follows that thorough debridement at the first attempt is of paramount importance.

When sodium hypochlorite (0.5–5.0%) irrigation supplements mechanical preparation, the frequency of negative cultures immediately after debridement increases to 25–98% of teeth (mean, 73%). Well-controlled clinical/microbiological studies have shown that the antibacterial effect is improved by mechanical preparation, sodium hypochlorite irrigation (alternated with ethylenediaminetetraacetic acid), the addition of ultrasonic activation and use of a calcium hydroxide dressing. The antibacterial actions reduce the number of bacteria from an initial range of 10^2–10^8 cells/ml to 10^1–10^3 cells/ml after initial debridement, further reducing recoverable cells after inter-appointment dressing with calcium hydroxide. However, culture reversals are reported when an active antibacterial dressing is not used in the root canal system between appointments. Reversals may be attributed to regrowth of residual bacteria or recontamination by bacterial leakage around the access cavity dressing.

Inter-appointment intracanal medication

The main rationale of this step is to help to degrade residual microbial biofilm and organic tissue and to kill remaining bacteria. The medicament should, therefore, also prevent bacterial recolonization of the root canal system, from either bacteria left behind after preparation or new invaders from lateral communications or the coronal access. In addition, it would be useful if the medicament possessed a range of other properties that would suppress pain and facilitate apical healing. An ideal root canal medicament should, therefore:

- be able to kill all root canal bacteria
- have long-lasting antibacterial effects
- not be inactivated by the presence of organic material
- be able to help to degrade residual organic tissue
- be able to help to degrade residual microbial biofilm and bacteria
- not be irritating to periapical tissues or have systemic toxicity
- be able to induce regeneration of periapical tissues
- have anodyne properties.

No single root canal medicament has proved capable of meeting all these requirements, and it is, therefore, not surprising that a vast range of different materials have been tried.

The collective antibacterial action during root canal preparation has not been shown to cause persistence of specific bacteria. A negative culture result before obturation can increase treatment success by an average of 12% (range, 0–26). The bacteria in such cultures would include *Enterococcus*, *Streptococcus*, *Staphylococcus*, *Lactobacillus*, *Veillonella*, *Pseudomonas* and *Fusobacterium* species and yeasts. A number of factors have led to the gradual abandoning of the culture test in clinical practice. The clinical outcome is especially compromised when a positive culture combines with the presence of a periapical lesion.

Root canal obturation and coronal seal

Obturation of the root canal system and coronal restoration helps to prevent bacterial recontamination by establishing a barrier to the passage of microorganisms and their products. In the past, the main emphasis was on establishing an apical 'seal.' However, in recent years, the importance of the coronal seal has been appreciated more fully, and it is now believed that the coronal restoration is as important, if not more important, than the apical seal. The aims and objectives of the obturation are to establish a barrier to the passage of microorganisms from the oral cavity to the periradicular tissues, 'entomb' and isolate any microorganisms that may survive the cleaning and shaping process, prevent leakage of potential nutrients into the canal system that would support microbial growth and reduce the risk of bacterial movement or fluid percolation into the canal system space from the gingival sulcus or periodontal pockets. The concept of a 'hermetic' or 'airtight' seal in endodontics is erroneous as it is now understood that all restorative materials leak to some extent. It suffices to say that all efforts should be made to hinder the ingress and growth of microorganisms.

As the primary goal of root canal preparation is to eradicate bacteria from the root canal system, there should be a suitable measure of this end point, but available methods rely on cultures, which take time and laboratory support. In the absence of a pre-obturation culture test, judgement about the readiness for obturation is made clinically by absence of pain, swelling, sinus, tenderness to percussion and palpation of adjacent soft tissues and persistent exudate in the canal.

Completion of the treatment in a single visit has a number of advantages for both the patient and the clinician, including the fact that the root canal system will never be 'cleaner' than immediately after shaping and debridement. The counter-argument is that this requires considerable efficiency, and obturation may hinder access to the root canal system should residual bacteria be left behind.

Ideally all root-filling material should remain within the confines of the root canal system. The apical extent of the root canal system is designated by the cementodentinal junction, which is approximately 0.5–0.7 mm from the external aspect of the apical foramen. It is difficult to determine this position radiographically, but electronic apex locators are a great aid. In practice, the extrusion of small amounts of sealer beyond the confines of the root canal system does not appear to have an adverse affect on success, and it is viewed by some endodontists as a desirable indication of the adequacy of obturation of the entire root canal system. It is important to appreciate the difference between overfilling and overextension of an obturation. An overextended obturation is one that has been extruded beyond the confines of the root canal system but does not completely fill the root canal system, while an overfilled canal is completely obturated and has, in addition, been extended beyond the confines of the root canal system. Difficulties frequently arise in root canal systems with incomplete apices or where resorption, incomplete apical development or iatrogenic causes have destroyed the normal apical anatomy. In these situations, modifications may have to be made during both the preparation and the obturation of the root canal system.

A variety of materials capable of being thermoplasticized and adapted to the root canal system have been advocated and used. These are mainly of gutta-percha formulation and, more recently, of other synthetic polymers. The modes of delivery vary from cold placement and then intracanal heating and adaptation, to heating outside and delivery by injection or on a carrier system. Most require technical skills and practice to manipulate satisfactorily. There is no difference in healing rates associated with different materials.

Periapical healing and outcomes

It is impossible to sterilize the root canal system and fortunate that sterility is not a precondition to successful outcome of root canal treatment; in fact,

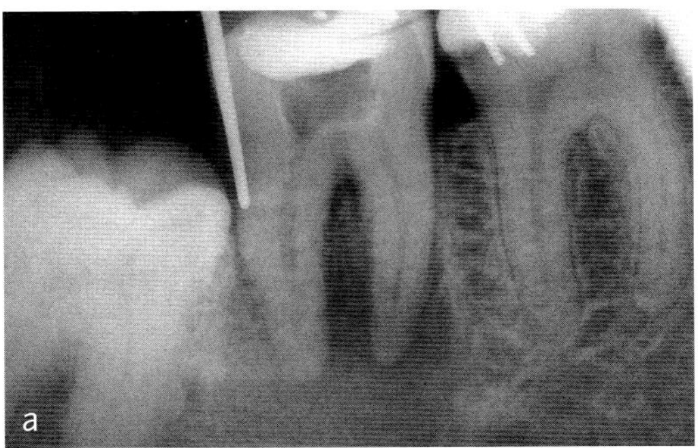

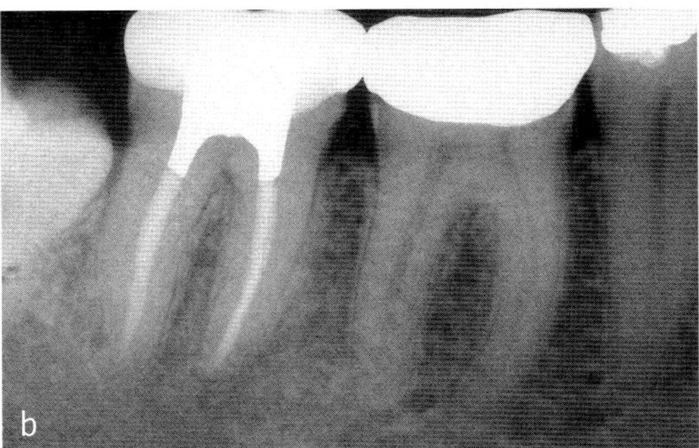

Fig. 7-12 A periapical lesion. **(a)** Preoperative radiographic view of the presenting lesion. **(b)** Postoperative radiographic view of periapical healing less than one year following root canal treatment.

the series of procedures act as permissive factors. Root canal treatment procedures work because the reduction in microbial content, together with its collective pathogenicity, is sufficient to promote periradicular healing. In rare and unusual cases, it has been demonstrated that a mere change in the coronal restoration, without active root canal treatment, may be sufficient to alter the pathogenicity of the flora to facilitate periapical healing. Even in teeth with conventional root canal treatment using contemporary protocols, survival of an intact bacterial biofilm has been demonstrated in the apical anatomy. The precise mechanisms by which this residual intraradicular apical biofilm is brought under control are not understood. Intuitively, the outcome must be a function of the interaction between the mechanical, chemical and obturation components of treatment, the nature of residual flora and the host's defense reactions. The length of time required for periapical healing (one to three years) (Fig. 7-12) suggests an ongoing interaction between the host immune system and residual bacterial flora. The healing process after root canal treatment has not been fully researched. It may be conceptualized using 'Fish's zones' of infection, contamination, irritation and stimulation in a chronic inflammatory lesion. The removal of bacteria and their products from the canal results in elimination of the zones of infection and contamination, allowing macrophages from the zone of irritation to invade the previous zones of infection and contamination to remove dead cells and debris. This process may then make way for osteoblasts, fibroblasts, new blood vessels and nerve fibers from the outermost and active zone of stimulation to proliferate into the zone of irritation. In this way, gradual healing may occur from the boundary of the lesion inwards until a normal periodontal ligament is established. Provided that the periodontal tissues have not been irreversibly damaged, ideal healing would eventually result in the formation of cementum over the apical foramen, isolating the root canal system completely from the periapex, but this is not an inevitable end result. Incomplete removal of the infection may reduce but not eliminate the inflammatory area. Healing may be modified and delayed by the treatment procedures and materials used, particularly if extruded out of the root into the periapical tissues.

Clinical judgement of the outcome of treatment is dependent upon the absence of signs of infection and inflammation, such as pain, tenderness to percussion of the tooth, tenderness to palpation of the related soft tissues, absence of swelling and sinus and radiographic demonstration of healing of the periapical lesion, with a completely normal periodontal ligament space. Absence of signs and symptoms of periapical disease but a persistence of a periapical radiographic radiolucency may indicate either healing by fibrosis or persistent chronic inflammation. Only time and an acute exacerbation will identify the latter, whereas the former should remain asymptomatic.

Table 7-2 Pooled weight success rates of root canal treatment based on strict criteria for determination of success by period of publication

Period (Year)	Number of studies	Mean success rate (%)
Before 1960	2	68
1961-1970	2	80
1971-1980	9	79
1981-1990	9	75
1991-1999	10	77

Systematic review and meta-analysis of the factors affecting root canal treatment outcome have revealed that, in the absence of apical periodontitis, the mean success rate of vital pulpectomy is 95%. This reduced to 85% when the root canal treatment was aimed at eradicating infection associated with an established periapical lesion. The factors having a major impact on root canal treatment outcome are:

- presence and size of periapical lesion
- presence of a sinus tract
- apical extent of root canal treatment in relation to radiographic apex
- outcome of culture test before obturation
- quality of root canal treatment judged by radiographic appearance of root filling
- quality of the final coronal restoration.

Factors having a minimal effect on root canal treatment outcome are age, gender and health of the patient, and root canal treatment technique other than length control. The improvements in techniques of mechanical and chemical canal preparation have not resulted in increases in success rates over the last century (Table 7-2).[43]

Bacteria associated with failed root canal treatment

The species recovered from root-treated teeth reside in accessory canals, in dentinal tubules or in the main canal alongside the root filling. They are a subset of those found in untreated teeth, though the diversity and quantity is reduced. The recovered bacteria include *Eubacterium*, *Lactobacillus*, *Propionibacterium*, *Actinomyces*, *Peptostreptococcus*, *Streptococcus*, *Bacteroides*, *Fusobacterium*, *Selenomonas* and *Veillonella* species. Unlike untreated teeth, treated teeth appear to contain few mixed cultures, often only three, two or single species are found, with a mean of only 1.7 species per tooth. Teeth with poor root fillings have the highest bacterial counts (10^3–10^5 CFU/mL) with a maximum of three to six species per canal and a diversity that resembles that of untreated teeth, perhaps reflecting poor primary treatment technique. *Enterococcus faecalis* is the commonest species. It is easily eliminated when it is present in small numbers in the primary infection, but it is difficult to eradicate if it infects in large numbers. Although specific bacterial species have not been implicated as being resistant to treatment in longitudinal studies, the presence of specific groups of bacteria in root-treated teeth suggests that, other than being survivors from the preexisting infection, they may be contaminants introduced during treatment. This may occur through inadequate tooth isolation, poor asepsis, leakage around the access dressing and the access cavity being left open for drainage. All of these factors, therefore, represent poor practice.

Outcome of retreatments

When root canal treatment fails to resolve periapical disease, it is often considered appropriate to retreat the tooth using conventional approaches, in particular when the previous treatment is technically deficient. This requires removal of the previous root-filling material and any other material placed for restorative reasons. Correction of any iatrogenic procedural errors may also be required, if possible. All material must be removed in its entirety to ensure delivery of antibacterial agents to the entire surface of the root canal. The success rates of retreatment may be lower than with primary treatment[44] (66%) because of obstructed access to the apical infection and possibly a more-resistant bacterial flora. However, when procedures are completed satisfactorily, the success rates of secondary treatment may be equal to that of primary treatment (76%).[45]

Periapical surgery and retrograde seal

In a small proportion of cases, the conventional chemomechanical approach alone does not resolve the problem, because of poor access to the site of infection within or beyond the root apex or because of host defense factors, as yet uncharacterized. In these instances, a surgical approach to the periapex may be required in addition to the conventional approach. Extraradicular infection cannot be diagnosed before primary treatment. It is rather a differential diagnosis arrived at by initial conventional treatment of the intraradicular infection. The healing process in such cases follows a more complicated pathway. Initially, there may be attempts at healing because of the removal of the primary source of infection, so there may be a reduction in the size of the periapical lesion. The persistent extraradicular infection would, however, frustrate attempts at complete healing. The surgical procedure, consisting of the incisional and dissectional wounds and concluding with the apical resection of the root, would then inflict additional trauma to the site and change the histologic picture altogether. The procedure would hopefully remove the causative factors, leaving a wound to heal by a process that is different from that in response to conventional root canal treatment. The healing essentially involves epithelial and connective tissue resolution, processes that are interdependent. The first step is the formation of an epithelial seal, which matures with the nutrient support from the developing underlying connective tissue. Reattachment of the mucoperiosteal flap may be compromised by the presence of periodontal disease. Further connective tissue healing consists of removal and organization of the clot into periosteum, alveolar bone, cementum and periodontal ligament. The apical root resection creates a surface of exposed dentin with a root canal outline that is large and filled with a material of variable toxicity. The exposed dentinal surface may become covered with cementum if the tubules are not infected, but none forms over the root canal over which fibrous tissue develops. If a retrograde filling material, such as mineral trioxide aggregate is used, its osteogenic potential may allow better coverage of the root end by regeneration of tissues than can be achieved by repair.

Effect of root canal treatment on the mechanical properties of teeth

A combination of factors inherent in root canal treatment may weaken teeth, including loss of proprioceptive function from the pulp, loss of intracoronal and intraradicular dentin and loss of organic and inorganic components from dentin.[46] Such processes can alter the rigidity and flexure of teeth. Whether this is sufficient to allow fracture has not been proven and may be dependent upon adequate amounts of remaining dentin. Restoration of teeth after root canal treatment should ideally involve conservation of as much dentin as possible, together with optimal distribution of stresses through appropriate design of restorations. Factors affecting tooth survival after root canal treatment include:[47]

- patient history of diabetes or systemic steroid therapy
- preoperative evidence of deep periodontal defect
- pain, sinus tract or cervical resorption
- pre- and intraoperative evidence of tooth perforation
- patency at canal terminus
- root filling extrusion
- number of adjacent teeth
- tooth morphological type

- type of restoration after treatment
- use of cast post and core for support and retention of restoration
- teeth serving as prosthesis abutments.

Much more research needs to be undertaken to clarify the modes and mechanisms of tooth failure and to find ways to resolve these problems to ensure longevity of endodontically treated teeth as functional, esthetic and pain-free units in the mouth.

Alternative concepts for root canal treatment

The philosophy adopted by some operators, though not one approved by the vast majority of endodontic societies or universities worldwide, has been that the root canal system anatomy is so complex that adequate biomechanical debridement is impossible and time consuming. Consequently, such 'alternative' practitioners advocate the use of chemical agents to destroy and fix the organic pulp tissue together with the bacteria, with a reduced emphasis on asepsis and mechanical preparation. A variety of materials (N2, Endomethasone, Spad) all containing formaldehyde as the fixative agent has been recommended. When used together with some degree of mechanical preparation and confinement of the material within the root canal system, the technique may in some instances provide successful results. There is, however, no scientific body of evidence to substantiate this practice as a predictable procedure. Furthermore, it has been demonstrated that the fixed pulp tissue is antigenically altered and can stimulate an immune response on its own, whereas unfixed necrotic tissue cannot. When such root-filling material is inadvertently extruded, there are serious consequences. The toxicity of the material can cause necrosis and can alter nerve function. The clinical manifestations of these include severe pain, paresthesia and profound anesthesia, especially when the material is extruded into the inferior dental canal. Of course, the same sequelae are likely if other materials are extruded into the nerve canal, but most of these resolve spontaneously over time, while such recovery is less probable with formaldehyde-containing materials.

Vision 2020

The historical and contemporary accounts of management of pulpal and periapical diseases demonstrate progression in the approaches used. Despite the vast improvements in treatment modalities, they remain far from perfect, revealing potential for further improvements in both efficacy and efficiency. Predicting the future development pathways is a hazardous exercise, in particular when the time frame is constrained. It is impossible realistically to account for life events and the hurdles they may create. Nevertheless, setting such time constraints aside does enable a better flow of imagination to envision a future for a biologically and scientifically driven endodontic discipline in 2020.

Prevention of pulpal and periapical disease

Pulpal, and either sequential or simultaneous periapical, inflammation can only come about as a result of direct or indirect injury. The sources of injury are related to damage to the hard tissue and subsequent invasion by bacteria. It is impossible to prevent many of these injuries because they relate to lifestyle choices, which are notoriously difficult to influence. Means of preserving teeth through fluoridation or use of probiotics to reduce the pathogenicity of the oral bacterial flora is also likely to remain subject to individual choices. It is, therefore, unlikely that a significant change will come about in preventive strategies in the next 10–12 years. Educational programs would need to be implemented and monitored for outcome, such as television advertisments promoting awareness of tooth surface loss, usually through the medium of cosmetic awareness, the one saleable quantity in contemporary life. At the same time, the population should be made aware of the disadvantages of cosmetic procedures that require removal of, let alone damage to, tooth tissue.

After disease, wear and tear and cosmetic procedures, a major risk factor in the development of pulpal disease is microbial leakage around restorations, which causes dentin sensitivity, marginal staining, degradation of restorative material and secondary caries. It had been hoped that adhesive dentistry, together with the development of tooth-colored restorations, could provide the solution to this problem; however, the method appears flawed and results so far have not substantiated the optimism surrounding it. Although adhesion to dentin has improved significantly, the formation of a leak-proof seal around the entire circumference of the restoration margin has proved to be a more profound challenge. The causative factors include lack of adequate adaptation of the material, dimensional changes upon placement and curing and, most importantly, tooth deformation. The long-term survival of the bonds is compromised by their hydrolysis in the oral environment and the constant and perpetual interfacial stress challenge of tooth flexure. Placement of large composites remains a technique-sensitive procedure that can often result in sensitivity and pulpal problems. So far, it has proved impossible to produce materials predictably capable of sealing the margins of restorations. An alternative approach to pulp protection may be to find ways to seal dentinal tubules artificially or to stimulate dentinal tubule sclerosis: that is, to mimic natural defensive mechanisms. The challenge will be to control the process so that it can be switched off at the completion of an adequate seal. Other methods reliant on knowledge of bacterial colonization mechanisms will need to be developed to inhibit ingress of bacteria into marginal gaps.

Pulpal and periapical disease diagnosis

The early diagnosis of pulpal and periapical disease is confounded by the fact that the tissues are not directly visible and the principal disease consists of chronic inflammation, which is notoriously poorly correlated with clinical signs and symptoms. The outcomes of both pulp therapy and root canal treatment are significantly influenced by the nature of the underlying disease process. The ability to diagnose the pulpal status and its sequel, periapical disease, non-invasively yet accurately would be a significant step forward.

The problem is to find an imaging system that can 'see' beyond the hard tissues yet elicit a strong and clean enough signal from the soft tissues within teeth to be able to distinguish normal and diseased tissues. The adoption of optical methods (laser Doppler flowmetry, pulse oximetry), while initially promising, has failed to yield a definitive solution. Trials with other electromagnetic radiation may possibly lead to visual clues in the future. Meanwhile, in the shorter term, the use of molecular technology to detect moieties associated with inflammation may prove helpful, as already tried in pulp capping, albeit in the case of exposed pulps.

Pulpal capping and dentin regeneration

Innovation has led to three main new approaches to pulp therapy. One is the extension of adhesive dentistry to pulp capping. It has been suggested that several of the adhesive agents are biocompatible with the pulp tissue that survives following capping. However, these studies are limited to short-term observations and while the approach shows promise there is potential for later failure through microbial leakage, as discussed above. Given the extensive clinical data currently available for contemporary approaches, it is premature to abandon them in favor of new methods that have little evidence base to support them. Long-term follow-up may yield further insight about their true potential.

Another approach is the use of mineral trioxide aggregate as a pulp-capping agent, given its biocompatibility with periapical tissues; relatively short-term trials on healthy human teeth have shown favorable histological results. The approach opens the question of how it works and, again, the secret would appear to lie in the fact that, like calcium hydroxide, it solubilizes the dentin matrix and releases growth factors.

A more promising future approach lies in the recruitment of natural growth factors harvested from dentin matrix or mass produced through biotechnology. These could be incorporated into filling materials to allow slow release and stimulate the production of a replacement pulp-dentin complex. Early experiments show the method may have promise, but clinically proven techniques will require some time in development; it is difficult to predict the time frame for such development.

Pulpal regeneration

Thought has been given to regeneration of the dental pulp, when inflamed and necrotic, in particular in the case of immature roots. An interesting case report has illustrated the natural healing potential of tissues when harnessed by biomimetic approaches; namely the use of scaffolds, growth factors and stem cells.[48] Again, this is a neophytic idea with much future potential but yet to be properly evaluated and developed into a predictable procedure.

Tooth germ generation and implantation

Given that endodontics has come under some threat from implant dentistry and that some dental clinicians now consider the predictability of such an approach outweighs the preservation of natural teeth (even though the imputation is unproven[49]), thoughts have turned to the possibility of growing natural teeth in the laboratory for implantation in humans. This possibility has not only been mooted but also laboratory tested, with interesting initial results; the approach, however, requires considerable work before it can develop into viable clinical procedures.[50]

Root canal treatment

The challenge to improve success rates with root canal treatment lie not in the management of pulpitis but in managing an established root canal infection, manifest as a periapical lesion. The fact that the range of procedures carried out over the world, spanning a century, do not show an improvement in success rates, despite improvements in instruments, techniques and materials, suggests that the principles rather than the procedures need to be overhauled. The problem, which has acted as the buffer to technological advances, is residual apical infection. Improvement of success rates would, therefore, logically require the invention of novel methods of controlling the unique and resistant infection at the terminus of the tooth roots.[51] This will require a two-pronged approach: to develop an effective means of delivering antibacterial agents to this complex anatomy and to develop bioactive root-filling materials capable of killing residual bacteria and facilitating regeneration of the periapical tissues, including cementum, periodontal ligament and bone.

Recognition of the biofilm nature of root canal infection will lead to alternative strategies for treatment, as such bacteria are more resistant to killing because:

- the exopolysaccharide matrix restricts diffusion of antibacterial agents to the bacterial cells
- multiple layers of bacterial cells act as barriers to diffusion
- some bacterial cells grow slowly or are dormant and are, therefore, more resistant to killing
- cells may exhibit specific resistance mechanisms
- biofilm phenotypes may be inherently resistant.

A better understanding of the physiology of root canal system biofilms will enable the targeting of key quorum-sensing, virulence gene and other survival molecular systems, which will form the basis of a specific root canal treatment protocol. This, however, will need to be preceded by characterization of key pathogens and development of chairside sensors to inform the clinician of the specific nature of the infection in a given tooth. A computer-based device will be able to match a cocktail of molecular agents to target the specific microbial flora, and this will be delivered by electromagnetic-driven mechanisms into the root canal system.

Apical infection versus host response

Root canal treatment outcome[41,52] and clinical/histological data[49] show that contemporary root canal treatment procedures fail to disrupt mechanically or chemically the apical-most bacterial biofilm in the majority of teeth, implying that contemporary root canal treatment procedures act as a permissive factor only. The many technical facets of treatment perceived to be important pale into insignificance; the key treatment factors include the length to which canals are debrided and filled, and the effectiveness of bacterial debridement in the mechanically prepared part of the canal. It also implies that, beyond satisfactory execution of the procedure, the failure of root canal treatment is beyond the control of the operator. Periapical lesion resolution or persistence must intuitively be associated with the nature of the interaction between the host and the residual bacteria. Future studies may find that the host defenses play a crucial role in periapical healing. The fact that the presence and size of periapical lesion, the presence of a sinus tract and apical resorption are important prognostic factors, suggest powerful biological factors at play in the outcome. It is known that all of the above preoperative prognostic factors are correlated with microbiological factors. Future improvements in root canal treatment success will be closely allied to research into host-microbial interactions.

Access and canal preparation

The majority of the technological improvements in root canal treatment over the past 20 or so years have been in the instruments and techniques available to cut and prepare the access cavities into the crown and the root, namely, root canal preparation. The chief advances have been the development of non-ISO taper nickel-titanium instruments used in a continuous rotary motion and capable of negotiating curved canals while maintaining this curvature with respect to the root curvatures. While, the use of these instruments requires a certain skill-set, they can nevertheless be said to be a great stride forward in at least partially eliminating the skill barrier that has so far prevented effective and efficient delivery of this service. The whole purpose of preparing a tapered shape is to deliver the antibacterial irrigants to the apical part of the root canal anatomy. To be able to do so effectively requires a cavity of predefined shape and size. Contemporary instruments using rotary motion inevitably cut a cavity of circular cross-section. Unfortunately, most root canals, in particular those in molars, do not have a circular cross-section; rather they are ribbon shaped in cross-section. Contemporary instruments, therefore, remove dentin from the root in areas where there is risk of root weakening and perforation. New developments in instruments and instrumentation techniques in the future should attempt to address this deficiency by developing instruments that enlarge root canals uniformly around their circumference and retain the original anatomical configuration, rather than the artificial shape machined by current instruments. Although some studies and operators reckon that larger canal preparations allow better apical debridement and microbial reduction, the problem is that more dentin removal requires better apical irrigation to flush out the generated dentin debris. Without proper irrigation, the dentin particles turn into a sticky sludge capable of blocking undebrided apical exits, leading to a decrease in success rates rather than an increase. This is indeed exactly the trend revealed by outcome studies.

The ultimate root canal treatment technique would involve the most minimal access cavity with minimal or no canal preparation. This almost came to fruition with the non-instrumented technique,[53] but the remaining problem was effective delivery of the irrigant to the apical anatomy.

Delivery of irrigants

The single most important problem in root canal treatment is the lack of an effective, predictable and reliable method to deliver the antibacterial agents to the canal terminus in sufficient concentration. A major reason for inadequate apical disinfection is that the tapering drilled holes are too small to allow free fluid motion within them; the fluid environment is viscously dominated. This makes the mixing of the fluid difficult owing to the absence of turbulence to provide mixing. Many of the problems are similar to those found in microfluidic devices, though in those cases they can be overcome by the use of wall obstacles, a solution not possible in root canal treatment. Dwell times are also important because disinfection only takes place successfully when the disinfectant is in direct contact with the bacterial biofilm and is constantly replenished. Currently, the irrigant is replenished and mixed by 'recapitulation,' where after the use of each new instrument; the fluid occupying the canal is agitated using a smaller file after each new drilling. This also prevents the fluid becoming progressively more and more debris laden, viscous and turning into a sludge, which may block the lateral exits in the complex apical anatomy. The time-consuming procedure of recapitulation and frequent irrigant replenishment is of paramount importance to the success of the procedure, yet it is perhaps the most poorly performed part of the operation, because it is not well understood by practitioners. Future developments in root canal treatment will be informed by better understanding of the science of fluid dynamics.

In addition to fluid dynamics, the interaction between antibacterial agents, apical anatomy and bacterial biofilms is poorly understood. Some, as yet unknown, functions of these interactions are surely responsible for helping to eliminate the bacterial biofilm better in some teeth than in others. The problem of root canal treatment in 2020 may, therefore, be defined not by the canal preparation and obturation, which has so far dominated it, but by attention specifically to the apical infection.

Slow-release antibacterial agents

It is apparent from the foregoing discussion that residual bacterial biofilm is a highly likely occupant of the apical anatomy after irrigation has been completed. Reaching it with agents in sufficient concentration may require gels capable of concentrating the active moieties in the relevant area from which it can act as a slow-release device, in the inter-appointment period. Such a gel could also be active in releasing analgesics or ions capable of providing a favorable environment for the chronic inflammatory process to be tipped more towards the healing element.

Delivery of bioactive root filling materials

Contemporary root fillings have traditionally been inert space-filling materials that are deemed effective only if they seal the apical exits of the canal terminus. The role of root canal obturation is undergoing somewhat of a re-evaluation. The prime purpose is to help to complete the task of infection control by depriving bacteria of further nutrition and, second, to prevent recolonization of the root canal walls and space. Such requirements call for altogether different types of material. It may also be considered that the role of root canal obturation should be extended to aiding the process of apical healing. This description calls for a retrievable material that may be placed in an aqueous environment yet creates a seal through ionic precipitation and, by the same process, is able to act as an antibacterial agent, as well as promote healing. Such experimental materials are already under investigation and could conceivably be available by 2020.

Final restoration

Having controlled the apical infection and thereby the periapical healing, it is necessary to ensure that the root canal system does not become reinfected. Antibacterial barriers or sealants may be important considerations. One of the problems of achieving such a seal is the nature of flexure of such weakened teeth. The greater flexure makes it difficult to create a permanent seal.

It may be important to consider ways to return the tooth back to its original state of resilience. This would require the invention of suitable materials compatible with dentin and able to provide a better bond than current materials. Ultimately, it is necessary that the tooth survives as long as possible, so it is necessary to investigate the factors affecting tooth survival.[47]

Tooth survival

The survival of root-treated teeth is influenced by a range of systemic and local conditions that affect perioapical healing, pain experience and mechanical failure. Tooth survival is influenced by many factors: medical factors, tooth type, periodontal and apical disease progression and healing, presence of cracks or fractures, excessive loss of tooth substance, cervical resorption, tooth perforation, cast restorations, post and cores, occlusal support characterized by presence of adjacent teeth and abutment function, patency at the canal terminus and root-filling extrusion. A better understanding of biomechanical processes and disease progression or healing will be key factors in improving survival of teeth in the future.

Summary

Endodontic procedures of the future will be underpinned by biological and biomechanical insight and application. The practitioner will have a thorough biological understanding as well as be adept at the technical and clinical skills underpinning the discipline.

References

1. European Society of Endodontology. Quality guidelines for endodontic treatment: consensus report of the European Society of Endodontology. Int Endod J 2006;39:921-930.
2. Rowe AHR. An historical review of material used for pulp treatment up to the year 1900. Int Endod J 1968;2:30-32.
3. Rowe AHR. An historical review of material used for pulp treatment up to the year 1900. Part two. Int Endod J 1968;2:47-48.
4. Francke OC. Capping of the living pulp: from Philip Pfaff to John Wessler. Bull History Dent 1971;19:17-23.
5. Bellizze R, Cruse WP. Endodontic historical perspective. A historical review of endodontics, 1689-1963, part 3. J Endod 1980;6:495-499.
6. Cruse WP, Bellizze R. Endodontic historical perspective. A historical review of endodontics, 1689-1963, part 1. J Endod 1980;6:576-580.
7. Cruse WP, Bellizze R. Endodontic historical perspective. A historical review of endodontics, 1689-1963, part 2. J Endod 1980;6:532-535.
8. Tsao T-F. Endodontic treatment in China. Int Endod J 1984;17:163-175.
9. Zias J, Numeroff K. Operative dentistry in the second century BCE. J Am Dent Assoc 1987;114:665.
10. Hunter W. The role of sepsis and of antisepsis in medicine. Lancet 1911;i:79-86.
11. Shandalow SL. Oral focal sepsis in relation to systemic disease. Dent Cosmos 1928;70:609-618.
12. Johnson CN. The problem of the pulpless tooth as seen by the general practitioner of dentistry. J Am Dent Assoc 1926;13:546-552.
13. Callahan JR. Sulfuric acid for opening root-canals. Dent Cosmos 1894;36:957-959.
14. Prinz H. Electro-sterilization of root-canals. Dent Cosmos 1917;59:373-381.
15. Hinman T. The interpretation of X-ray picture of apical granulations, giving differential diagnosis of cases favourable and cases unfavourable of treatment and root-canal filling. J Natl Dent Assoc 1921;8:83-87.
16. Blayney JR. The clinical results of pulp treatment. J Natl Dent Assoc 1922;16:198-208.
17. Johnston HS. Pulp-canal opening and filling by diffusion. Technique and results of electrolytic medication. Dent Cosmos 1923;65:277-285.
18. Crane B. The pulpless tooth problem. J Am Dent Assoc 1926;13:179-189.
19. Puterbaugh PG. Pulp canal therapeutics. J Am Dent Assoc 1926;Oct:1384-1391.
20. Rhein ML, Krasnow F, Gies WJ. A prolonged study of the electrolytic treatment of dental focal infection: a preliminary report. Dent Cosmos 1926;68:971-981.
21. Coolidge ED. A discussion of clinical results of root canal treatment and filling. Dent Cosmos 1927;69:1280-1288.
22. Appleton JLT. A study in experimental and applied electrosterilization. J Dent Res 1931;12:311-319.
23. Buchbinder M. A statistical study of root-canal therapy. Dent Cosmos 1936;78:20-26.
24. Auerbach MB. Clinical approach to the problem of pulp canal therapy. J Am Dent Assoc 1938;25:939-942.
25. Rhein RL. Oral sepsis. Dent Cosmos 1912;54:529-534.
26. Hall EM. Pulpless teeth. Dent Cosmos 1928;71:145-150.
27. Noyes FE. The clinical results of pulp treatment. J Natl Dent Assoc 1922;16:198-208.
28. Naidorf IJ. Inflammation and infection of pulp and periapical tissues. Oral Surg Oral Med Oral Pathol 1972;34:486-497.
29. Gulabivala K, Aung TH, Alavi A, Ng Y-L. Root and canal morphology of Burmese mandibular molars. Int Endod J 2001;34:359-370.

30. Ng Y-L, Aung TH, Alavi A, Gulabivala K. Root and canal morphology of Burmese maxillary molars. Int Endod J 2001;34:620-630.
31. Alavi AM, Opasanon A, Ng Y-L, Gulabivala K. Root and canal morphology of Thai maxillary molars. Int Endod J 2002;35:478-485.
32. Gulabivala K, Opasanon A, Ng Y-L, Alavi A. Root and canal morphology of Thai mandibular molars. Int Endod J 2002;35:56-62.
33. Shovelton DS, Friend LA, Kirk EE, Rowe AH. The efficacy of pulp capping materials. A comparative trial. Br Dent J 1971;130:385-391.
34. Haskell EW, Stanley HR, Chellemi J, Stringfellow H. Direct pulp capping treatment: a long-term follow-up. J Am Dent Assoc 1978;97:607-612.
35. Cvek M. A clinical report on partial pulpotomy and capping with calcium hydroxide in permanent incisors with complicated crown fracture. J Endod 1978;4:232-237.
36. Baume LJ, Holz J. Long term clinical assessment of direct pulp capping. Int Dent J 1981;31:251-260.
37. Santini A. Assessment of the pulpotomy technique in human first permanent mandibular molars. Use of two direct inspection criteria. Br Dent J 1983;155:151-154.
38. Horsted P, Sandergaard B, Thylstrup A, El Attar K, Fejerskov O. A retrospective study of direct pulp capping with calcium hydroxide compounds. Endod Dent Traumatol 1985;1:29-34.
39. Mejàre I, Cvek M. Partial pulpotomy in young permanent teeth with deep carious lesions. Endod Dent Traumatol 1993;9:238-242.
40. Caliskan MK. Pulpotomy of carious vital teeth with periapical involvement. Int Endod J 1995;28:172-176.
41. Barthel CR, Rosenkranz B, Leuenberg A, Roulet JF. Pulp capping of carious exposures: treatment outcome after 5 and 10 years: a retrospective study. J Endod 2000;26:525-528.
42. Al-Hiyasat AS, Barrieshi-Nusair KM, Al-Omari MA. The radiographic outcomes of direct pulp-capping procedures performed by dental students: a retrospective study. J Am Dent Assoc 2006;137:1699-1705.
43. Ng Y-L, Mann V, Rahbaran S, Lewsey J, Gulabivala K. Outcome of primary root canal treatment: systematic review of the literature. Part 1. Effects of study characteristics on probability of success. Int Endod J 2007;40:921-939.
44. Hepworth MJ, Friedman S. Treatment outcome of surgical and non-surgical management of endodontic failures. J Can Dent Assoc 1997;63 364-371.
45. Ng Y-L, Mann V, Gulabivala K. Outcome of secondary root canal treatment: systematic review of the literature. Int Endod J 2008;41:1026-1046.
46. Gulabivala K, Patel B, Evans G, Ng Y-L. Effects of mechanical and chemical procedures on root canal surfaces. Endod Topics 2005;10:103-122.
47. Ng Y-L. Factor affecting outcome of non-surgical root canal treatment. PhD Thesis, Oregon Health and Science University. Portland, OR, 2008.
48. Banchs F, Trope M. Revascularization of immature permanent teeth with apical periodontitis: new treatment protocol? J Endod 2004;30:196-200.
49. Torabinejad M, Anderson P, Bader J, Brown LJ, Chen LH, Goodacre CJ et al. Outcomes of root canal treatment and restoration, implant-supported single crowns, fixed partial dentures, and extraction without replacement: a systematic review. J Prosthet Dent 2007;98:285-311.
50. Ohazama A, Modino SA, Miletich I, Sharpe PT. Stem-cell-based tissue engineering of murine teeth. J Dent Res 2004;83:518-522.
51. Nair PN, Henry S, Cano V, Vera J. Microbial status of apical root canal system of human mandibular first molars with primary apical periodontitis after 'one-visit' endodontic treatment. Oral Surg Oral Med Oral Pathol Oral Radiol Endod 2005;99:231-252.
52. Ng Y-L, Mann V, Rahbaran S, Lewsey J, Gulabivala K. Outcome of primary root canal treatment: systematic review of the literature. Part 2. Influence of clinical factors. Int Endod J 2008;41:6-31.
53. Lussi A, Nussbächer U, Grosrey J. A novel noninstrumented technique for cleansing the root canal system. J Endod 1993;19:549-553.

CHAPTER 8

Implant dentistry

Steven E. Eckert

Definition

Implant dentistry is classically defined as the 'field of dental art and science concerned with diagnosis and treatment planning for implant-supported restorations, surgical placement of implants, and the restorative treatment and subsequent maintenance procedures.'[1]

Although this definition clearly describes the use of implants to support dental prostheses, it is equally clear that all the principles of dentistry continue to apply to implant dentistry. Patient goals continue to be the provision of comfortable, functional and esthetic restorations that will serve the patient for many years, with minimal intervention for maintenance during that time. The primary objective is to provide dental prostheses that mimic nature for patients who have lost one or more of the natural teeth.

Although the field of implant dentistry has been referred to as 'implantology,' this term is considered to be a misnomer as it describes the very limited study of a specific device, the dental implant. Instead, implant dentistry demands an understanding of the physiologic response of biologic tissue and alloplastic device. Furthermore, this understanding must transcend the device itself and instead consider the interaction of the implanted device with the dental prosthesis in a patient.

Historical milestones

Throughout history, humans have sought to replace missing or lost teeth. Ancient civilizations, as demonstrated through archeological artefacts, rewarded some members of society with tooth replacements after death. This postmortem replacement of missing teeth may have been an effort to make the person whole for transition into the afterlife. Clearly, there is an emphasis on tooth replacement that goes beyond simple cosmetic concerns.

Tooth replacements can be accomplished using prostheses that are inserted in, and removed from, the oral cavity by the patient; these are known as removable dental prostheses. Other replacements may be permanently connected to the remaining dentition and are termed fixed dental prostheses. Although most dental prostheses depend upon oral mucosa or residual teeth to provide prosthesis support, dental implants are devices that are placed beneath the oral soft tissue or within the jawbone to provide the support.

Early dental implants were made from a variety of different materials. In some instances, teeth from other animals or humans may have been implanted in the hope that these could provide the same service as the natural dentition. Historically, dental implants were not terribly reliable; however, scientific investigation in the twentieth century led to dramatic improvements in the predictability of long-term service from these devices. Today, the use of dental implants to support and retain dental prostheses is a relatively common procedure. The reason for the adoption of implant support is related to the increase in predictability coupled with a decreasing incidence of adverse outcomes subsequent to implant failure.

In the first half of the twentieth century, physicians, dental clinicians and scientists developed an understanding of the factors that influence the body's acceptance of alloplastic devices. With time, a better appreciation of biocompatibility began to emerge. Recognition developed that the placement of materials within bodily tissue induced minimal adverse response as long as the materials were resistant to corrosion, the patient possessed normal healing capacity and there were no allergies to those specific materials. Although some materials were relatively inert and resistant to corrosion, this did not necessarily ensure a favorable biologic response.

The era of modern implant dentistry coincided with the recognition that non-corrosive biocompatible alloplastic materials could be used within the body to support dental prostheses. Early dental implant designs were either placed within the osseous structure or upon the underlying bone beneath the periosteum. The therapeutic goal with these implants was to use them to support dental prostheses, with the clinical recognition that the adjacent bone would gradually deteriorate secondary to functional loading. These early implant designs underwent a process known as 'fibrointegration' whereby fibrous connective tissue aligned

Table 8-1 Success criteria for dental implants outlined at the consensus conference between the National Institute of Health and Harvard University

Type	Criteria
Subjective	Adequate function
	Absence of discomfort
	Patients believe in the treatment and emotional and psychological attitudes are improved
Objective	Good occlusal balance and vertical dimension
	Bone loss no greater than one third of the vertical height of the implant, with an absence of symptoms and functionally stable after five years
	Gingival inflammation amenable to treatment
	Immobility of < 1 mm buccolingual, mesiodistal and vertically
	Absence of symptoms and infection associated with the implant
	Absence of damage to adjacent tooth or teeth and their supporting structures
	Absence of paresthesia or violation of mandibular canal, maxillary sinus or floor of nasal passage
	Healthy collagenous tissue without polymorphonuclear infiltration

From the US Department of Health and Human Services (1977),[2] Schnitman & Shulman (1980)[3] and Schnitman & Shulman (1979).[4]

parallel to the implant surfaces. Unlike the suspension mechanism of teeth in alveolar bone, the parallel fiber alignment provided little resistance to bacterial ingress. These early implant designs exhibited only short-term clinical success, primarily because the implant exhibited a large area of surface contact. Long-term maintenance depended upon a favorable biologic response on the part of the individual patient, or an ever-increasing dependence upon antibiotic therapy to combat the low-grade infective response to the embedded implant. It was often recognized that the biologic advantages achieved by the provision of a dental restoration supported by implants were often offset by the adverse consequences associated with a foreign body reaction within the tissues.

A consensus conference was conducted jointly between the National Institute of Health and Harvard University in 1978 to assess the clinical performance of implants of that era.[2] That conference stated that 'to be considered effective and successful, a dental implant should provide functional services for five years in 75% of cases.' In addition to absolute implant survival, other criteria were described to define clinical 'success' (Table 8-1).[2–4]

Unfortunately, these early implant approaches depending on fibrointegration did not routinely achieve the described success rate. One of the reasons for this was the technical difficulty of the procedure, which demanded an exceedingly high level of skill. A further issue was that the concept depended upon a fibrous encapsulation of the implant and this capsule invariably led to ingress of bacteria, which caused infection.

A variety of different implant shapes and approaches were used but all appeared to suffer from the fundamental problem associated with fibrous encapsulation. Indeed, although natural teeth are suspended in the alveolus by a periodontal ligament, the fibrous capsule surrounding endosseous implants did not mimic this situation. For this reason implants of early design remained in limited use.

Clinical investigation into alternative methods of implant connection was, however, being conducted in the mid-1960s and 1970s. One approach was a direct bone-to-implant contact, known as osseointe-

Table 8-2 Factors required for osseointegration

Area of importance	Factors
Host	Patient health status suitable for surgical intervention
	Adequate bone quality
	Adequate bone quantity
	Psychologically predisposed to desire the intervention
	Patient committed to the oral hygiene needed to maintain prostheses
Implant	Biocompatible material for implant
	Appropriate shape of implant (macrostructure)
	Appropriate surface of implant to allow bone to implant contact (microstructure)
Surgical procedure	Gentle handling of soft and hard tissues
	Careful consideration of critical bone temperatures (< 43°C)
	Primary closer of soft tissue
	Undisturbed healing
	Rigid fixation of implants in final prosthesis

gration or functional ankylosis.[5,6] The process of osseointegration was identified though a serendipitous chain of events. Researchers studying the healing of injuries created in bone discovered that titanium chambers placed within the bone to protect optical lenses appeared to bond to the surrounding bone in some instances. The researchers eventually described the phenomenon of bone-to-implant contact and identified its application in clinical dentistry.

The process of osseointegration was dependent upon the use of a biocompatible implant that was placed in a receptive host using an atraumatic surgical procedure and with minimal disturbance during the early healing periods. Once biologic healing had occurred, such implants are thought to be relatively resistant to physiologic degradation.

A number of requisite factors for osseointegration have been described (Table 8-2). One factor is a period of undisturbed healing within bone. Depending upon bone quality, this healing period was considered to be three months in bone that had a thick cortex and a moderate amount of marrow, as typically found in the mandible, or six months when little or no cortex was evident and the trabecular pattern within the marrow was relatively loose, as typically seen in the maxilla. The approach of undisturbed healing was in direct contradiction to the approach used with the fibro-integrated implants that were common at that time. Fibrointegrated implants were functionally loaded soon after placement and were often connected to the surrounding natural teeth.

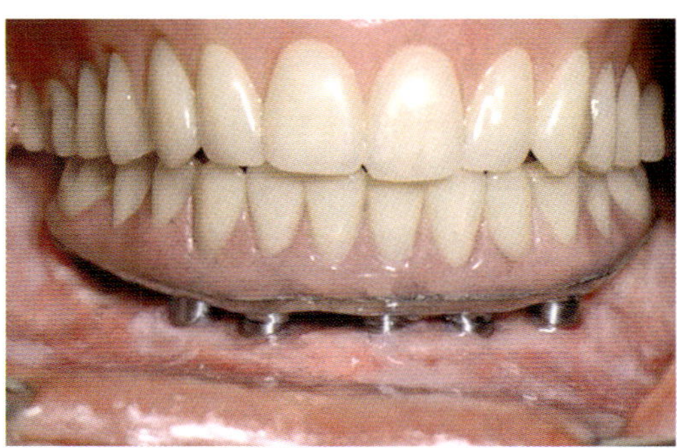

Fig. 8-1 An implant-supported mandibular prosthesis.

The primary advantage associated with osseointegration was its predictability. In contrast to implants placed by previous methods, those integrated by ossoeintegration were reliably successful if the clinicians followed a specific surgical and prosthetic protocol. Likewise, once achieved, osseointegration appeared to remain stable over long periods of time. Once long-term studies had documented the clinical performance of implants using these methods, the standing of implant dentistry changed dramatically, as reasonably prudent clinicians following well-defined protocols could anticipate clinical success that exceeded that of previous implant designs. In fact, the success criteria described in the previous era were quickly abandoned in favor of a more rigorous approach, as proposed by Albrektsson and co-workers:[7]

- an individual, unattached implant is immobile when tested clinically
- radiographic examination does not reveal any periimplant radiolucency
- after the first year in function, radiographic bone loss is < 0.2 mm per annum
- the individual implant performance is characterized by an absence of signs and symptoms such as pain, infections, neuropathies, paresthesiae or violation of the inferior dental canal
- as a minimum, the implant should fulfill the above criteria with a success rate of 85% at the end of a five-year observation period and 80% at the end of a 10-year period.

Treatment concepts

Osseointegration has now become the goal of implant dentistry. Implants that fail to achieve the requisite union between bone and alloplastic material are thought of as clinical failures.

Early descriptions of the use of osseointegrated implants limited their use to cases of complete edentulism in patients who were unable to use conventional dental prostheses (Fig. 8-1). Early clinical success with implant support in these situations led to expansion of the technique. Today, implants are used in the management of all types of edentulism, whether restoration of a single tooth or of all teeth in an edentulous arch. Furthermore, although early restorations were designed to provide function with relatively little regard for esthetic tooth replacement, conventional therapy now includes restorations that are esthetically pleasing.

Before discussing the current state of implant dentistry, it might be appropriate to describe the development of implant dentistry specifically as it relates to osseointegration. As mentioned above, osseointegration was not a specific research goal, but was a clinical finding derived from research into bone healing.

Adell and co-workers[8] described the results from up to 15 years of endosseous implants in the treatment of edentulous jaws. Survival in this monumental study was reported at 91% in the mandible and 81% in the maxilla at the described time period. During a similar time frame, Schröder and co-workers[5] conducted parallel research, with the observation that implants could achieve 'functional ankylosis'. In essence, these two groups were using different terms to describe the same phenomenon, which today is referred to universally as osseointegration.

Since dental rehabilitation of the edentulous jaw was a daunting task, depending upon close adaptation of a carefully fashioned methyl methacrylate denture base to underlying mucosa, this became the first target for implant rehabilitiation. Brånemark[6] described the use of five or six implants placed in the anterior mandible between the mental foramina. These implants were placed in a surgical procedure designed to minimize trauma to the bone and to eliminate movement of the implant during the early healing periods. With appropriate clinical management, the implant healed predictably, allowing it to support a prosthesis. The early prosthetic designs, using implants placed in the anterior mandible, depended upon posterior cantilevered prostheses to allow the replacement of the majority of the teeth in the edentulous arch.

In an approach that differed from that espoused by Brånemark and colleagues, Schröder and colleagues[5] used an implant design that passed through the tissue at the day of surgical placement. It should be stressed, however, that this implant, although described as a one-stage implant, was not placed in occlusal function until healing had occurred. In essence, both groups favored a healing time to ensure successful osseointegration.

The initial application of implants in the anterior mandible appears to have been a fortuitous choice of anatomic location. Bone in this portion of the jaw typically has a dense superior and inferior cortex surrounding a cancellous bone core. Once implants were successful in the mandible, the technology was applied to the edentulous maxilla. This transition was not simple, as the bone in the maxilla differs from that of the mandible. Maxilllary bone typically possesses a thin cortex with a large volume of cancellous core. In addition, although the maxilla might possess a cortex at the ridge crest, there is only limited thickness of cortical bone at the nasal and sinus floor. Indeed, it is possible that the difference in bone quality between maxilla and mandible led to the lower implant survival in the maxilla during the early experiences in implant-supported rehabilitation of this jaw. Ultimately, however, the survival rate of implants in the maxilla gradually improved with clinical experience to the point that there is now no significant difference in survival between the maxilla and the mandible.

The combination of advances in surgical technique, implant designs and prosthetic components, together with an ever-increasing knowledge base, has allowed implant dentistry to make the transition from an approach of limited application to one that offers broad opportunities for the clinician. Indeed, implant dentistry represents a paradigm shift in the thinking of many clinicians. During the early years of the osseointegration approach, there was a perception that implants should be reserved only for otherwise terminal dentitions. Restorations were only offered after all other options had failed to create acceptable results. It was not uncommon for patients to maintain their dentition with advanced stages of periodontal breakdown rather than removing diseased teeth and relying on dental implants to serve as root analogs. Similarly, patients with advanced dental caries, fractured and missing teeth and complex defective restorations were treated with complex fixed dental prostheses. Unfortunately, these two categories of patient, those with advanced periodontal disease and those with heavily restored compromised dentitions, frequently experienced ongoing deterioration, leading to ever more complex needs.

Patients with advanced dental disease are often provided with prostheses to compensate for loss of function. Since the predictability of dental implants has improved so dramatically, many of these patients are now treated with implants as the primary means of intervention. The effect of this treatment approach has been therapeutically and economically advantageous to patients, as complicated transitional prostheses are now routinely avoided in favor of the more predictable implant-supported prostheses.

Restoration of the dentition with dental implants differs somewhat from traditional therapy. Dental implants exhibit appreciably less movement within the alveolus than do natural teeth. In fact, implants move so little as to be described as immobile. Technically this description is incorrect as implants do have a small amount of mobility, but this mobility is so much less than that of natural teeth that most clinicians describe it as non-existent.

Compensation for lack of physiologic mobility, as seen with natural teeth, must be considered.[9–11] When endosseous implants are used to support prostheses, these implants will carry the majority of the physiologic load if the prothesis is placed in the same level of occlusal contact as the remaining natural teeth. Consequently, suggestions have been made to place implant-supported restorations in slight infraocclusion relative to the remaining natural dentition. Recommendations suggesting infraocclusion of 100 μm are found in the literature; however, the methods used to achieve this level of occlusion precision are not routinely available. Use of shim stock, articulating paper, tactile sensation or even occlusal tracking devices such as the 'T-Scan' remain somewhat subjective. Clearly, clinicians benefit from experience in achieving appropriate infraocclusion, but it is unlikely that the target of 100 μm is reliably achieved.

Recently, there has been renewed interest in the time to loading of endosseous implants. Although the early protocols used machined implants that required undisturbed healing times of three to six months depending on the quality of bone, changes in implant surfaces allowed the recruitment of increased numbers of multipotential cells (pre-osteoblasts) adjacent to the implant surface, which ultimately leads to increased numbers of osteoblasts and more rapid healing of bone to the implant surface. This surface technology change allowed more rapid loading of implants, reducing it to around three to six weeks.

In addition to the advantages achieved with surface changes to implants, it was also recognized that reduction of the micromovement of implants could allow osseointegration to occur even if functional loading occurred immediately following implant placement. An early attempt to limit this movement was described by Brånemark and colleagues for the Novum system.[12–14] In this treatment, three endosseous implants are placed in a predetermined arrangement. Since the implants are placed using a rigid surgical template that allows placement in only one position, a preformed prosthetic framework can be connected to the implants to allow support of a prosthesis while simultaneously limiting movement of the implants. The key to the success of this treatment is the rigid fixation of the implant, which allows loading while osseointegration is occurring. Other authors have described similar rigid fixation approaches with favorable clinical results.[15,16]

Currently, there are a number of approaches that utilize immediate restoration of endosseous implants. Most reports describe immediate placement of provisional restorations that are slightly out of occlusion; however, even if implant-supported restorations are not in occlusion in a static condition, they will be placed in occlusion under functional loading as the food bolus contacts the restoration. The forces generated will be primarily vertical in nature. Elimination of static contact will eliminate non-axial loading associated with parafunctional activity, which might be the critical issue in the survival of these implants.

Many authors have discussed the need for immediate stabilization of implants and high insertion torque values if implants are to be loaded immediately. To a great extent, implant stability is a function of the quality and quantity of supporting bone together with the sufficiency of the surgical technique used to place the implant. Insertion torque is influenced by the surgical technique and the design of components. When an osteotomy is prepared, the dimensions of the preparation relative to the diameter of the implant will influence the insertion torque. If there is a relatively narrow osteotomy with an implant of relatively wide diameter, the insertion torque will be increased; however, this must be balanced by awareness that the implant is being placed within biologic tissue and the insertion torque must not be so extensive as to overly compress tissue to the point of tissue damage. At this time, there is no definitive clinical research to establish the ideal insertion torque of the implant system that ensures osseointegration. This is an area that demands future attention as identification of these critical values is mandatory to ensure continuing success of dental implants.

Implant designs and surfaces have been modified in an ongoing effort to increase the amount and tenacity of bone-to-implant contact. The changes have affected implant shape, thread pattern, length and diameter. Surfaces of implants have been modified in a variety of ways, including coating of implants with hydroxyapatite or titanium oxide spray, abrasive spraying, anodizing or machine turning. Although most surface modification has been performed with the intention of creating an appropriately a roughened at the level of 0.5–10 μm, there is a renewed interest in surface modification in the nanometer range, as 'nanotechnology' is thought to influence molecular activity surrounding an implant. Finally, creation of polished or laser-modified surfaces in specific locations on the implant has been proposed to enhance soft tissue adherence at the coronal aspect of the implant. There are also hypotheses that specific roughening of the implant surface may influence the soft tissue response.

Given the large number of potential variations in the design and surface technology, the only clear statement that can be made is that this is evolving technology. It appears that the trend is towards roughened surfaces on implants as this modification appears to recruit cellular activity adjacent to the implant, but the ideal level of 'roughness' remains a nebulous concept. Cellular recruitment, although a valuable early response, may or may not influence long-term clinical performance. Unfortunately, there is a paucity of sufficiently detailed long-term clinical research that can be used to determine 'ideal' characteristics. This leaves the clinician involved in implant research in the precarious position of being reliant on theories that have yet to be validated.

It is important to understand that the primary desire of the patient is not for the acquisition of a dental implant, but is for the replacement of missing teeth. Towards this end, the clinician must have a variety of methods to allow dental prostheses to be connected to an implant.

The first generation of implants used a prosthesis that was attached to the implant through the use of a screw. Screw-retained restorations addressed a few critical issues. The first was the need to protect the implant. A small screw used to secure the prosthesis could also provide a 'fail-safe' mechanism in the event that occlusal or masticatory forces reached a level that could jeopardize the osseointegration process. Should excessive force be applied to the prosthesis, the prosthesis-retaining screw would fail rather than the implant losing integration or fracturing.

Alternative implant designs utilized larger implants, some of which were formed from titanium alloy, which possesses a much higher resistance to

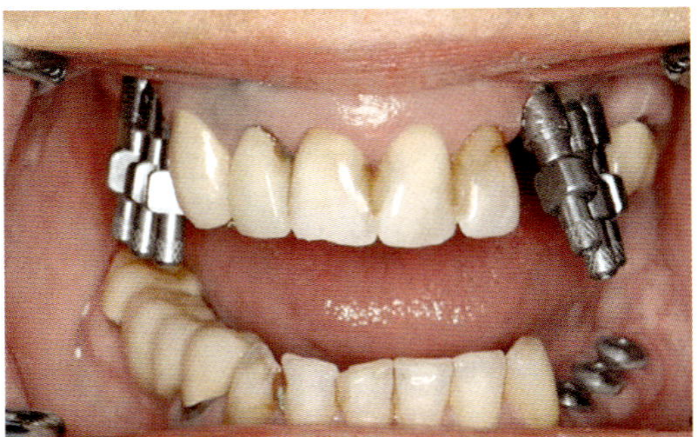

Fig. 8-2 Implants placed too far to facially in left maxilla.

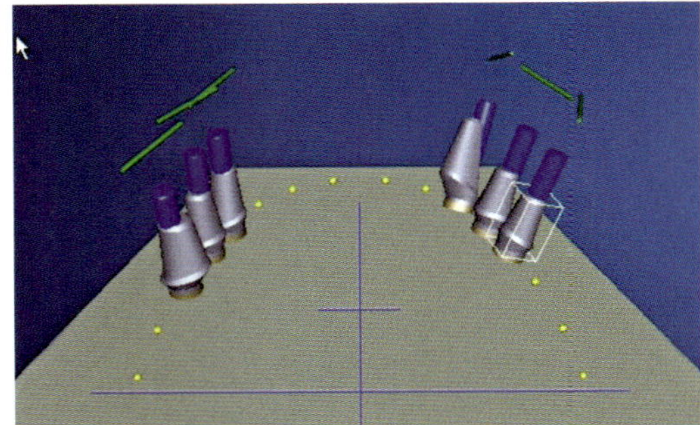

Fig. 8-3 Virtual design of custom abutments using computer-assisted design technology. Computer-assisted manufacturing will be used remotely to construct the custom abutments.

fracture. When such implants are used, the need for the fail-safe system may be less critical, as the strength of the implant is sufficient to withstand excessive forces without being subject to fracture. Assuming that the bone-to-implant contact is sufficiently robust to withstand functional loading, even excessive functional loading, it may be possible to consider the use of prostheses that are retained by dental cement. Indeed, this approach has gained popularity, as cement retention eliminates the need for a screw access and may provide a level of compensation for slight misfit that may be undetectable by the human eye.

The second consideration associated with screw retention of dental prostheses relates to the ability to retrieve a prosthesis in the event of material wear, fracture, or the need for future modification of a dental prosthesis.

Prosthesis retrieval followed by modification and re-insertion is one of the most critical justifications for implant-supported restorations, as this approach provides more flexibility to the clinician and also provides a more economical approach to ongoing management of the patient's state of edentulism.

It is ultimately necessary for implant-supported prostheses to address all concerns of the patient, specifically the need to restore comfort, function and esthetics. Early use of implants to support prostheses relied primarily on restoration of function and comfort. In this regard, the early prosthetic designs were esthetically adequate, but were clearly not beautiful. With time, however, the transmucosal elements of the implant were improved to the point where cosmetically acceptable restorations are now the norm rather than the exception. These components are now available in a variety of angles, heights and dimensions. In addition the use of computer-assisted design (CAD) software, coupled with computer-assisted manufacturing (CAM), allows components to be customized to address the specific needs of the individual patient (Figs 8-2 and 8-3).

Ultimately the success of a dental implant is judged only after years of clinical function. An implant that exhibits progressive bone loss may ultimately fail in its provision of support for a dental prosthesis. Likewise, an implant system that cannot reliably maintain prosthetic support secondary to repeated screw joint complications will not be deemed successful for the individual patient.

The use of implants in support of dental prostheses has taken dramatic strides since the 1970s, but this observation should not lead to complacency. This field has many areas that merit investigation. In this regard, the ongoing development of implant dentistry is likely to provide enormous opportunity for future research.

Vision 2020

Dental implant research has centered primarily on the bone-to-implant interface. Efforts to recruit more rapid and tenacious contact between bone and implant are ongoing. In the next decade. it is likely that research will provide better understanding of the biologic aspects of osseointegration. This will lead to an appreciation of the shortest healing period necessary to achieve this effective osseointegration. Ultimately, nature may be accelerated but it cannot be replaced. Accepting this comment, it behooves investigators to understand the limits of accelerated healing. This should be well defined in the coming decade.

It may be possible to enhance the surface of implants through the application of biologic materials. Today the material that is discussed most often is bone morphogenetic protein, but this is expensive to produce, and this expense has limited its general use. It is possible that technologic advances in gene therapy will identify methods to provide bone morphogenetic protein in a more affordable package. Once again, it must be stressed that this material is an enhancement , not a substitute for normal bone healing, a biologic phenomenon that requires time. It is likely that other materials will be identified to further enhance the biologic response. Current research in this field is ongoing and breakthroughs are likely.

Implant design will continue to be refined. Thread patterns on implants will ultimately be optimized to achieve improved stability within bone, while resisting ongoing bone loss. Indeed, it is recognized today that immediate implant stability and insertion torque are highly influenced by the matching of the osteotomy dimensions with the implant design. Although it is unlikely that the profession will suddenly agree that any design has been maximized, it is likely that some underperforming designs will be eliminated over time.

The understanding of implant surfaces and their influence on the biologic response is a field of interest. There are suggestions that specific S-ratios, representing the microscopic peak-to-valley ratio over a defined area, are more favorable than others in respect of early restoration of endosseous implants. In the next decade, this area of investigation will continue to be an exciting one. Assessment of surface enhancements to induce molecular responses should also continue to be a critical area.

Implant-loading protocols will continue to undergo refinement. At present, there are no reliable presurgical markers that identify the likelihood that an implant can be reliably loaded. One proposed approach is to assess the density of bone in the area of anticipated implant placement.

The degree of attenuation of X-rays by tissue when computerized tomography is used, measured by Hounsfield units, describes the radiodensity of a tissue as a pixel density, and this has been discussed as a potential marker of bone density. However, the method remains to be validated.[17-19] This will likely occur before 2020.

It is possible that no implants will require a healing period before being functionally loaded, but given the history of implant dentistry, this seems unlikely. Instead, it appears that some implants perform exceptionally well when loaded immediately, while others are miserable failures under similar conditions. Current evidence suggests that insertion torque may be a reliable predictor of an implant's potential for early or immediate loading. Unfortunately, such a predictor is not as valuable as a presurgical marker, as a predictor at the time of surgery (especially one for an inability of a dental implant to take an immediate loading) creates a situation of practice inefficiency for the clinician scheduled to place the dental prosthesis.

Immediate loading of individual implants will continue to be the most perplexing problem for clinicians involved in implant dentistry. With restorations supported by multiple implants, there is a greater opportunity for the implants to be mechanically locked (splinted), thereby reducing micromotion and improving overall performance when loaded immediately. Single implants placed in immediate function, by comparison, lack the capacity to be splinted. For single implants, the stability of the implant within the osteotomy is critical to the survival of the implant. It is likely that implant designs will be modified to address this issue, as a large-diameter implant in a narrow-diameter osteotomy will achieve a much higher insertion torque than would a matched implant–osteotomy complex. Of course, the critical issue in respect of insertion torque is the amount of trauma to surrounding bone when the implant is placed. High insertion torque depends upon high compression to surrounding bone. If bone compression is too high, it can lead to irreparable damage to the bone and a failure of the residual cells or the recruited cells to achieve integration.

Osseointegration is a biologic phenomenon that depends upon cellular recruitment, with differentiation of cells into osteoblasts and then maturation into osteocytes. While this is occurring, there is also a need for osteoclastic activity, as this is essential in ongoing wound repair and remodeling. Medications such as the bisphosphonates target the osteoclast to address diseases of bone mineral density such as osteoporosis.[20] The bisphosphonates reduce osteoclastic action, thereby reducing loss of bone mineral. Unfortunately, this leaves the bone susceptible to necrotic lesions as the body's normal defense mechanism is reduced as the osteoclast is not participating in the bone-remodeling process. It has been suggested that serum markers of bone metabolism may provide valuable information regarding the risks for specific patients, but these markers appear to vary widely in the population. In the coming decade, it is likely that the current marker, serum CTX (serum C-telopeptide of type I collagen), or others will be thoroughly investigated to determine their value in management of bone-healing capacity.

Restoration of dental implants will continue to be a critical issue as patient expectations of esthetic restorations grows. It is likely that ongoing emphasis will be placed on the use of CAD/CAM technology, as this allows each patient to be treated in a customized fashion befitting the unique nature of each situation. In addition, this technology is economically appropriate for the dental implant manufacturers, as it reduces the need for inventory maintenance and provides only the product that the customer (dental clinician) desires, thereby resulting in reduced waste as implant components pass expiry dates.

CAD/CAM technology will gradually replace traditional lost wax techniques used in the construction of dental prostheses. With CAD/CAM, dental laboratory technicians will be able to create virtual restorations based upon a library of natural and restored teeth. The virtual tooth forms will be created on the computer; the forms will be modified virtually to provide sufficient reduction for ceramic application while simultaneously providing sufficient support for the veneering ceramic material. The form for the ceramic application, can then be duplicated and used in a pressed ceramic application to the underlying metal coping. Production time will be minimized, thereby allowing more restorations to be created in shorter time periods with higher quality.

Physical impressions of implants will be replaced by optical or laser impressions of implants within the dental arch. This technology will be much simpler to apply to dental implants than to prepared teeth, as the implant represents a predetermined geometric pattern that is not seen in the natural dentition. The technology to perform these impressions is already available, but the cost is relatively high at present. It is likely that this situation will be corrected as demand for scanning devices grows.

Today, guided surgery using intraoral guides made from information gathered using computerized tomographic imaging is already common. It is likely that such devices will undergo further refinement, ultimately becoming the 'state of the art' in implant dentistry.

Materials used in implant dentistry need to be continuously scrutinized. The use of commercially pure titanium in the production of dental implants has been quite successful. The current methods used to handle the raw titanium stock have resulted in an increased strength of the material. Addition of titanium alloys has been beneficial in terms of reducing the risk for implant fracture. Ceramic implants have been described in the current literature and further use of such implants in situations of high esthetic demand is likely to increase.

Dental prostheses supported by implants have an entirely different mobility pattern to that of natural teeth, and yet the materials used to restore implants remain the same. Ultimately, this situation will change with development of specific materials for use on functionally immobile implants.

Biologic substitutes for the natural dentition using stem cell technology on the horizon. Within the next 10 years, biologically created teeth will likely become available.

Summary

The use of dental implants to support and retain prostheses was stimulated by the need to address a physical disability related to tooth loss. Edentulism remains one of the most common conditions known to mankind, and implant-supported restorations offer an opportunity to manage this condition. Ideally, the use of implants needs to become a routine part of the practice of dentistry. Rather than routinely employing technically demanding and failure-prone procedures associated with fixed prosthodontics to address issues of tooth loss, it is suggested that implant dentistry should be expanded and developed as a matter of priority.

References

1. Academy of Prosthodontics. Glossary of prosthodontic terms, 8th edn. J Prosthet Dent 2005;94:1-104.
2. US Dept. Health and Human Services. Dental Implants: Benefit and Risk. A NIH-Harvard Consensus Development Conference. Bethesda, MD: US Department of Health and Human Services, 1977, NIH Pub. No. 81-1531.
3. Schnitman P, Shulman L. Dental Implants: Benefit and Risk. Bethesda, MD: US Department of Health and Human Services, 1980.
4. Schnitman PA, Shulman LB. Recommendations of the consensus development conference on dental implants. J Am Dent Assoc 1979;98:373-377.
5. Schröder A, van der Zypen E, Stuch H, Sutter F. The reactions of bone, connective tissue, and epithelium to endosteal implants with titanium-sprayed surfaces. J Maxillofac Surg 1981;9:15-25.
6. Brånemark PI. Osseointegration and its experimental background. J Prosthet Dent 1983;50:399-410.
7. Albrektsson, T, Zarb G, Worthington P, Eriksson A. The long-term efficacy of currently used dental implants: a review and proposed criteria of success. Int J Oral Maxillofac Implants 1986;1:11-25.
8. Adell R, Lekholm U, Rockler B, Brånemark P-I. A 15-year study of osseointegrated implants in the treatment of the edentulous jaw. Int J Oral Surg 1981;10:387-416.
9. Schulte W, Kleineikenscheidt H, Lindner K, Schareyka R. [The Tubingen immediate implant in clinical studies.] Dtsch Zahnarztl Z 1978;33:348-359.
10. Schulte W, Kleineikenscheidt H, Schareyka R, Heimke G. [Concept and testing of the Tubingen immediate implant.] Dtsch Zahnarztl Z 1978;33:319-325.
11. Babbush CA, Kirsch A, Mentag PJ, Hill B. Intramobile cylinder (IMZ) two-stage osteointegrated implant system with the intramobile element (IME): part I. Its rationale and procedure for use. Int J Oral Maxillofac Implants 1987;2:203-216.
12. Brånemark PI, Engstrand P, Öhnell L-O, Gröndahl K, Nilsson P, Hagberg K, et al. Brånemark Novum: a new treatment concept for rehabilitation of the edentulous mandible. Preliminary results from a prospective clinical follow-up study. Clin Implant Dent Relat Res 1999;1: 2-16.
13. Engstrand P, Nannmark U, Martensson L, Galéus I, Brånemark PI. Brånemark Novum: prosthodontic and dental laboratory procedures for fabrication of a fixed prosthesis on the day of surgery. Int J Prosthodont 2001;14: 303-309.
14. Parel SM. A system for definitive restoration of single-stage implants in one day. Dent Today 2002;21:106-111.
15. Balshi TJ, Wolfinger GJ. Immediate loading of dental implants in the edentulous maxilla: case study of a unique protocol. Int J Periodontics Restorative Dent 2003;23: 37-45.
16. Balshi TJ, Wolfinger GJ. Teeth in a day for the maxilla and mandible: case report. Clin Implant Dent Relat Res 2003;5:11-16.
17. Shahlaie M, Gantes B, Schulz E, Riggs M, Crigger M. Bone density assessments of dental implant sites: 1. Quantitative computed tomography. Int J Oral Maxillofac Implants 2003;18:224-231.
18. Shapurian T, Damoulis PD, Reiser GM, Griffin TJ, Rand WM. Quantitative evaluation of bone density using the Hounsfield index. Int J Oral Maxillofac Implants 2006;21: 290-297.
19. Turkyilmaz I, Tumer C, Ozbek EN, Tzm TF. Relations between the bone density values from computerized tomography, and implant stability parameters: a clinical study of 230 regular platform implants. J Clin Periodontol 2007;34: 716-722.
20. Marx RE, Sawatari Y, Fortin M, Broumand V. Bisphosphonate-induced exposed bone (osteonecrosis/osteopetrosis) of the jaws: risk factors, recognition, prevention, and treatment. J Oral Maxillofac Surg 2005;63: 1567-1575.

CHAPTER 9

Orthodontics

Efthimia K Basdra

Introduction

Orthodontics, less commonly referred to as dentofacial orthopedics, was recognized as a specialist branch of dentistry more than a century ago. Together with otolaryngology, orthodontics is one of the oldest specialties in healthcare.

Historic milestones

Archeological evidence indicates that ancient people attempted to treat malocclusions, having discovered that teeth may be moved by means of applying loads to them.

Orthodontic tooth movement is made possible by the capacity of alveolar bone to remodel. The first investigation of orthodontic tooth movement dates back more than 100 years, with the purpose of the research being to explain the sequence of events that occur in the tissues of the jaws when teeth are loaded.[1,2]

The association between loading and bone shape, whereby the shape of bone can be reformed by loading, was known as far back as the ancient Chinese, through the process of feet binding, but it was not the subject of any scientific publications until 1892, when Wölff's law was published.[3]

Gradually techniques were developed to use the association between loading and bone shape in orthodontics. Loads were applied to teeth by different systems, progressing to the present-day use of wires and, typically, brackets temporarily fixed to teeth. The forces generated by the applied loads are transmitted through the tooth and the suspensory periodontal ligament to the supporting alveolar bone. Studies of bone biology provided insight into the series of biological events involved in orthodontic tooth movement. A system of cells and extracellular processes respond to the forces, resulting in remodeling of the alveolar bone and, in turn, tooth migration. Although these biological events are somewhat complex,[4] they can explain clinical events and outcomes.

Treatment concepts

In common with biological systems in general, form in the dentition is largely determined by the adoption of shapes influenced by environmental factors, including stresses and strains associated with naturally occurring forces and applied loads.

Base modeling

Since the formulation of Wölff's law,[3] it has been clear that bone remodeling is an ongoing, lifelong, hormone-dependent process of considerable impact and importance to general well-being, health and mobility, in particular in older individuals. It also has a major role in musculoskeletal conditions. The process is influenced by many factors, including functional and other loading.[5] Bony remodeling is made possible by the combined action and coordination of two cell systems: osteoblasts, which lay down new bone, and osteoclasts, which resorb old bone. As in bony remodeling in general, the combined osteoblast/osteoclast activity forms the basis of mechanisms that result in remodeling changes to the jaws and the arrangement of teeth in the jaws. When loads are applied to teeth and, as a consequence, to the supporting alveolar bone through the periodontal ligament, the well-orchestrated system of osteoclasts and osteoblasts makes possible tooth movement and associated reshaping of the dental arches.

The periodontal ligament

The periodontal ligament acts as a suspensory ligament linking the tooth to the supporting alveolar bone. The periodontal ligament plays a critical role in tooth movement. Osseointegrated implants, which lack a periodontal ligament, cannot be moved orthodontically. Similarly, ankylosed teeth with an obliterated periodontal ligament cannot be moved. More importantly, it would appear that the periodontal ligament is critical to the growth, development and, in particular, maintenance of the entire alveolar bone structure, as alveolar bone will not grow in the absence of teeth, and atrophy of the alveolar bone occurs following extraction. The periodontal ligament must, therefore, be considered a key structure both in terms of the presence and absence of alveolar bone and in the movement of teeth, including orthodontic tooth movement.[6] The periodontal ligament consists of cells, a rich extracellular matrix and an abundance of fibers. The ligament protects the tooth from excessive functional loading and provides proprioceptive information important to jaw function, in particular chewing and related activities.

The periodontal ligament is a highly specialized tissue that transforms the signal of mechanical loading to a biological response, including triggering the well-coordinated interplay between osteoblasts and cytokine-activated osteoclasts, causing apposition and resorption of bone in orthodontic tooth movement. In this process, the periodontal ligament serves the additional function of being a source of immature pre-osteoblasts, which are required to help balance osteoblast/osteoclast activity.[6]

The cells of the periodontal ligament are primarily fibroblasts. In the presence of certain induction and signaling mechanisms, fibroblasts have the ability to differentiate into pre-osteoblasts or cementoblasts or to produce fibers, and thus can enter the bone remodeling process.

Periodontal ligament fibroblasts when isolated and cultured have the abilities of osteoblast-like cells: production of alkaline phosphatase, expression of osteocalcin and the ability to respond to 1α, 25-dihydroxyvitamin D_3.[6] Furthermore, under certain cell culture conditions, periodontal ligament cells can form mineralized structures: nodules in contact with collagen fibers. Electron microscope examination of these nodules indicates that their microstructure resembles that of immature bone tissue,[7] indicating that cells of the periodontal ligament have the capacity under certain conditions, such as extracellular signaling related to orthodontic tooth movement, to differentiate into pre-osteoblasts, which then mature into osteoblasts.

Recent studies have shown that the periodontal ligament is a source of stem cells, with a regenerative role including the production of cementum and periodontal ligament-like tissues.[8] Transplantation of these cells, which are readily accessible and capable of culture, may find application in the future in tissue regeneration techniques.

Alveolar bone

The response of the alveolar bone to loading is central to orthodontic tooth movement and associated bony remodeling. The response involves complex tissue dynamics, including distortion of the alveolus, resorption and the deposition of bone. The extent and nature of the response depends on the direction, duration and magnitude of the load. While the precise sequence of biological events causing the response is still obscure, the sequence in orthodontic tooth movement differs from the sequence in the skeleton, which is mainly osteogenic.[9] This difference in response is linked to the existence of the periodontal ligament between tooth and alveolar bone.

Orthodontic tooth movement

When an orthodontic force is applied to a tooth, the periodontal ligament space on the side away from the force is compressed, while the ligament on the side of the force is expanded. Where the periodontal ligament space is expanded, the periodontal ligament fibers are put under tension. Where the periodontal ligament is compressed, the fibers are also compressed. The clinical observation of this phenomenon gave rise to the classical theory of compression and tension.[1,10,11] In the early 1950s, investigations undertaken by Kaare Reitan provided new understanding of the reaction of alveolar bone to externally applied loads of different types, continuous or intermittent, and magnitude.[12–14] It became apparent that different tooth types moved in different ways under loading, reflecting differences in the configuration and surface areas of roots. This gave rise to the concept of differential loading and, as a consequence, differential force application.[15] Concurrently, optimum values for loading and resultant forces to maximize the rate of tooth movement were investigated:[16] 150–250 g for canines and 400–600 g for molar teeth, given the greater root surface areas of these teeth. Today, the optimum force is intended to achieve the maximum rate of tooth movement without damaging the tissues or causing discomfort to the patient. The force is characterized by its magnitude and its nature: continuous versus intermittent, constant versus declining, tipping versus bodily. As these two parameters may vary from patient to patient, and for different types of teeth, comparisons between patients and for different types of treatment are difficult. Future investigations of optimum tooth-moving forces should focus on the variation in patient factors and of the distribution of stresses and strains in the periodontal ligament space.[17]

The classic theory of compression and tension assumes that the effects of tension and compression are similar, in that both consequences of loading result in bone remodeling. This is incorrect as in that compression results in bone resorption, while tension causes bone deposition. Contrary to what is observed in alveolar bone remodeling during orthodontic tooth movement, mechanical loading in bone biology has an osteogenic rather than a resorptive effect.[9,18] The reason for this difference may be found in considering tension and compression effects in the loaded periodontal ligament. To date, there is inconclusive evidence that similar stresses and strains are generated in different parts of the loaded periodontal ligament, in particular given that stretching of the principal fiber bundles of the periodontal ligament does not appear to generate tension.[3] To explain resorption and apposition mechanisms during orthodontic tooth movement, it is attractive to consider the phenomenon of piezoelectricity.[19] This phenomenon fails, however, to provide a cause and effect relationship for all types of remodeling, given the influence of the periodontal ligament interface. It is, therefore, apparent that the explanation of orthodontic tooth movement mechanisms lies within the periodontal ligament interface and its contents.

Orthodontic force signaling

The reactions of cells in the periodontal ligament to the forces generated by loading, and the associated mechanisms, attracted early attention in basic research in orthodontics. A variety of investigations were undertaken to study the cellular responses. A mouse model developed to examine regulation of osteoblast- and cementoblast-associated genes under conditions of mechanical loading suggested that the primary responses to osteogenic loading are the induction of differentiation and an increase in cell function.[20,21] The osteoblast phenotype predominates, without the initial proliferative response, indicating that mechanical loading has a targeted effect on osteoblast precursors responsive to environmental signaling. Bone markers such as alkaline phosphatase and bone sialoprotein may be detected after loading for 24 h, followed by stimulation of osteocalcin and type 1 collagen at 24–48 h. Deposition of osteoid may be observed after 72 h. It would appear that a well-defined temporal pattern of cell-specific gene regulation exists in periodontal ligament pre-osteoblasts. This regulation operates after mechanical stimulation has triggered the pre-osteoblasts to differentiate and deposit bone matrix.

Organ culture of mouse molar explants has provided a useful experimental design to study orthodontic tooth movement.[22,23] Given the similarities between fibrous sutures and the periodontal ligament, researchers have also investigated the loading of organ culture systems from cranial sutures.[24,25] The mouse model provided new insight into remodeling mechanisms. Protein and collagen synthesis increased after 6 h. The type of collagen synthesized differed between stressed and unstressed sites; unstressed sites synthesized type I collagen, while stressed sites were characterized by the synthesis of 20% more type III collagen. Moreover, the model revealed that enzymes relating to collagen and the degradation of extracellular matrix, including matrix metalloproteinases, collagenase and stromelysin, were stimulated after mechanical deformation.[26-28] By using cDNA probes and antibodies to human, mouse and rat proteins, the various findings were confirmed both *in vitro*[29] and *in vivo*.[30] Very soon thereafter, various cell culture systems were developed to mimic the effects of orthodontic forces *in vivo*. Human periodontal ligament fibroblasts were cultivated in collagen substrates and subjected to stretching. Another system involves culturing the cells in culture dishes with flexible bases. The base of these culture dishes can be distorted to stretch the culture by placing them on top of a spheroidal template. The amount of stretching can be varied and controlled by placing different weights on the cover of the dish. Biochemical analysis of stretched periodontal ligament cell cultures has revealed that prostaglandin[31-35] and cyclic AMP are implicated in the process.[36-39] Inositol phosphates are also increased,[40] and intracellular calcium may change subsequent to stretch activation of ion channels.[41,42]

Initial findings from cell culture systems related the mechanical loading of periodontal ligament cells to general signaling pathways, observed as cellular responses to other extracellular signaling. To provide more information in respect of the specific response of periodontal ligament cells to mechanical forces, a more molecular approach was attempted, mindful that when a signal reaches the surface of the cell it somehow needs to overcome the barrier of the cell membrane and then travel through the cytosol, by complex molecular reactions, before reaching the nucleus, where it exerts its action. In general, cells residing in tissues and in cell cultures are attached to extracellular matrix and the surrounding substrate. These attachments involve specialized sites, know as focal adhesions, that are especially sensitive to signals pertaining to motion, thereby resisting any attempt to violate the positional equilibrium of the cell. Proteins called integrins transverse the cell membrane and link cytoskeletal proteins to the extracellular matrix.[43] Integrins are composed of structurally distinct α- and β-subunits, forming heterodimeric receptors with specific binding for collagen, laminin and vitronectin. The integrin molecules extend outside the cell and expose their focal adhesion sites, where they can physically link cytoskeletal proteins with extracellular matrix[44] and adjacent cells. Disturbances in this link create responses that result in proliferation and differentiation.[45,46] When external mechanical forces are applied to cells, they cause pertubations in the cell-to-cell and

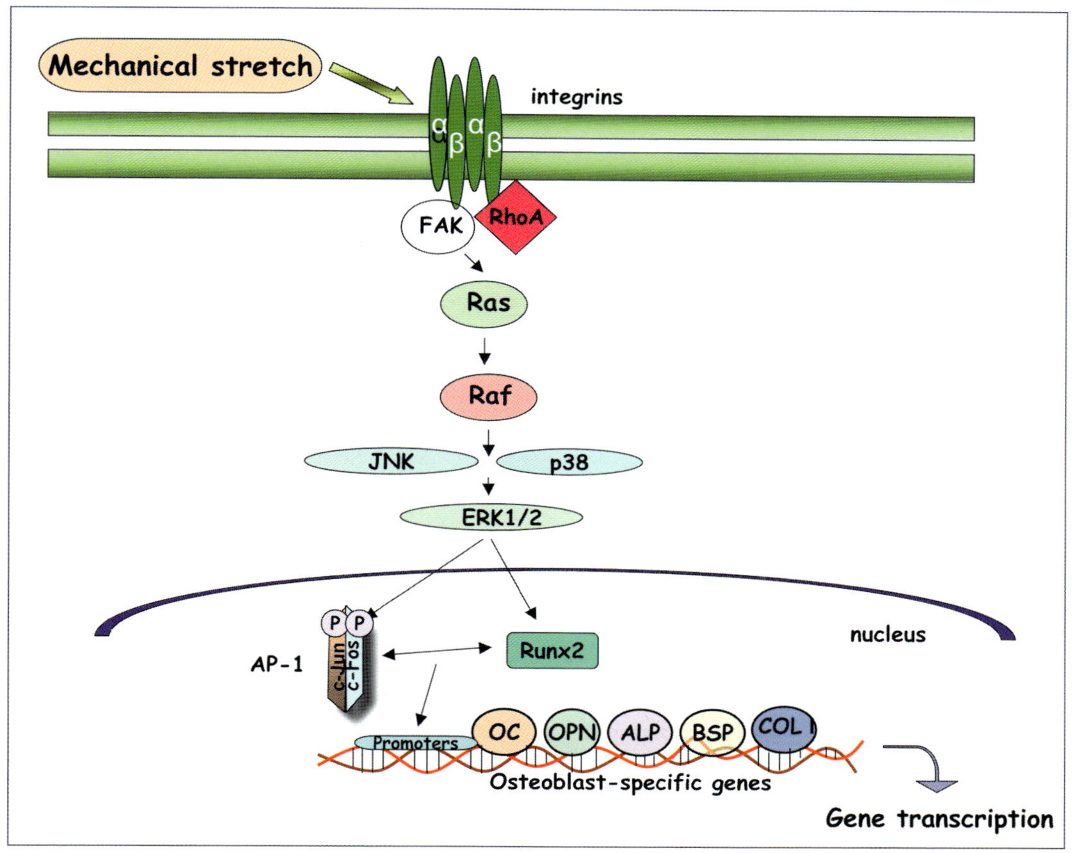

Fig. 9-1 Externally applied mechanical forces act on the pre-osteoblasts in the periodontal ligament, activate transcription factors and modulate the gene transcription machinery of the cell, thus modifying cell differentiation and function. FAK, focal adhesion kinase; RhoA, Ras homolog gene family, member A; Ras, rat sarcoma oncogene product, cellular homolog; Raf, a serine/threonine-specific kinase; OC, osteocalcin; OPN, osteopontin; ALP, alkaline phosphatase; BSP, bone sialoprotein; COL1, collagen type I; other abbreviations as in the text.

cell-to-extracellular matrix attachments. Such external signals generate a biomechanical cellular response through stress fibers, which transmit the applied forces, and integrins, which act as mechanoreceptors.[47] Mechanical signals are also transmitted by changes in the cyclic AMP signaling cascade and downstream gene transcription in a G protein-dependent manner.[48]

An increase mRNA for the β_1-integrin subunit can be detected after mechanical stimulation of bone cells.[49] Increases can also be shown in the small, low-molecular-weight GTP-binding proteins of the Ras-related GTPase family (Rab and Rho) and the mitogen-activated protein kinase subtypes (extracellular signal-regulated kinases [ERK] and c-Jun terminal kinase [JNK]) in mechanically stretched cells derived from human periodontal ligament membrane.[50-53] These are all components of the integrin-mediated signaling system. This signaling is vital in the early stages of osteoblast differentiation. Continuous low-level mechanical stimulation of osteoblast-like human periodontal ligament cells results in rapid induction of the principal constituents of the dimetric transcription factor activator protein 1 (AP-1: dimers c-Jun/c-Jun and c-Jun/c-Fos). Activation of AP-1 through ERK/JNK signaling augments the DNA-binding activity of the transcription factor for osteoblast-specific genes, modulating their pattern of expression. The effect is a shift towards differentiation and the onset of the osteoblast phenotype.[54–56] Recently, the role of the bone-specific transcription factor core-binding factor A1 (CBFA1; often known as Runx2) has been described. This factor binds to the osteoblast *cis*-acting element 2 found in the promoter regions of all major osteoblast-specific genes (ie osteocalcin, type I collagen, bone sialoprotein, osteopontin, alkaline phosphatase and collagenase type III) and controls their expression.

In this way, Runx2 production is a key factor in osteoblast differentiation and the process of skeletogenesis. Runx2 would appear to be an essential sensor of mechanical stimuli applied to osteoblast-like periodontal ligament cells. It has been shown that direct, low-level mechanical stimulation of periodontal ligament cells upregulates the expression and DNA-binding activity of Runx2. The effect is mediated by stretch-triggered induction of ERK, which was found to physically interact with and phosphorylate endogenous Runx2 *in vivo*, potentiating this transcription factor. This provides a molecular link between mechanostressing and the stimulation of osteoblast differentiation.[57,58] By following the cellular response of the human periodontal ligament cells to external applied mechanical forces, step by step, it is possible to observe (Fig. 9-1):

- disturbances in cell-to-cell and cell-to-extracellular matrix attachment through integrin involvement at focal adhesion sites
- transmission of these 'disturbances' to the cytoplasm via small GTP-bindng proteins (Rho and Rab) relating to the cell membrane
- activation of the mitogen-activated protein kinases (ERK, JNK) signaling pathway
- activation of the bone-specific transcription factor Runx2 and the bone-related transcription factor AP-1
- stimulation of the DNA-binding potential of Runx2 and AP-1 to specific genes associated with osteoblastic differentiation (alkaline phosphatase, osteocalcin, collagen type I)
- alteration in gene expression
- reprogramming towards the osteoblast phenotype: differentiation.

Differentiated periodontal ligament cells can produce cytokines that are able to induce osteoclast differentiation, commence bone-remodeling actions (resorption followed by apposition), change the architectural structure of the area and allow orthodontic tooth movement. This cycle of orthodontic force-induced alveolar bone remodeling is sustained throughout the periodontal ligament. The pluripotential periodontal ligament tissue acts as a cell resource, providing undifferentiated cells for the remodeling cycle. With mechanical stimulation, as occurs in orthodontic tooth movement, the undifferentiated cells differentiate to osteoblasts through the molecular mechanisms described above, producing cytokines that induce osteoclast differentiation and initiate bone resorption activities.

Cytokines are low-molecular-weight peptides or proteins (< 25 kDa) produced by many cell types, including connective tissue cells. They act as signaling molecules, being released from cells under stimulation and acting on receptors to initiate cells responses. Connective tissue cells (fibroblasts and osteoblasts) release cytokines that are pivotal in remodeling procedures and the interplay between osteoblasts and osteoclasts. These cytokines are involved in physiological bone turnover and remodeling by regulating or modifying the action of other cells in an autocrine or paracrine manner. Their synthesis and action are controlled by systemic hormones and mechanical signaling. A very important cytokine produced by osteoblast cells is the receptor activator of nuclear factor B ligand (RANKL; a member of the membrane-associated tumor necrosis factor ligand family). RANKL plays a crucial role in osteoclast formation and function.[59,60] Osteoclast precursors and osteoclasts express RANKL receptor (RANK).

RANKL binds to RANK and induces osteoclast differentiation. Another very important cytokine, also produced by osteoblast precursors and osteoblasts, is osteoprotegerin.[61] Contrary to RANKL action, osteoprotegerin inhibits osteoclast function by competing with RANKL for the membrane receptor RANK. Periodontal ligament cells produce RANKL and osteoprotegerin.[62] Culture media from mechanically stimulated periodontal ligament fibroblasts causes osteoclastogenesis in stromal cell cultures and upregulated RANKL mRNA expression.[63] The study of the interplay between these two cytokines in mechanically induced bone remodeling seems to be of pivotal importance for future pharmacologic intervention. Another key element in the study of orthodontic-induced bone remodeling is the inflammation phenomena relating to external force application. Manipulating the inflammatory process might provide solutions to controlling alveolar bone remodeling.

Vision 2020

Although orthodontics has been recognized as a specialist branch of dentistry for more than a century, the understanding of the mechanisms involved in orthodontic tooth movements, as described in this chapter, has only been realized through research performed over the last 20 years. The explosion in molecular biology research and the study of molecular mechanisms of disease have facilitated this research, together with research in respect of the growth and development of the condylar tissues.[64–67]

Solutions for more efficient means of orthodontic treatment will come from further research in molecular biology and materials science: mechanistic approaches to orthodontics having exhausted their potential. Following the innovations that led to the introduction of straight-wire appliances and different mechanistic methods, for example bioprogression, orthodontics is becoming static in terms of further improvements in treatment parameters, including treatment time, clinical outcomes, long-term stability and patient cooperation and satisfaction.

For many years, orthodontic treatment times have remained largely unchanged, despite some improvements realized through developments in the materials employed in treatment. The introduction of flexible and resilient archwires, including nickel-titanium and thermoplastic systems, has helped to rationalize the number of appointments required and to reduced treatment time. The use of frictionless brackets seems to hold promise, but evidence is required to justify the claims made in respect of function and outcomes. In an effort to reduce reliance on patient cooperation and compliance, there is a move to make orthodontics more invasive, through the use of implants. This development would appear to be contrary to the shift in the clinical practice of dentistry, and medicine in general, towards minimal interventive techniques. While there are indications for the use of implants in orthodontics, in particular adult orthodontics, it must be asked if orthodontics is moving in the correct direction with this development. Introducing the use of implants into the management of situations that have been successfully treated by conventional means for several decades may be viewed as a somewhat desperate attempt to involve orthodontics in implant dentistry, with little, if any, real benefit to patients – evidence failing to demonstrate improved stability with the use of implants.

In contrast, new knowledge and understanding in bone biology have shown that pharmaceutical interventions could usefully influence and control the interplay between osteoblasts and osteoclasts and, in turn, orthodontic tooth movement. Modulating, or in extreme cases stopping, bone remodeling, as utilized in metabolic bone diseases, may find application in orthodontics. Drugs that could be introduced into the periodontal ligament space might have a stimulating or inhibitory effect on orthodontic tooth movement. Through monitoring of such effects, alveolar bone remodeling and, as a consequence, tooth movement could be accelerated or impeded according to treatment needs.

In addition to the above, it is suggested that advanced products from innovations in biotechnologies will transform, if not replace, conventional materials and techniques. For example, useful high-strength fiber materials have recently become available, based on recombinant spider silk-like protein extracted from the milk of transgenic goats. These fibers, which have tenacities in the range of 2–3 denier and an elongation range of 25–45%, form lightweight, strong, versatile materials with a variety of applications,[68] possibly including an ingenious means of replacing steel archwires. Mindful of the miraculous properties of natural spider silk, this potential fiber replacement for steel archwires may help to revolutionize the clinical practice of orthodontics in the twenty-first century.

Orthodontics could be seen to be at a crossroads: it is either going to move forward in a creative scientific direction, in common with most other branches of dentistry and specialties in healthcare, or it is going to be left behind to become a technical, procedure-driven aspect of the clinical practice of dentistry. With investment in further research into the biological aspects of tooth movement and the development of novel materials and devices, orthodontics could be revolutionized. Treatment times could be significantly shortened; teeth might be selectively moved or prevented from moving, and the reliance on patient cooperation and compliance might be significantly reduced, if not consigned to the past. For such changes to occur, further research, including translational research, needs to be successfully completed, followed by a substantial element of retraining of the existing orthodontic workforce to allow the application of molecular, evidence-based, patient-customized orthodontic care.

Paraphrasing TS Elliot: 'Orthodontics should not cease from exploration. And the end of all its explaining will be to arrive where it started. And know the place for the first time.'

References

1. Sandstedt C. Einige Beiträge zur Theorie der Zahnregulierung. Nord Tandläkare Tidskrift 1904;5:236–256.
2. Sandstedt C.Einige Beiträge zur Theorie der Zahnregulierung. Nord Tandläkare Tidskrift 1905;6:1–25, 141–168.
3. Wölff JD. Das Gesetz der Transformation der Knochen. Berlin: von August Hirschwald, 1892.
4. Meikle MC. The tissue, cellular, and molecular regulation of orthodontic tooth movement: 100 years after Carl Sandstedt. Eur J Orthod. 2006;28:221–240.
5. Frost HM. Bone remodelling dynamics. Springfield, IL: Charles C Thomas, 1963.
6. Basdra EK. Biological reactions to orthodontic tooth movement. J Orofac Orthop 1997:58:2–15.
7. Basdra EK, Komposch G. Osteoblast-like properties of human periodontal ligament cells: An in vitro analysis. Eur J Orthod 1997;19:615–621.
8. Seo BM, Miura M, Gronthos S, Bartold PM, Batouli S, Brahim J et al. Investigation of multipotent postnatal stem cells from human periodontal ligament. Lancet 2004;364: 149–155.
9. Hrt J, Lisková M, Landa J. Reaction of bone to mechanical stimuli. Part 1. Continuous and intermittent loading of tibia in rabbit. Folia Morphol 1971;19:290–300.
10. Oppenheim A. Biologic orthodontic theory and reality. A theoretical and practical treatise. Angle Orthod 1935;5:159–211.
11. Schwarz AM. Tissue changes incidental to orthodontic tooth movement. Int J Orthod Oral Surg Radiol 1932;18: 331–352.
12. Reitan K. The initial tissue reaction incident to orthodontic tooth movement as related to the influence of function. An experimental histological study on animal and human material. Acta Odontol Scand 1951;9(Suppl 6):1–240.
13. Reitan K. Some factors determining the evaluation of forces in orthodontics. Am J Orthod 1957;43:32–45.
14. Reitan K. Effects of force magnitude and direction of tooth movement on different alveolar types. Angle Orthod 1964;34:244–255.
15. Storey E, Smith R. Force in orthodontics and its relation to tooth movement. Aust J Dent 1952;56:11–18.
16. Storey E. The nature of tooth movement. Am J Orthod 1973;63:292–314.
17. Ren Y, Maltha JC, van 't Hof MA, Kuijpers-Jagtman AM. Optimum force magnitude for orthodontic tooth movement: a mathematic model. Am J Orthod Dentofacial Orthop 2004;125:171–177.
18. Lanyon LE, Baggott DG. Mechanical function as an influence on the structure and form of bone J Bone Joint Surg 1976;58B:436–443.
19. Zengo AN, Pawluk RJ, Bassett CAL. Stress-induced bioelectric potentials in the dentoalveolar complex. Am J Orthod 1973;64:17–27.
20. Pavlin D, Gluhak-Heinrich J. Effect of mechanical loading on periodontal cells. Crit Rev Oral Biol Med 2001;12: 414–424.
21. Pavlin D, Zadro R, Gluhak-Heinrich J. Temporal pattern of osteoblast-associated genes during mechanically-induced osteogenesis in vivo: early responses of osteocalcin and type I collagen. Connect Tissue Res 2001;42:135–148.

22. Melcher AH, Turnbull RS. Organ culture in studies of the periodontium. In: Balls M, Monnickendam M (eds). Organ Culture in Biomedical Research. Cambridge, UK: Cambridge University Press, 1972:149-163.
23. Yen EHK, Melcher AH. A continuous flow culture system for organ culture of large explants of adult tissue. Effect of oxygen tension on mouse molar periodontium. In Vitro 1978;14:811-818.
24. Meikle MC, Reynolds JJ, Sellers A, Dingle JT. Rabbit cranial sutures in vitro: a new experimental model for studying the response of fibrous joints to mechanical stress. Calcif Tis Int 1979;28:137-144.
25. Meikle MC, Heath JK, Hembry RM, Reynolds JJ. Rabbit cranial suture fibroblasts under tension express a different collagen phenotype. Arch Oral Biol 1982;27:609-613.
26. Meikle MC, Sellers A, Reynolds JJ. Effect of tensile mechanical stress on the synthesis of metalloproteinases by rabbit coronal sutures in vitro. Calcif Tis Int 1980;30:77-82.
27. Meikle MC, Heath JK, Reynolds JJ. The use of in vitro models for investigating the response of fibrous joints to tensile mechanical stress. Am J Orthod 1984;85:141-153.
28. Green DD, Hembry RM, Atkinson SJ, Reynolds JJ, Meikle MC. Immunolocalization of collagenase and tissue inhibitor of metalloproteinases (TIMP) in mechanically deformed fibrous joints. Am J Orthod Dentofac Orthop 1990;97:281-288.
29. Bolcato-Bellemin AL, Elkaim R, Abehsera A, Fausser JL, Haikel Y, Tenenbaum H. Expression of mRNAs encoding for and β integrin subunits, MMPs and TIMPs in stretched human periodontal ligament and gingival fibroblasts. J Dent Res 2000;79:1712-1716.
30. Takahashi I, Nishimura M, Onodera K, Bae JW, Mitani H, Okazaki M et al. Expression of MMP-8 and MMP-13 genes in the periodontal ligament during tooth movement in rats. J Dent Res 2003;82:646-651.
31. Harell A, Dekel S, Binderman I. Biochemical effect of mechanical stress on cultured bone cells. Calcif Tis Res 1977;22:202-207.
32. Somjen D, Binderman I, Berger E, Harell A. Bone remodelling induced by physical stress is prostaglandin E2 mediated. Biochim Biophys Acta 1980;627:91-100.
33. Yeh C-K, Rodan GA. Tensile forces enhance prostaglandin E2 synthesis in osteoblastic cells grown on collagen ribbons. Calcif Tis Int 1984;36:S67-S71.
34. Farndale RW, Sandy JR, Atkinson SJ, Pennington SR, Meghji S, Meikle MC. Parathyroid hormone and prostaglandin E2 stimulate both inositol phosphates and cyclic AMP accumulation in mouse osteoblast cultures. Biochem J 1988;252:263-268.
35. Saito M, Saito S, Ngan PW, Shanfield J, Davidovitch Z. Interleukin 1 beta and prostaglandin E are involved in the response of periodontal cells to mechanical stress *in vivo* and *in vitro*. Am J Orthod Dentofac Orthop 1991;99: 226-240.
36. Rodan GA, Bouret LA, Harvey A, Mensi T. Cyclic AMP and cyclic GMP. mediators of the mechanical effects of bone remodeling. Science 1975;189:467-471.
37. Davidovitch Z, Shanfield JL. Cyclic AMP levels in alveolar bone of orthodontically-treated cats. Archiv Oral Biol 1975;20:567-574.
38. Ngan PW, Crock B, Vargese J, Lanese R, Shanfield J, Davidovitch Z. Immunohistochemical assessment of the effect of chemical and mechanical stimuli on cAMP and prostaglandin E levels in human gingival fibroblasts *in vitro*. Arch Oral Biol 1988;33:163-174.
39. Ngan PW, Saito S, Saito M, Shanfield J, Davidovitch Z. The interactive effects of mechanical stress and interleukin 1β on prostaglandin E and cyclic AMP production in human gingival fibroblasts *in vitro*: comparison with cloned osteoblastic cells of mouse (MC3T3-E1). Arch Oral Biol 1990; 35:717-725.
40. Sandy JR, Farndale RW, Meikle MC. Recent advances in understanding mechanically induced bone remodeling and their relevance to orthodontic theory and practice. Am J Orthod Dentofac Orthop 1993;103:212-223.
41. Davidson RM, Tatakis DW, Auerbach AL. Multiple forms of mechanosensitive channels in osteoblast-like cells. Pflugers Arch 1990;416:646-651.
42. McDonald F, Somasundaram B, McCann TJ, Mason WT, Meikle MC.Calcium waves in fluid flow stimulated osteoblasts are G protein mediated. Arch Biochem Biophys 1996;326:31-38.
43. Ingber DE. Integrins as mechanochemical transducers. Curr Opin Cell Biol 1991;3:841-848.
44. Sastry SK, Burridge K.2000 Focal adhesions: a nexus for intracellular signaling and cytoskeletal dynamics. Exp Cell Res 261:25-36.
45. Wang N, Butler JP, Ingber DE. Mechanotransduction across the cell surface and through the cytoskeleton. Science 1993;269:1124-1127.
46. Clarke EA, Brugge JS. Integrins and signal transduction pathways: the road taken. Science 1995;268:233-239.
47. Shyy Y-J, Chien S. Role of integrins in cellular responses to mechanical stress and adhesion. Curr Opin Cell Biol 1997;9:707-713.
48. Meyer CJ, Alenghat FJ, Rim P, Fong JH, Fabry B, Ingber DE. Mechanical control of cyclic AMP signaling and gene transcription through integrins. Nat Cell Biol 2000;2: 666-668.
49. Carvalho RS, Bumann A, Schwarzer C, Scott E, Yen EHK. A molecular mechanism of integrin regulation from bone cells stimulated by mechanical forces. Eur J Orthodont 1996;18:227-235.
50. Basdra EK, Huber LA, Papavassiliou AG. Rab and Rho GTPases are involved in specific response of periodontal ligament fibroblasts to mechanical stretching. Biochim Biophys Acta 1995;1268:209-213.

51. Basdra EK, Komposch G, Huber LA, Papavassiliou AG. Mechanically stretched periodontal ligament fibroblasts: identifying components of the mechanotransduction cascade. In: Davidovitch Z (ed.). Biological Mechanisms of Tooth Movement and Craniofacial Adaptation. Boston, MA: Harvard Society for the Advancement of Orthodontics, 1996:41-49.
52. Basdra EK, Kohl A, Komposch G. Mechanical stretching of periodontal ligament fibroblasts: a study on cytoskeletal involvement. J Orofac Orthop 1996:57:24-30.
53. Basdra EK Biological reactions to orthodontic tooth movement. J Orofac Orthop 1997;58:2-15.
54. Kletsas D, Basdra EK, Papavassiliou AG. Mechanical stress induces DNA synthesis in PDL fibroblasts by a mechanism unrelated to autocrine growth factor action. FEBS Lett 1998;430:358-362.
55. Kletsas D, Basdra EK, Papavassiliou AG. Effect of protein kinase inhibitors on the stretch elicited c-fos and c-jun up-regulation in human PDL osteoblast-like cells. J Cell Physiol 2002;190:313-321.
56. Peverali FA, Basdra EK, Papavassiliou AG. Stretch-mediated activation of selective MAPK subtypes and potentiation of AP-1 binding in human osteoblastic cells. Mol Med 2001;7:68-78.
57. Ziros P, Rochas-Gill AP, Georgakopoulos T, Habeos I, Kletsas D, Basdra EK et al. The bone specific transcriptional regulator Cbfa1 is a target of mechanical signals in osteoblastic cells. J Biol Chem 2002;277:-23934-23941.
58. Ziros P, Basdra EK, Papavassiliou AG. Runx2: of bone and stretch. Int J Biochem Cell Biol 2008;40:1659-1663.
59. Lacey E, Timms H, Tan M, Kelley C, Dunstan T et al. Osteoprotegerin ligand is a cytokine that regulates osteoclast differentiation and activation. Cell 1998;93:165-176.
60. Yasuda H, Shima N, Nakagawa N, Yamaguchi K, Kinosaki M, Mochizuki S et al. Osteoclast differentiation factor is a ligand for osteoprotegerin/osteoclastogenesis-inhibitory factor and is identical to TRANCE/RANKL. Proc Natl Acad Sci USA 1998;95:3597-3600.
61. Simonet W, Lacey D, Dunstan C, Kelley M, Chang M, Lüthy R et al. Osteoprotegerin: a novel secreted protein involved in the regulation of bone density. Cell 1997;89:309-319.
62. Ogasawara T, Yoshimine Y, Kiyoshima T, Kobayashi I, Matsuo K, Akamine A et al. In situ expression of RANKL, RANK, osteoprotegerin and cytokines in osteoclasts of rat periodontal tissue. J Periodont Res 2004;39:42-49.
63. Kanzaki H, Chiba M, Shimizu Y, Mitani H. Periodontal ligament cells under mechanical stress induce osteoclastogenesis by receptor activator of nuclear factor B ligand up-regulation via prostaglandin E2 synthesis. J Bone Min Res 2002;17:210-220.
64. Basdra EK, Huber L, Komposch G, Papavassiliou AG. Mechanical loading triggers specific biochemical responses in mandibular condylar chondrocytes. Biochim Biophys Acta 1994;1222:315-322.
65. Papachristou DJ, Pirttiniemi P, Kantomaa T, Papavassiliou AG, Basdra EK. JNK/ERK-AP-1/Runx2 induction 'paves the way' to cartilage load-ignited chondroblastic differentiation. Histochem Cell Biol 2005;24:1-9.
66. Papachristou D, Prittinemi P, Kantomaa T, Agnantis N, Basdra EK. Fos- and Jun-related transcription factors are involved in the signal transduction pathway of mechanical loading in condylar chondrocytes. Eur J Orthod. 2006;28: 120-126.
67. Papadopoulou AK, Papachristou DJ, Chatzopoulos SA, Pirttiniemi P, Papavassiliou AG, Basdra EK. Load application induces changes in the expression levels of Sox-9, FGFR-3 and VEGF in condylar chondrocytes. FEBS Lett 2007;581:2041-2046.
68. Lazaris A, Arcidiacono S, Huang Y, Zhou JF, Duguay F, Chretien N et al. Spider silk fibers spun from soluble recombinant silk produced in mammalian cells. Science 2002;295:472-6.

CHAPTER 10

Oral surgery

J. Thomas Lambrecht

Definition

Oral surgery, by definition, is closely allied to oral and maxillofacial surgery. It is principally intraoral surgery: dentoalveolar surgery in respect to the hard tissues and gingival/mucosal surgery in respect to the soft tissues of the oral cavity.

Oral surgery traditionally includes treatment of dental trauma, tumors, infections and any teeth-related complication that requires a surgical approach. In addition to these classical procedures, implant surgery has become a very important part of oral surgery, broadening the spectrum of the discipline.

Oral surgery is mostly performed under local anesthesia. Monitoring of pulse, blood pressure and oxygen saturation is strongly recommended. Some indications require conscious sedation, sometimes combined with an anesthesiologist on standby for patient safety or general anesthesia.

Oral surgery is established in Europe, together with orthodontics, as an acknowledged speciality in dentistry. Postgraduate training programs typically follow two or more years of postgraduate experience and include, with varying emphasis across Europe, implant surgery, oral radiology, oral medicine and oral pathology. They take a qualified dental clinician three to four years to complete.

Oral surgery research reflects the spectrum of the specialty, underpinned by a number of well-renowned national and international journals that document scientific progress in the field.

Historical milestones

The evolution of oral surgery across the world has two backgrounds: surgery and dentistry. It involved either dental clinicians becoming interested in surgery or surgeons becoming involved in the oral and maxillofacial region of the body.

In the USA it is, in all probability, Simon P. Hullihen (1810–1857) who can be considered to be the first oral surgeon. He had both a medical and a dental education. Around 1840 in Wheeling, West Virginia, he opened a specialized hospital for 'oral surgery.' The first hospital for oral surgery integrated into a dental college was directed by James Edmund Garretson (1828–1895), a medical physician and a dental clinician. He established oral surgery in the USA as an autonomous subject in the medical field. In 1869, he published the book 'A Treatise on the Diseases and Surgery of the Mouth, Jaws and Associate Parts,' which was published in six editions, latterly under the title 'A System of Oral Surgery'.[1] The Massachusetts General Hospital Oral and Maxillofacial Surgical Service originated in 1867, the same year that the Harvard Dental School (now the Harvard School of Dental Medicine) was founded.[2]

In Europe, the Frenchman Pierre Fouchard (1678–1761) and his younger German (Prussian) contemporary Philipp Pfaff (1713–1766) can be recognized as the first authors of oral surgery literature.[3] Carl Partsch (1855–1931), a surgeon as well as a dental clinician and the first director of the Dental School of the University in Breslau, is recognized as a father of oral surgery. He summarized his lifetime achievement: 'I gave the scalpel into the hand of the dental clinician'. The first textbook in German on oral surgery was published in 1914 by Paul Preiswerk (1879–1921) from Basel.[4] In 1928, this was followed by 'Guide through Operative Dentistry' by Robert Neumann.[5] In the textbooks from Wassmund (1934),[6] Pichler and Trauner (1948)[7] and Hofer et al. (1952),[8] oral surgery was anchored as an integral element of oral and maxillofacial surgery. This history reveals the knowledge and therapeutic possibilities 50 to 100 years ago. Topics including 'extraction of teeth', 'root cysts', 'follicular cysts' and 'removal of retained teeth' persist today with the same importance and treatment modalities. Other topics such as 'mishappenings during and after the operation' are now regarded in a different light, as intra- and postoperative complications. The traditional approach to oral surgery was dominated by surgical technique. In contrast, the modern approach to oral surgery has seen a shift to medical and biological considerations: basic principles of medicine, disturbances in wound healing and risk assessment being examples of considerations that are influencing clinical practice and the management of patients today.[9]

Milestones in the development of oral surgery are well established. It is difficult to conceive of many of the advances in oral surgery and dentistry in general being possible without the introduction of local anesthesia. It was not until 1905 that Brown synthesized procaine, which for many years was the most widely used local anesthetic. It was almost 40 years later that the more effective local anesthetics currently in use, including lidocaine and mepivacaine, became available. More modern agents such as bupivacaine provide profound long-lasting local anesthesia, offering the opportunity of a comfortable postoperative period for the patients.

Another great discovery of the twentieth century that had a profound influence on the surgical management of patients, in particular those with life-threatening infections, was the identification of penicillin by Fleming in 1928. Other pharmacologic discoveries in the twentieth century have also had a significant impact on the ability of oral surgeons to offer a better service to their patients. Non-steroidal anti-inflammatory drugs first became available in the late 1970s. Subsequent research has provided the oral surgeon with a wide variety of narcotic and non-narcotic analgesics for a pain-free postoperative recovery.[10]

The introduction of improved imaging techniques was yet another significant milestone in the development of both oral and maxillofacial surgery. The advent of panoramic radiography in the 1960s made it possible to view the entire dentition, together with the maxilla and mandible, in one radiograph, allowing simultaneous evaluation of potential pathology affecting the teeth and jaws. Computerized tomography (CT) and magnetic resonance imaging (MRI) were technologies developed in the late twentieth century. These technologies have further improved the diagnostic ability of the oral surgeon. The application of CT has been extended by special reformatted views for the maxillofacial region. Three dimensional viewing, volume rendering and the construction of three-dimensional models have been valuable spin-offs from CT imaging.[11] MRI is valuable for soft tissue diagnosis, including assessments of the fibrocartilagenous disk of the temporomandibular joint, tumors and early diagnosis of osteomyelitis of the

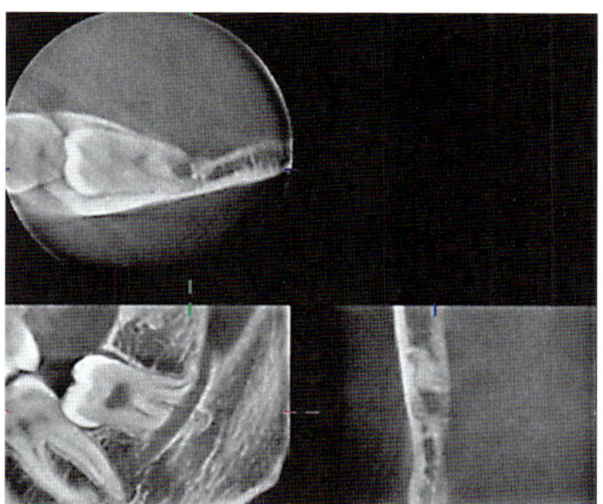

Fig. 10-1 Cone beam computerized tomography illustrating a close topographical relationship between the inferior dental alveolar nerve and a third molar tooth. (From Lambrecht [2008][25] with permission.)

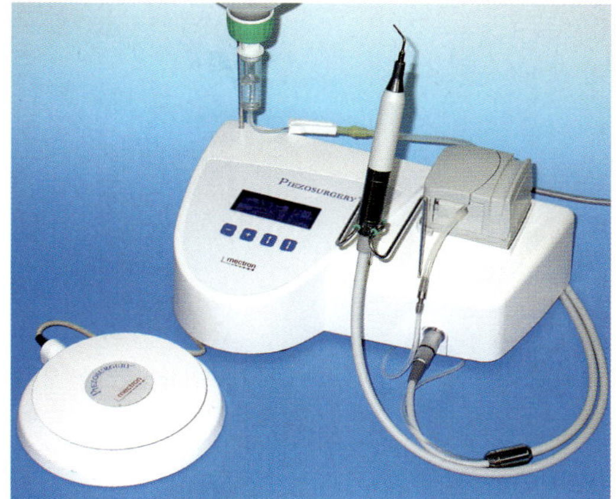

Fig. 10-2 Piezoelectric apparatus for bone surgery with minimal damage to adjacent soft tissues. (From Lambrecht [2008][25] with permission.)

jaws. Most recently, cone beam CT (CBCT; also known as digital volume tomography) is revolutionizing three-dimensional dentomaxillofacial imaging (Fig. 10-1).

Innovations in instrumentation since the mid-twentieth century have altered the ways in which many oral surgery procedures are now performed. For example, the development of miniaturized saws and piezoelectrical surgical instruments (Fig. 10-2) has had a great impact on modern approaches to oral surgery involving the hard tissues. Concurrently, lasers have replaced the scalpel in the execution of many routine procedures in intraoral soft tissue surgery (Fig. 10-3).

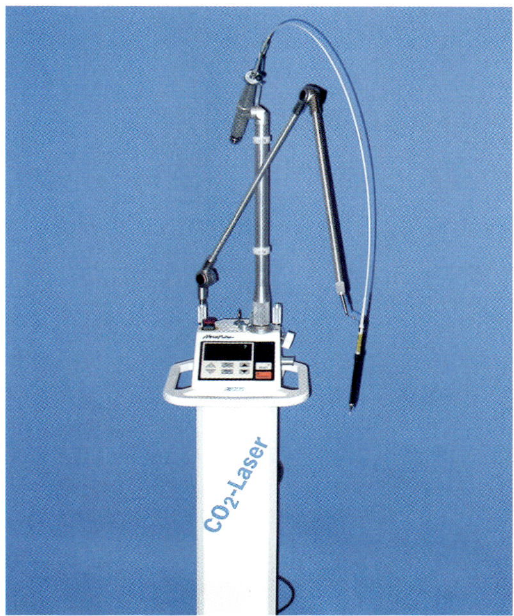

Fig. 10-3 A mobile CO_2 laser for use in oral surgery procedures. (From Lambrecht [2008][25] with permission.)

Arguably, developments in the twentieth century that have changed, and will continue to influence, the practice of oral surgery are those involving implant osseointegration. Patients are now able to have fixed prostheses in situations in which such restorations were formerly impossible. As a consequence, the use of osseointegrated implants has changed concepts in preprosthetic surgery. There is now a greatly reduced need for procedures such as vestibuloplasty, alveolar ridge augmentation and the removal of tori to enhance denture-bearing areas. Patients are, therefore, able to select to have long-term oral rehabilitation by means of implant-

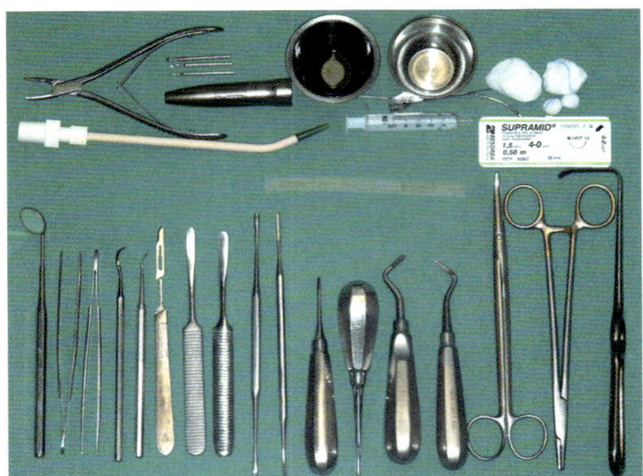

Fig.10-4 Basic instrumentation set for the removal of third molar teeth. (From Lambrecht [2008][25] with permission.)

supported prostheses without the need for complex extensive or multiple preprosthetic surgical procedures.

Treatment concepts

Informed consent

Before oral surgery procedures can be undertaken, the patient must understand the nature of the surgery, the likelihood of success and the risk of possible adverse outcomes. Armed with this information, the patient must give informed consent to the proposed procedure. For consent to be valid, the diagnosis needs to be accurate and the details of the condition, the proposed surgery and its likely outcome and risks effectively communicated to the patient. The patient must also be given reasonable time and opportunity to decide whether or not to agree to undergo the surgery. Failure to obtain informed consent prior to undertaking a surgical procedure runs the risk of costly medicolegal complications.

Instrumentation

Instruments have to be prepared in sterile sets. A basic set of instruments (Fig. 10-4) can be added to for specific surgical procedures such as soft tissue surgery or endodontic surgery. Atraumatic suture materials are typically standard.

Infection control

Good infection control is necessary to protect the patient and the team performing to surgical procedures. Infection control, including clinical dressings, hand hygiene and protection, the decontamination and sterilization of instrumentation and preparation of the surgical site, must comply with all relevant standards and requirements and be subject to effective quality control.

Devices

Besides basic and any necessary supplemental instrumentation, there is typically the need to prepare one or more medical devices. For hard tissue surgery, a surgical motor, handpiece and cooling system are necessary, together with an appropriate selection of surgical burs. For endosseous implant surgery, a site-preparation system with specific characteristics in terms of velocity, torque and water cooling is necessary. Piezo equipment (Fig. 10-2) may be a useful adjunct for hard tissue surgery. For root-end preparation in endodontic surgery, an ultrasonic preparation and cleaning system may be advantageous. Use of a CO_2 laser is increasingly considered routine for intraoral soft tissue surgery, given that it offers the opportunity to have a bloodless operating field, with minimal postoperative pain and limited risk of infection.

Further equipment may well include a surgical operating microscope and equipment to monitor the patient's reaction to the surgery. Monitoring equipment typically takes the form of a pulse-oximeter, but may include other equipment to monitor a range of physiological parameters.

Medication

Pre-, intra- and postoperative medications, including sedative agents, local anesthetics, analgesics

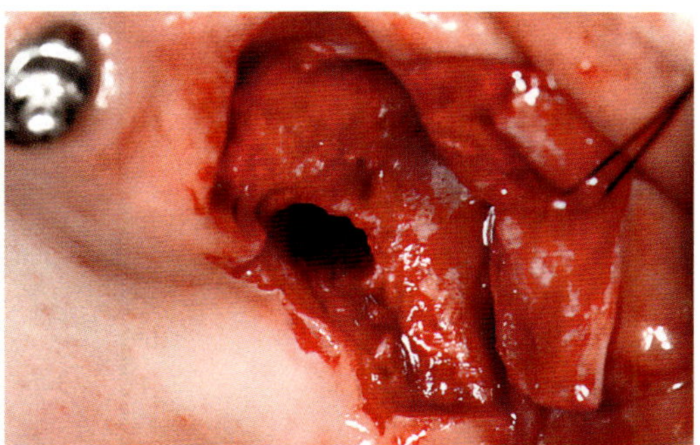

Fig. 10-5 Mobilized mucoperiosteal flap (Rehrmann flap) to close an antraoral fistula. (From Lambrecht [2008][25] with permission.)

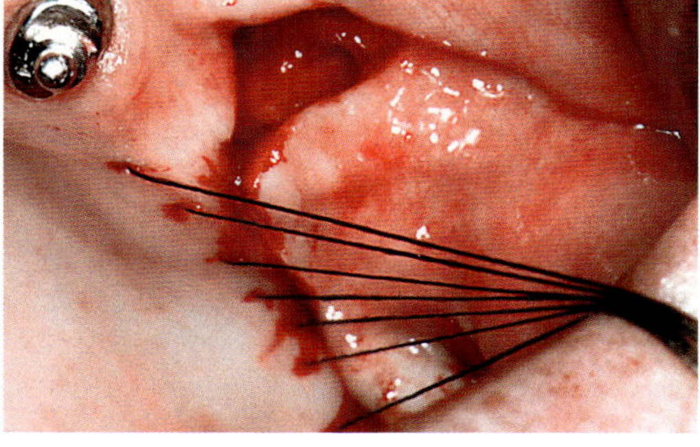

Fig. 10-6 Palatal mattress sutures for flap fixation. (From Lambrecht [2008][25] with permission.)

and antibiotics, should be readily available. Medications should be administered according to the nature of the surgical procedure and the specific needs of the patient, possibly in consultation with the patient's physician and according to preexisting conditions and the patient's medical and dental history.[12]

Extraction of teeth

The extraction of teeth, typically under local anesthesia, is a routine element of the clinical practice of oral surgery. The procedure may entail the use of a chlorhexidine mouthwash preoperatively; judicious removal of the tooth, with care being taken to ensure that the tooth is intact and the expansion of the alveolus has been reduced; management of the soft tissues, with the removal of any undesirable tags; control of the bleeding; and any other postoperative measures indicated clinically, including the prescription of any necessary medication.

With the increasing likelihood of the extraction of diseased and damaged teeth being followed by some form of implant dentistry, great care must be taken to preserve bone in the process of extracting teeth - the surgeon takes the tooth, the patient keeps the bone. By preserving the buccal and lingual (palatal) cortical plates to contain the blood clot, the loss of bone following extraction should be limited, particularly by the time the site has healed sufficiently to accept an implant for osseointegration. Alternative approaches to ridge preservation continue to be developed, based on atraumatic techniques for the extraction of teeth.

Complications associated with the routine extraction of teeth continue to include damage to adjacent teeth; root fractures; thermal trauma caused by rotary instruments with insufficient cooling; nerve damage, both direct and indirect; and damage to the jaws, including the creation of an antraoral fistula in the maxilla (Figs 10-5 and 10-6). Further complications include the displacement of teeth, or more commonly fragments of teeth and bone, into the soft tissues and a 'dry socket' developing postoperatively. Such complications are better treated sooner rather than later, typically with immediate effect.[13]

Removal of impacted and displaced teeth

Third molar surgery

In the way that appendectomy is the most common procedure for the general surgeon, the removal of third molar (wisdom) teeth is the procedure most commonly undertaken by the oral surgeon.

In the event of a third molar tooth being associated with an acute soft tissue infection, typically a pericoronitis, the infection must be managed prior to there being any consideration of surgery. This management is normally conservative. This may

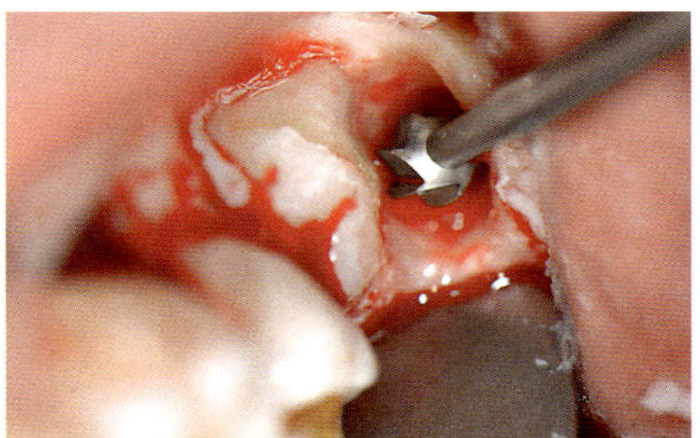

Fig. 10-7 Bone removal to facilitate the removal of a third molar tooth. Note the protection of the lingual nerve. (From Lambrecht [2008][25] with permission.)

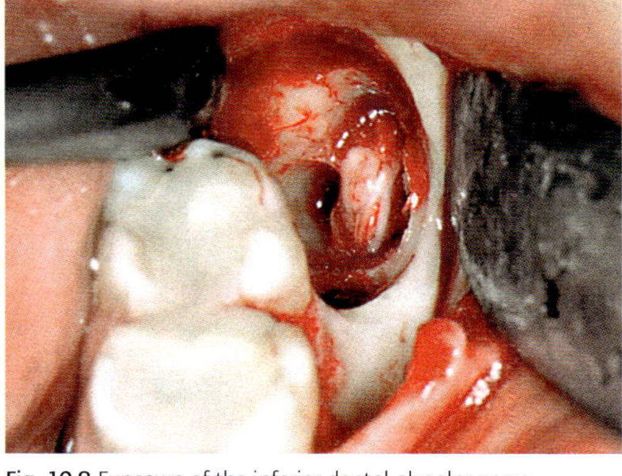

Fig. 10-8 Exposure of the inferior dental alveolar nerve following removal of a third molar tooth. (From Lambrecht [2008][25] with permission.)

involve local debridement with an antibacterial agent such as chlorhexidine and the prescription of antibiotics, particularly if there is a risk of a spreading infection. In severe infection, incision and drainage may be necessary.

In subsequent considerations as to whether to remove a third molar following resolution of an infection, the risk of complications when the tooth is removed must be weighed against the risk of complications if the tooth is left in situ. Sailer and Pajarola[14] introduced the 'SAC' classification to assist in such matters.

- *Simple.* The routine extraction of a non-impacted third molar tooth in a healthy patient, which can be performed by a general practitioner or other qualified dental clinician.
- *Advanced.* The operative procedure for removal of an impacted third molar tooth, possibly in a medically compromised patient, which should be performed by an oral surgeon or a dental clinician who has received postgraduate training in oral surgery.
- *Complex.* Removal of an impacted third molar tooth, with anticipated complications such as the possibility of nerve damage or fracture of the jaw, which needs to be undertaken by an oral or maxillofacial surgeon.

In all surgery procedures for third molars, special attention is required to avoid perforating the buccal and lingual periosteum and to limit trauma to adjacent tissues. The lingual nerve must be protected at all times (Fig. 10-7). In addition to protecting the lingual nerve, care must also be taken to avoid damage to the inferior dental alveolar nerve (Fig. 10-8). The risk of damaging the inferior dental alveolar nerve can be minimized by thorough preoperative radiological assessment involving panoramic radiography or, when the third molar tooth is in close anatomical relationship with the mandibular canal, CBCT (Fig. 10-1).

Further complications of third molar surgery include postoperative infection, damage to the distal surface of the adjacent second molar tooth, bony fractures, perioperative bleeding, nerve damage during infiltration of the local anesthesia, intraoperative root fractures and postoperative swelling and pain.

The possible complications associated with a retained third molar tooth include recurrent pericoronal infections, caries in the distal surface of the adjacent second molar tooth and the development of other pathology, including odontogenic cysts, which may, in time, increase the risk of facture of the mandible. Similar complications may be associated with the retention of maxillary third molar

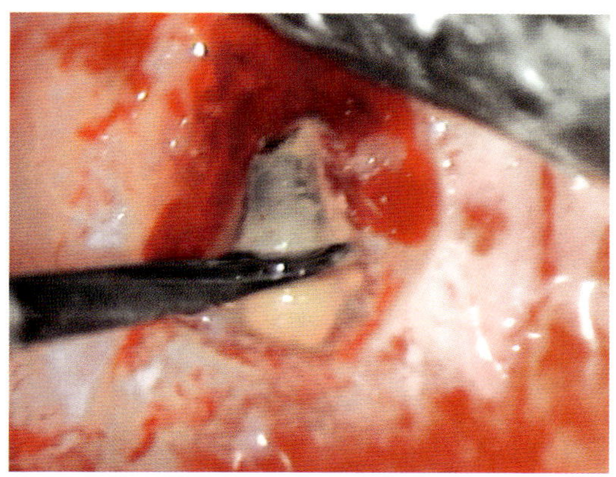

Fig. 10-9 Apicoectomy: separation of the apex of the root. (From Lambrecht [2008][25] with permission.)

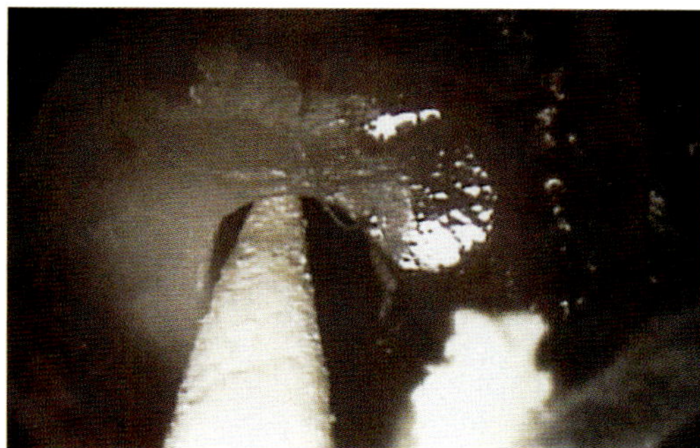

Fig. 10-10 Retrograde filling of the root canal (×16 magnification). (From Lambrecht [2008][25] with permission.)

teeth, with the development of associated pathology running the risk of fracture of the maxillary tuberosity or involvement of the maxillary sinus.

Displaced teeth

Displaced teeth, notably displaced maxillary canine teeth, may be removed, repositioned or exposed. The techniques and complications involved in the removal of such teeth are similar to those for other displaced and impacted teeth. Repositioning or exposure, typically to facilitate subsequent orthodontic alignment, requires surgical skills aimed at minimizing trauma to the teeth and adjacent tissues. Failure to exercise extreme care in such procedures may result in resorption of the tooth and its subsequent loss, or at least a compromised clinical outcome.[15]

Surgical preservation of teeth

Periradicular surgery may involve periapical curettage, the removal of a cyst (cystectomy) or apicoectomy and the placement of a retrograde root-end filling. The goal of periradicular surgery is to preserve the tooth, typically following endodontic treatment that has failed to achieve a successful outcome. The classic indication for periradicular surgery is chronic or recurrent periapical periodontitis, with or without associated infection and other pathology.

Further indications for periradicular surgery include incomplete orthograde root fillings, the fracture of an endodontic instrument beyond the apex of the tooth, and the extrusion of root canal filling material, typically endodontic sealer, into the periapical tissues.

Periradicular surgery involves a mucoperiosteal flap to expose the bone overlying the apex of the affected tooth. Once a window has been created in the bone over the apex, the apex may be exposed and assessed together with the adjacent tissues or associated lesion such as a cyst. If granulation tissue is present, it is removed together with any other lesion and foreign body that may be present periapically, and the apex of the tooth is sealed (Fig. 10-9). Methylene blue (1%) may be used to assess for any fracture of the retained root. The use of a surgical microscope or endoscope is advisable. Retrograde preparation of the root canal, using ultrasonic instrumentation, precedes the placement of the root-end filling (Fig. 10-10). To conclude the procedure, the mucoperiosteal flap is replaced and sutured. Postoperative recalls, including radiographic assessments, should extend over a period of several years. Such recalls may be undertaken by the referring practitioner.

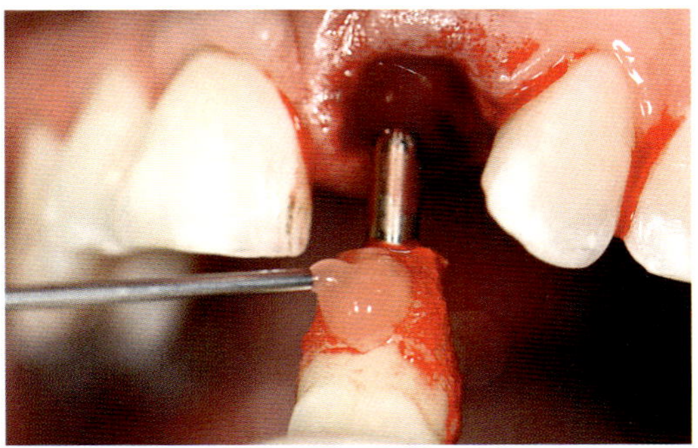

Fig. 10-11 Intentional replantation: application of Emdogain with relocation of the tooth. (From Lambrecht [2008][25] with permission.)

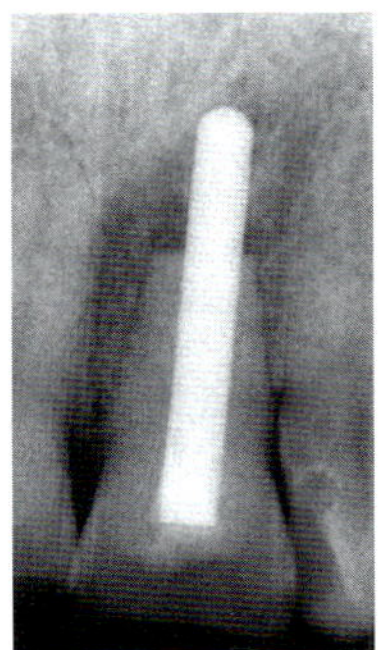

Fig. 10-12 Postoperative radiograph following intentional replantation. (From Lambrecht [2008][25] with permission.)

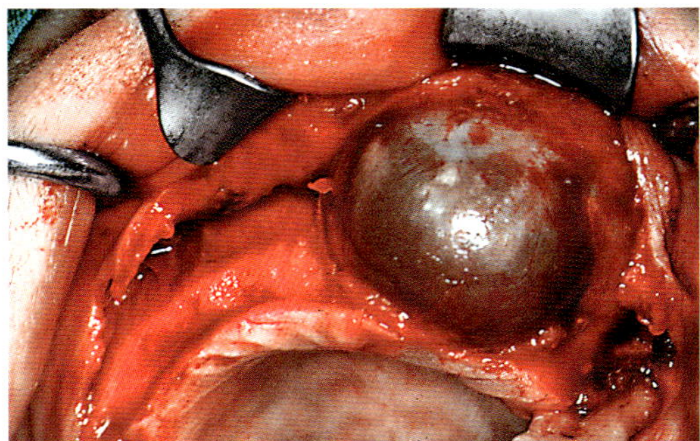

Fig. 10-13 Exposed follicular cyst in the anterior segment of an edentulous maxilla. (From Lambrecht [2008][25] with permission.)

Replantation is a further form of surgical preservation of teeth. The technique involves the removal and endodontic treatment of a tooth and its replacement in the jaw (Figs 10-11 and 10-12). Replantation may be indicated if periradicular surgery is contraindicated or impossible to undertake.[16]

Autotransplantation, hemisection, root amputation and other procedures, including crown lengthening and other soft tissue procedures, are further forms of the surgical preservation of teeth.

Cysts, bony lesions and odontogenic tumors

Odontogenic cysts include Epstein pearls, dentigerous cysts, eruption cysts, lateral periodontal cysts, gingival cysts and glandular odontogenic cysts. Non-odontogenic cysts include nasopalatine duct cysts, nasolabial cysts and fissural cysts. Cysts of infectious origin include radicular cysts, residual radicular cysts, residual follicular cysts (Fig. 10-13), inflammatory collateral cysts and surgical ciliated cysts, according to the most recent World Health Organization classification.

The treatment strategies for cysts are classically twofold:

- *Cystostomie (marsupialization).* The cyst is opened and emptied, with the removal of part of the cyst wall for pathohistological diagnosis, leaving the cyst open to reduce in size during healing. This technique is indicated when neighboring anatomical structures would be endangered by performing a cystectomy.
- *Cystectomy.* The whole cyst is removed in one operative procedure, with primary wound closure (Fig. 10-14). If indicated, autogenic alloplastic or synthetic filling materials can be used to enhance bone regeneration to infill the cyst cavity.

Osteolytic lesions include subperiosteal giant cell tumors, Stafne cavities and extravasation cysts.

Osteoplastic lesions can be differentiated into osteomas and exostoses (tori).

The most common odontogenic tumors are odontomas and the keratocystic odontogenic tumor.[17]

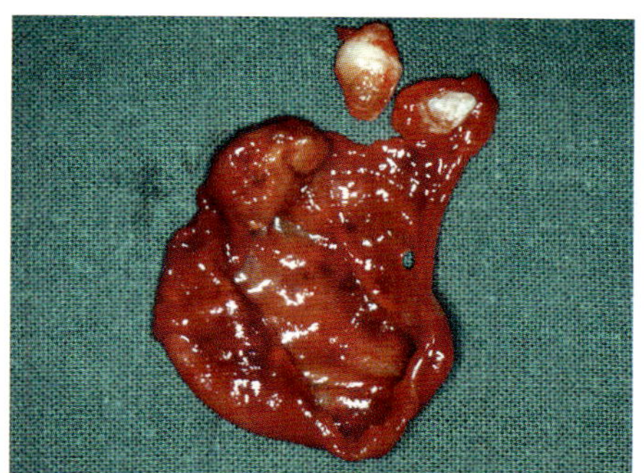

Fig. 10-14 Excised follicular cyst with associated tooth. (From Lambrecht [2008][25] with permission.)

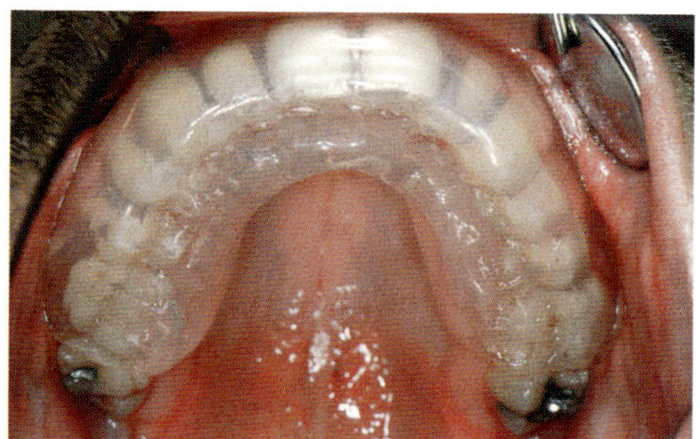

Fig. 10-15 A customized mouthguard. (From Lambrecht [2008][25] with permission.)

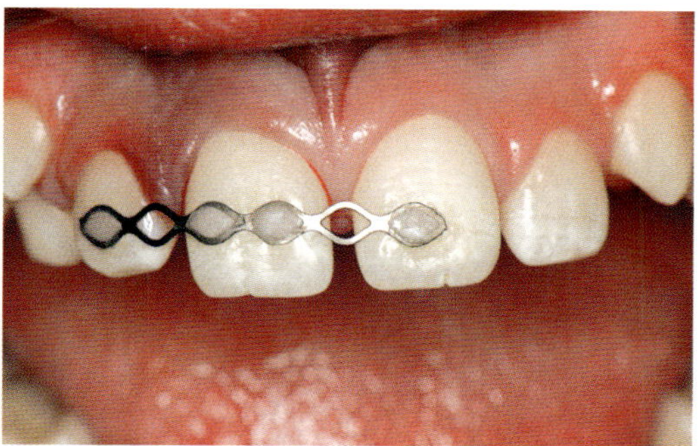

Fig. 10-16 Fixation of an avulsed maxillary right central incisor using a titanium trauma splint. (From Lambrecht [2008][25] with permission.)

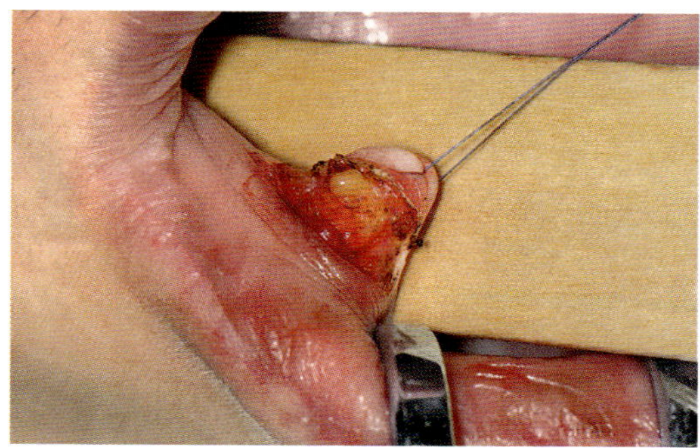

Fig. 10-17 Intraoral fibroma: intraoperative situation during removal using a CO_2-laser: Note the absence of bleeding. (From Lambrecht [2008][25] with permission.)

Dental traumatology

High-risk, 'trendy' sports have led to a considerable increase in dental injuries. Inline skating, kick-boarding and similar precarious sports are strongly associated with dental trauma, let alone other injuries. The dental trauma tends to be largely inflicted in the maxillary anterior segment of the mouth, with maxillary central incisors tending to be the teeth most commonly affected. Prevention is possible when protective headgear and multilayer mouthguards are worn (Fig. 10-15). The training of sports coaches and referees, together with information and instruction sheets as part of first-aid facilities at sports locations, may help to minimize the impact of the common forms of dental injuries: loosening, fracture and chipping, dislocation, intrusion and avulsion of teeth, together with alveolar fractures and associated trauma to the circum- and intraoral soft tissues and lips.

Treatment of dental trauma must follow well-established, evidence-based protocols for the purpose of achieving the most favorable clinical outcome.

Strategies such as immediate replantation (Fig. 10-16) may be aimed at preserving alveolar bone and dental arch form until such time as facial growth has been completed and implant-supported rehabilitation can be undertaken.[18]

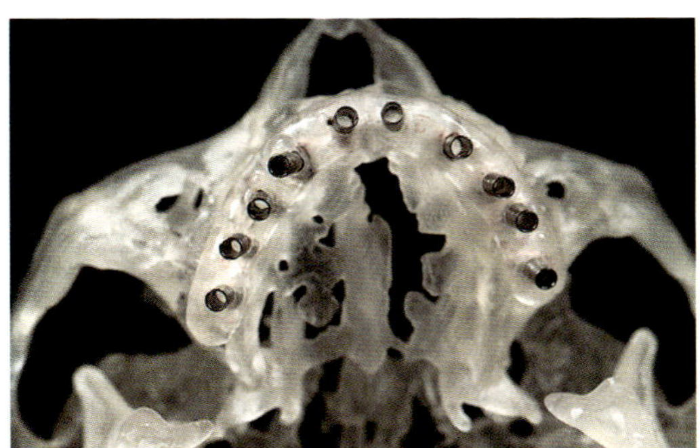

Fig. 10-18 Planning implant placement in a three-dimensional stereolithographic model. (From Lambrecht [2008][25] with permission.)

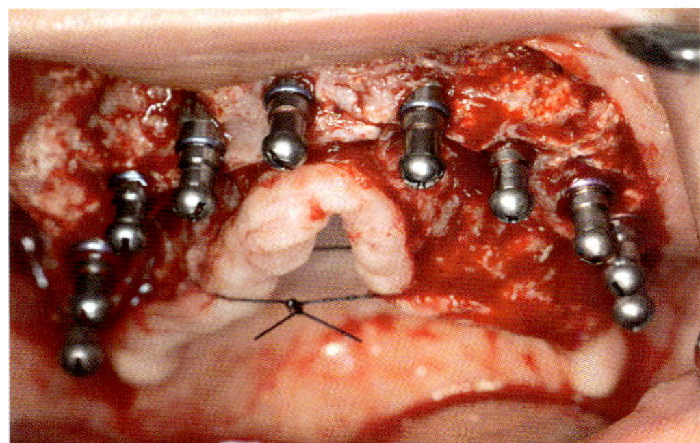

Fig. 10-19 Postoperative appearance following the insertion of 10 implants using a template constructed in the process of preoperative planning. (From Lambrecht [2008][25] with permission.)

Intraoral soft tissue surgery

Biopsies for the histopathologic examination of intraoral tumors and other lesions may be incisional, punch or of the brush type, depending on the nature, history and location of the lesion. Periodontal surgery, including gingivectomy, mucogingival surgery and flap procedures, and various forms of preprosthetic soft tissue surgery are increasingly being applied as adjunctive surgery to implant dentistry. Surgery of the small minor salivary glands is mostly performed with a CO_2 laser, which also finds application in the excision of benign tumors (Fig. 10-17) and hyperplastic gingival tissues. All practicing dental clinicians, oral surgeons and practitioners with a special interest in oral surgery must be especially vigilant to recognize and make arrangements for the early treatment of premalignant and malignant lesions of the orofacial soft tissues.[19] The management of intraoral abscesses and other acute swellings remains an important element of intraoral soft tissue surgery. The outcome of such surgery is highly dependent on meticulous attention to detail and atraumatic techniques. Distortion and excessive postoperative scarring of the circum- and intraoral soft tissues may have a significant impact on patient satisfaction and subsequent oral healthcare provision.

Implant surgery

In the 1980s, implant surgery was a minor part of the clinical practice of oral surgery. In the intervening time, it has become a major element, given the exceptional success rates (> 95%) of osseointegrated dental implants. A key factor in successful implant surgery and, in turn, implant dentistry is effective diagnostic imaging as an integral element of patient assessment and treatment planning. Diagnostic imaging prior to implant surgery may include panoramic radiographs, reformatted CT scans and three-dimensional CBCT. Navigated and template-guided procedures (Fig. 10-18) are also crucial to favorable clinical outcomes (Fig. 10-19). Considerations of facilitated osseointegration, the delay, if any, prior to loading and aspects of soft tissue management continue to be subjects of research and debate. The surgical approach and procedures tend to be influenced by the nature of the implant dentistry: restoration of a bonded edentulous space, the management of free-end distal-extension removable partial dentures or the rehabilitation of a typically resorbed edentulous arch (Figs 10-20 and 10-21).

Bony defects may be treated by augmentation procedures, guided regeneration, ridge preservation, bone splitting and filling, grafts (inlay and onlay) and osteogenic distraction procedures, or by combinations of two or more of these techniques. Many of the techniques continue to be developed and refined.

Mini-implants have been developed as an alternative or adjunct to other forms of implant dentistry. Mini-implants may find application for transitional

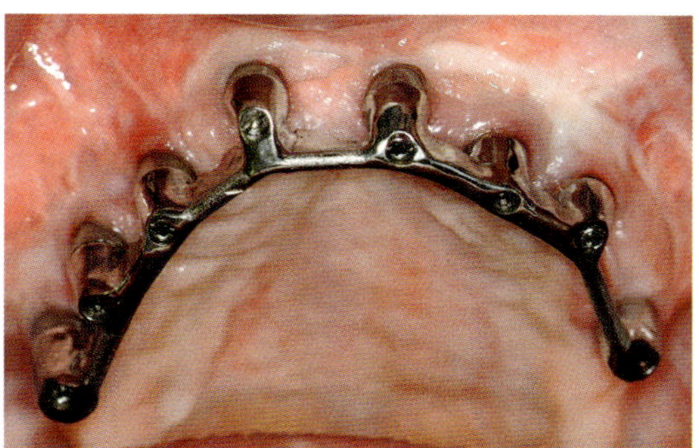

Fig. 10-20 Implants eight years after placement. (From Lambrecht [2008][25] with permission.)

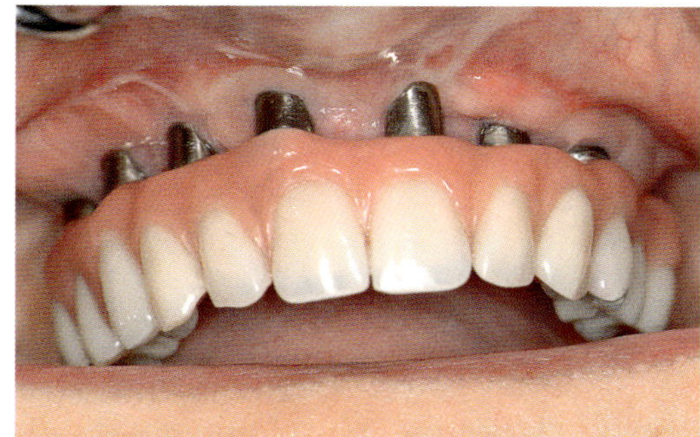

Fig. 10-21 Prosthetic rehabilitation after nine years in clinical service. (From Lambrecht [2008][25] with permission.)

use in the immediate prosthetic rehabilitation of endentulous areas or arches and in orthodontic situations requiring additional or atypical anchorage.

Failures in implant surgery may be early or long term. Early failures are typically caused through inadequate planning or inappropriate techniques. Long-term failures often relate to the development and failure to manage to peri-implantitis: recall protocols and procedures are important to the long-term success of osseointegrated implants.[20]

Vision 2020

Dental conditions requiring surgical intervention have not changed greatly over time and, as a consequence, the *raison d'être* for oral surgery is set to continue. The pattern and extent of the major dental diseases, caries and periodontal disease, will, however, continue to change and result in changes in the clinical practice of dentistry, including the clinical practice of oral surgery. Increasing emphasis will be placed on prevention, including preventive surgical intervention, rather than the treatment of disease. This, in time, will lead to many more people retaining increasing numbers of teeth into old age, with steady growth in needs and expectations in terms of maintaining functional dentitions. Implant dentistry, including implant surgery, will expand to help to meet these needs and expectations.[21]

Oral surgery will undoubtedly exist in 2020; however, it will change with time. As indicated above, the need for traditional forms of oral surgery, in particular the extraction of teeth, may decline, but this will be more than compensated for by the anticipated growth in implant and related surgery. Concurrently, new innovative techniques and devices may be developed to further simplify operative techniques, and to contribute to success in terms of favorable long-term clinical outcomes.

The new era in oral surgery caused by the growth in implant dentistry, with the related developments in transplants, allografts, growth factors, guided tissue regeneration and new materials and techniques, may well still be in its infancy. There are good reasons to believe that there is much more to come. The use of navigation systems and operating robots may well offer greatly enhanced accuracy and consistency in the planning and execution of implant osteotomies and placements. Concurrently, further developments in the field of computer-aided three-dimensional imaging will improve diagnostic capabilities, as recently evidenced by the introduction of CBCT.

Regarding autogenous bone grafting, which is still considered the gold standard of bone grafting, research in respect of osteoconduction and osteoinduction is opening up new opportunities. While osteoconduction uses the regenerative capacity of local bone, osteoinduction is characterized by the differentiation of pluripotent and mesenchymal cells into cartilage- and bone-forming precursor cells under the influence of bone morphogenetic proteins. Several different types of these proteins have been isolated, and it has been possible to produce them using gene technology. It should not be an unrealistic expectation that, in the future, new bone will be formed both at the site of defects and at distant sites for transplantation into the oral region. Similar research is being undertaken in respect of cartilage, skin and mucosa. This field of tissue engineering will play a large part in the further development of oral surgery.[21]

New methods will be supported by further developments in instrumentation. This will accelerate the trend towards minimally invasive surgical procedures, supported by flexible and rigid endoscopes, surgical microscopes of ever-increasing sophistication and 'high-tech' navigation tools for exact targeting and precision surgery.

Lasers will be further developed for hard tissue surgery (HF Zeilhofer 2008, personal communication), probably competing, sooner rather than later, with further advances in minimally invasive piezoelectric surgery.[22]

Oral surgery has traditionally been provided largely on an ambulatory care basis. These arrangements are set to expand, with further reductions in inpatient management, despite the likelihood of increasing numbers of patients with special needs and an anticipated shift towards more challenging forms of, in particular, implant surgery. These trends in the provision of oral surgery, which will be reflected across surgery in general, will be accompanied by further, more rigorous quality control processes. Clinicians with less favorable surgical outcomes will be identified for retraining, or possibly even exclusion from surgical practice.

Oral surgery is closely linked to oral radiology, oral medicine and oral pathology. Oral radiology and oral pathology are clinical diagnostic sciences critical to patient assessment and treatment planning. Oral medicine dovetails with oral surgery in the management of a large variety of soft tissue and other orofacial conditions, including, for example, diseases of the salivary glands and the management of atypical facial pain. With a growing population of aging patients with increasing morbidity, risk factors in oral surgery are increasing, and the management of such patients is becoming more multidisciplinary, with collaborative working between oral surgeons and colleagues in oral medicine (oral physicians) and medicine in general. An increasingly large proportion of the patients seen by oral surgeons will comprise those undergoing radiotherapy or chemotherapy, with immunosuppression subsequent to organ or bone marrow transplantation, or with other complex medication regimens.

An increasing number of drugs are known to have a direct impact on oral surgery, either in the form of unwanted complications or requiring significant considerations in the planning of surgery. For example, with the increasing incidence of osteoporosis and the high incidence of breast cancer in females and prostate cancer in males, all of which may involve treatment with bisphosphonates at some stage, bisphosphonate-induced osteonecroses of the mandible or maxilla will be seen more commonly by oral surgeons. Drug-induced hyperplasia of the gingivae and xerostomia will also become increasingly common. Further conditions that may increase in incidence in the next decade and may impact directly or indirectly, given treatment strategies and medication regimens, include hypertension, diabetes mellitus, chronic obstructive pulmonary disease, viral diseases (notably hepatitis B and C and human immunodeficiency virus), allergies, asthma, neurodegenerative diseases and chronic polyarthritis.

There will also be greatly increased patient expectations, with patients knowing much more about their conditions through, in particular, the Internet. They will seek second and third opinions and will expect favorable, long-term clinical outcomes that resolve their condition together with good functional and long-lasting esthetic qualities. Anticipation of such expectations, let alone increased risks of medicolegal challenges, will drive up the need for more documentation, auditing and other quality assurance processes; this will make the administrative load all the more burdensome for the clinician.

Although surgery is considered an 'imperfect science,' surgical practice, including the practice of oral surgery, will need to become much more evidence-based. This will inevitably lead to standardization and the possibility of patients feeling that they are not being assessed and treated as individuals, with unique sets of presenting problems and concerns.

Education in oral and maxillofacial surgery will be cost linked and driven by patient demands. While it will be necessary to maintain a network of dual qualification oral and maxillofacial surgeons, according to Laskin[23] the singly (dental) qualified oral surgeon will play an increasingly important role in dentally related surgical services. Furthermore, integrated patient care and research in modern medical centers will demonstrate the value of dentistry, including oral surgery, to the health professions and the success of academic health science centers of the future.[24] For the benefit of patients and the further development of dentally related surgical services, there needs to be reconciliation and cooperation rather than animosity and competition between oral and maxillofacial surgery and oral surgery.

Good scientific and clinical training must be provided to the surgeons of the future. Surgical skills alone will not, however, suffice. The surgeons of the future, including the oral surgeons of tomorrow, must have, in addition to expert clinical skills, advanced knowledge and understanding of the business of clinical service provision, relevant computer technologies, medical ethics and healthcare professionalism.

References

1. Härle F. Die Entwicklung der Arbeitsgemeinschaft für Kieferchirurgie. Dtsch Zahnärztl Z 1989;44:924-931.
2. Guralnick WC. History of Harvard/MGH Oral and Maxillofacial Surgery. J Mass Dent Soc 2000;49:36.
3. Pfaff P. Abhandlung von den Zähnen des menschlichen Körpers und deren Krankheiten. Berlin: Haude Spener, 1796.
4. Preiswerk P. Lehrbuch und Atlas der zahnärztlichen-stomatologischen Chirurgie. Munich: Lehmann, 1914.
5. Neumann R. Führer durch die operative Zahnheilkunde. Berlin: Berlinische Verlagsanstalt, 1928.
6. Wassmund M. Lehrbuch der praktischen Chirurgie des Mundes und der Kiefer. Leipzig: Meusser, 1934.
7. Pichler H, Trauner R. Bücher für die zahnärztliche Praxis, Vol. 12: Mund-und Kieferchirurgie. Munich: Urban & Schwarzenberg, 1948.
8. Hofer O, Reichenbach E, Kreudenstein TS, von Wannenmacher E. Lehrbuch der klinischen Zahn-, Mund- und Kieferheilkunde. Leipzig: Barth, 1952.
9. Lambrecht JTH. Dentoalveoläre Chirurgie. Mund Kiefer Gesichts Chir 2000;4:265-269.
10. Laskin DM. Oral and maxillofacial surgery: a century of progress. Alpha Omegan 2001;93,40-43.
11. Lambrecht JTH. 3-D Modeling Technology in Oral and Maxillofacial Surgery. Chicago, IL: Quintessence, 1995.
12. Dunsche A. Aufklärung, OP: Vorbereitung, Medikation. In: Lambrecht JTH (ed.). Zahnärztliche Operationen. Berlin: Quintessenz, 2008:1-20.
13. Kreusch T, Lambrecht JTH. Die Entfernung nicht retinierter Zähne. In: Lambrecht JTH (ed.). Zahnärztliche Operationen. Berlin: Quintessenz, 2008:21-47.
14. Sailer FH, Pajarola GF. Orale Chirurgie. In: Rateitschak KH, Wolf HF (eds). Farbatlanten der Zahnmedizin 11. Stuttgart: Thieme, 1996.
15. Lambrecht JTH, Hoffmeister B. Operative Entfernung retinierter und verlagerter Zähne. In: Lambrecht JTH (ed.). Zahnärztliche Operationen. Berlin: Quintessenz, 2008:50-80.
16. Lambrecht JTH, Filippi A. Zahn erhaltende Operationen. In: Lambrecht JTH (ed.). Zahnärztliche Operationen. Berlin: Quintessenz, 2008:81-119.
17. Wangerin K. Zysten, Knochenläsionen, odontogene Tumoren. In: Lambrecht JTH (ed.). Zahnärztliche Operationen. Berlin: Quintessenz, 2008:121-167.
18. Filippi A. Traumatologie bleibender Zähne. In: Lambrecht JTH (ed.). Zahnärztliche Operationen. Berlin: Quintessenz, 2008:171-223.
19. Dunsche A, Lambrecht JTH. Chirurgie der intraoralen Weichgewebe. In: Lambrecht JTH (ed.). Zahnärztliche Operationen. Berlin: Quintessenz, 2008:225-270.
20. Ewers R. Implantatchirurgie. In: Lambrecht JTH (ed.). Zahnärztliche Operationen. Berlin: Quintessenz, 2008: 271-420.
21. Hausamen J-E. The scientific development of maxillofacial surgery in the 20th century and an outlook into the future. J Craniomaxillofac Surg 2001;29:2-21.
22. Reichwein A, Lambrecht JTH, Schicho K, Undt G, Ewers R. Clinical experience with piezosurgery. In: Bell WH, Guerrero CAG (eds). Distraction Osteogenesis of the Facial Skeleton. Hamilton NJ: BC Decker, 2007:229-231.
23. Laskin DM. The past, present, and future of oral and maxillofacial surgery. J Oral Maxillofac Surg 2008;66:1037-1040.
24. Assael LA. Changes in dental education: dictating the future of the specialty. J Oral Maxillofac Surg 2008;66: 837-838.
25. Lambrecht JTH (ed.). Zahnärztliche Operationen. Berlin: Quintessenz, 2008.

CHAPTER 11

Dentistry tomorrow

Nairn Wilson

Introduction

Good as dentistry is today,
it should be a step-change better by 2020.

The concluding sections of the various chapters of this book set out subject-specific ways in which the principal elements of the clinical practice of dentistry are anticipated to change by 2020. In addition, there will also be very significant developments in other aspects of dentistry in the next 10 years or so. Such developments may stem, for example, from further evidence of associations between dental diseases and systemic health;[1] from developments in salivary and other dental diagnostics, including risk assessment methodologies;[2] and from the increasing involvement of dental practitioners in facial cosmetic medicine and surgery. Given such possibilities, which some would say are probabilities, change is not only inevitable, but inevitably is going to be substantial.

Changes in dentistry of the type forecast will have far-reaching implications, spanning the regulation of the profession, dental education at all levels, the skill mix of the dental team and, in turn, the qualities and aspiration of those recruited for the purpose of future workforce development. As systems for regulation, education and workforce development take time to change, typically several years, those responsible for such systems should be at least planning, if not introducing, systems better suited to future needs. Failure to act sooner rather than later will, in all probability, run the risk of delaying, if not stifling, change, much of which will benefit patients. More of the same type of regulation, education and arrangements for workforce development is unlikely to suffice the needs that will exist by 2020, if not before.[3,4]

As indicated by all the contributors to this book, it is anticipated that progress will have been made by 2020 in respect of the prevention and control of the principal dental diseases - dental caries and periodontal disease - to a much greater extent than has proved possible to date, both in developed and developing countries. It is hoped also that other forms of orofacial disease, including both mouth cancer and the less life-threatening but potentially disabling forms of oral mucosal disease, may be better understood. This, in turn, may lead to prevention or at least control in ways that improve prognosis and give affected patients a better quality of life. Furthermore, it is hoped that conditions such as chronic orofacial pain, xerostomia and pathological toothwear may be better understood and managed more effectively. Assuming such things are achieved, the dental practitioner as leader of the dental team will become as much an oral physician as a dental surgeon, spending an increasing proportion of patient contact time helping to maintain oral health rather than treating disease.[5] Such change will, amongst other influences, have a profound effect on the patient–practitioner relationship, in particular if circumstances, including the arrangements for the funding of dental services, encourage longitudinal care.

For the patient, there is the hope of freedom from dental pain and discomfort and a move to 'teeth for life.' When dental operative intervention is indicated, it will be minimally interventive with little if any iatrogenic damage and, as a consequence, greatly improved clinical outcomes. These goals may not be fully realized by 2020, but dentistry should set itself the challenge to make substantial inroads into meeting the anticipated expectations of patients. Above all else, it is suggested that moves to more minimally interventive, atraumatic techniques, with reduced levels of operator variability, should be high on the agenda to improve clinical care in dentistry.[5]

Attitude to oral health

Over the next 10 years, it is to be hoped that there will be a major shift in public attitude to oral health. Many more people will hopefully come to terms with the concept that they have responsibility to maintain their oral health, with some help and support from their dental team, rather than the dental team looking after their teeth with some self-help and limited patient involvement. This, together with effective oral health campaigns targeted at achieving behavioral change, could herald a new era of continuous improvements in oral health around the world. As with other challenges in effecting improvements in health, a key to success is a positive change in the attitude of the population.[5]

Translation of modern science into practice

In looking forward, an area of great uncertainty comprises the timing of the translation of new knowledge in craniofacial development and biomolecular oral health sciences into the clinical practice of dentistry.[6] Predictions on this front could be overly optimistic given the potential difficulties in getting certain novel treatment modalities into clinical trials, let alone into accepted general use in clinical practice. Further barriers to progress on this front may be affordability and favorable cost benefits. As and when such barriers can be overcome, it is apparent that novel forms, for example of regenerative dentistry and bioengineering, will have a substantial if not profound impact on dentistry as it is known and practiced today. The translation into practice of developments in dental biomaterials science and related processes, for example novel ceramic systems and sophisticated forms of computer-assisted design/computer-assisted milling, should be less problematic than taking forward breakthroughs in biosciences, but the former may lack the qualities and cost benefits necessary to allow widespread application. Many approaches and techniques that are presently experimental may be possible by 2020, but utility and cost consequences must be attractive to achieve market acceptance and common use in clinical practice; low-cost, high-efficacy solutions are needed to address common problems.

Care of the older patient

As a consequence of anticipated changes in population demographics, the dental team can anticipate caring for a greater number of older patients in years to come. This, together with the trend towards older patients retaining more of their teeth through to the end of life, will account for a substantial increase in treatment needs in aging patients. Meeting the dental treatment needs of older patients can be challenging, involving a range of advanced skills, tempered by experience. Given that gerodontology is not presently a subject area of great interest to younger practitioners and students, ways need to be found to improve the appeal of this important and professionally fulfilling aspect of the clinical practice of dentistry. Very often, the successful care of older patients is more about managing the person than nuances in the technicalities of treatment. That said, the successful care of older patients can be very time consuming and, as a consequence, relatively expensive, given that the most expensive element of dental care tends to be the cost of the oral healthcare professionals' time. Such considerations need to be factored into schemes for the future provision of oral healthcare, mindful that many older patients may have special needs and fall into the category of the socially disadvantaged in evolving societies.[7]

Futurology and the future

Predicting the future is fraught with uncertainty. Critics decry 'futurologists,' citing many examples of failed predictions. In contrast, futurology is a recognized key skill of strategists, who may be called upon to assist in decision making that may affect whole populations. While 'futurity' should rightly be viewed with some caution, and suffers the effects of unforeseen events, it is important in mapping out the way forward. To discard all anticipations and predictions as speculation and work from day to day without vision is not a realistic option in today's world.

Given the above, this book serves an important function beyond being an authoritative, thought-provoking source of reference. Above all else, through the commonality of the views of the various contributors, this book highlights that dentistry is undergoing substantial changes, which in all probability will gather momentum through at least 2020. Faced with this situation, members of the dental team must be prepared to learn and adopt new concepts and ways of working, if for no other reasons they are best to serve their patients. Standing still and being reluctant to grasp new opportunities as they arise fails patients and compromises the profession. Time lost in a period of substantial and, in many ways, fundamental change may never be recouped. So, even the sceptics amongst those who read this book are encouraged to reflect on its contents and plan ahead accordingly.

All said and done, the future, barring unforeseen events, is what we make it. Given the building blocks available to the profession, dentistry has the opportunity to create a great future as an integral element of modern, mainstream healthcare.

References

1. Williams RC, Barnett AH, Claffey N, Davis M, Gadsby R, Kellett M et al. The potential impact of periodontal disease on general health: a consensus view. Curr Med Res Opin 2008;24:1635-1643.
2. Wong DT. Salivary diagnostics: enhancing disease detection and making medicine better. Eur J Dent Ed 2008;12 (Suppl 1):22-29.
3. Eaton KA, Reynolds PA, Grayden SK, Wilson NHF. A vision of dental education in the third millennium. Br Dent J 2008;205:261-271.
4. Wilson NHF, Gallagher JE. The future dental workforce. Br Dent J 2009; in press.
5. Wilson NHF. Minimally Invasive Dentistry. London: Quintessence.
6. Ford P, Seymour G, Beeley JA, Curro F, DePaola D, Ferguson D et al. Adapting to changes in molecular biosciences and technologies. Euro J Dent Ed 2008;12(Suppl 1):40-47.
7. Kandelman D, Petersen PE, Yeda H. Oral health, general health, and quality of life in older people. Spec Care Dentist 2008;28:224-236.

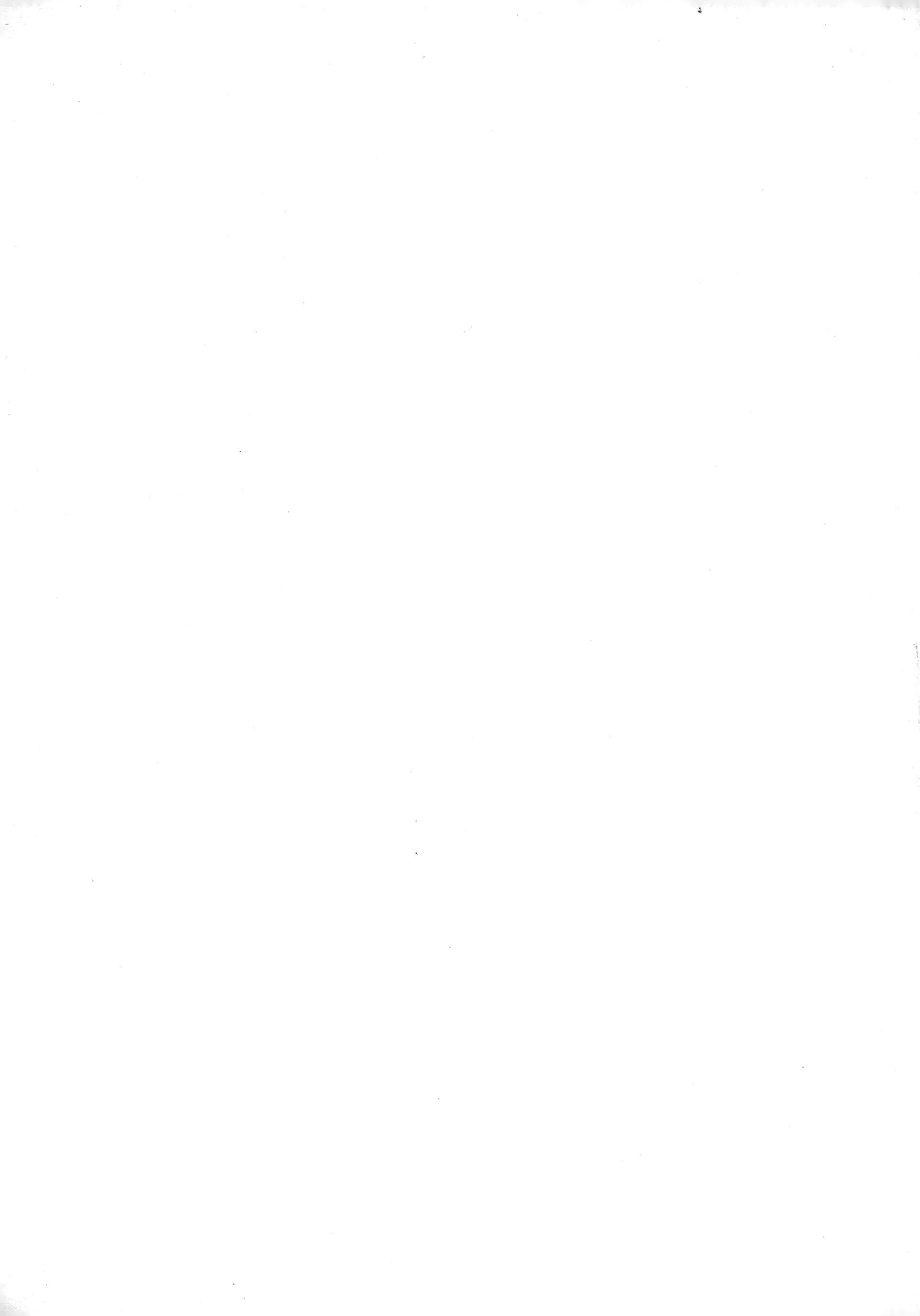